A HANDBOOK OF RESEARCH FOR THE HELPING PROFESSIONS

A HANDBOOK OF RESEARCH FOR THE HELPING PROFESSIONS

CAROLE SUTTON

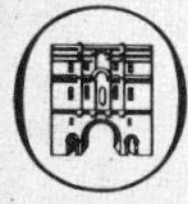

Routledge & Kegan Paul
London and New York

First published in 1987 by
Routledge & Kegan Paul Ltd
11 New Fetter Lane, London EC4P 4EE

Published in the USA by
Routledge & Kegan Paul Inc.
in association with Methuen Inc.
29 West 35th Street, New York, NY 10001

Set in Linotron Sabon and Helvetica
by Input Typesetting Ltd, London SW19 8DR
and printed in Great Britain
by Richard Clay Ltd
Bungay, Suffolk

Library of Congress Cataloging in Publication Data

Sutton, Carole.
A handbook of research for the helping professions.

Includes bibliographies and index.
1. Social service—Research. I. Title.
HV11.S868 1987 361'.0072 86–21961
ISBN 07102–0502–3
British Library CIP Data also available

ISBN 0–7102–0502–3

To 'Gran', Dorothy Nye, who knew without the need for any research that people need encouragement and appreciation.

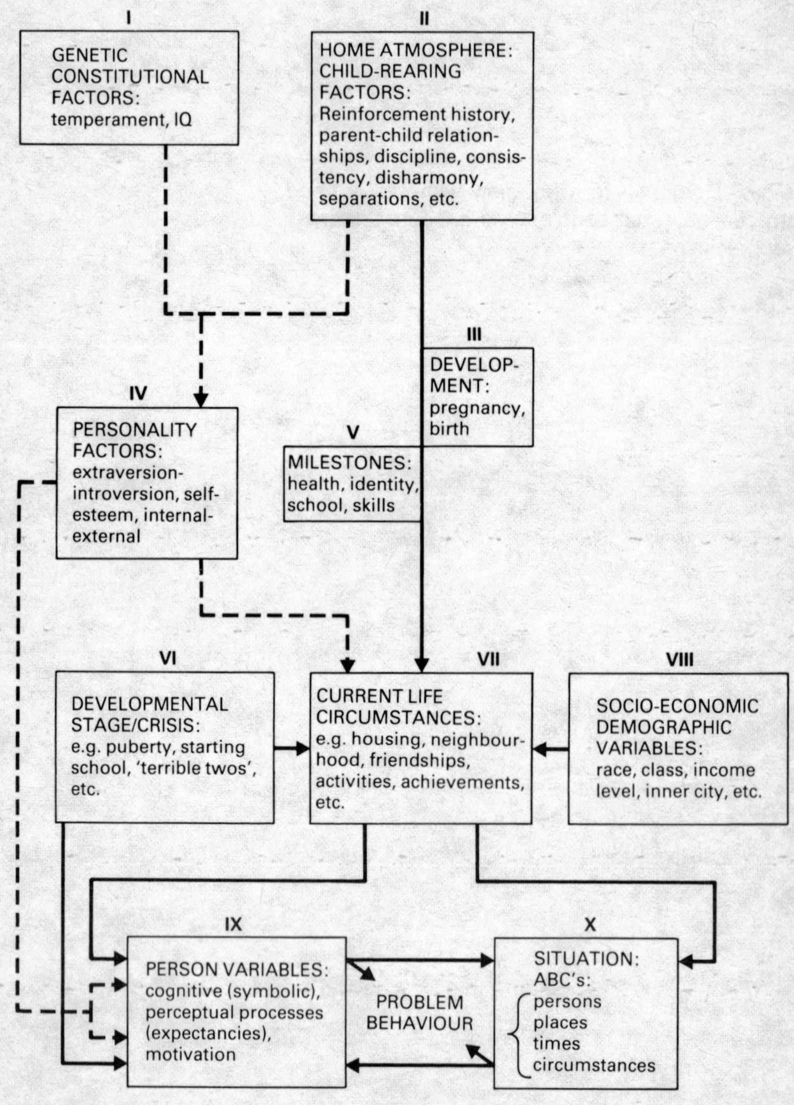

FRONTISPIECE The ten-factor clinical formation (Herbert, 1981, adapted from Clarke, 1977) This can be seen as a 'systems' formulation.
The dotted line represents indirect pre-disposing contributory factors.

CONTENTS

	List of figures and tables		x
	Acknowledgments		xiv
	Introduction		1
PART 1	**Principles and concepts of working within the human social system**	*Consultant*	7
1	Three disciplines within a 'systems' approach: sociology, psychology and psychiatry		9
2	The empirical approach in the social sciences: gathering verifiable data		18
3	The empirical approach in the social sciences: evaluation of intervention		27
4	Community work and community development	Paul Taylor	35
5	Managing organizational or inter-group conflict		43
6	Small group work	Dr Michael Argyle	51
7	Problem-solving and decision-making group work	Dr Michael Argyle	58
8	Therapeutic group work and sensitivity training	Dr Peter Smith	64
9	Social learning theory and goal-setting approaches	Professor Martin Herbert	71
10	Counselling and brief psychotherapy		79
11	General management skills	Hilary Unwin	86
PART 2	**Research concerning people experiencing particular stress and disadvantage**		97
12	Research concerning people in poverty and at social disadvantage		99
13	Research concerning unemployed people		107
14	Research concerning people from ethnic minorities	Usha Prashar	117

15 Research concerning people with physical handicaps — 127

PART 3 Research concerning youth work and the youth service — 139

16 Research concerning youth work and the youth service — Ray Fabes — 141

PART 4 Research concerning women's issues — 149

17 Research concerning women's experience of violence, including rape — 151

PART 5 Research concerning the family and family life — 161

18 Research concerning aspects of family life, marriage and divorce — Dr Jack Dominian — 163

19 Research concerning one-parent families — Dr Carol Smart — 172

PART 6 Research concerning young people in difficulties — 181

20 Research concerning young people and emotional disorders — Professor Michael Rutter — 183

21 Research concerning young people and conduct disorders — Professor Martin Herbert — 195

22 Research concerning bed-wetting (enuresis) — Professor Martin Herbert — 205

PART 7 Research concerning services and settings with statutory implications — 211

23 Research concerning aspects of statutory child care, including residential care — Chris Payne — 213

24 Research concerning child abuse and child sexual abuse — Raymond Castle — 225

25 Research concerning fostering — Tony Hall — 238

26 Research concerning adoption — Tony Hall — 247

27 Research concerning the residential care of the elderly, the physically handicapped, the mentally handicapped and the mentally ill — Chris Payne — 257

PART 8 Research concerning young people and adults in trouble with the law 267

28 Research concerning young offenders — Professor Michael Rutter — 269
29 Research concerning differing approaches to young offenders including Intermediate Treatment — Professor Norman Tutt — 280
30 Research concerning probation — Professor Martin Davies — 287
31 Research concerning custodial and other responses to offenders — Dr Ken Pease — 294

PART 9 Research concerning aspects of mental health and mental handicap 303

32 Research concerning anxiety and forms of anxiety: phobias and obsessive disorders — Dr Anthony C. Carr — 305
33 Research concerning depression — Dr Jack Dominian — 315
34 Research concerning suicide and parasuicide — Dr Norman Kreitman — 323
35 Research concerning schizophrenia — Professor John Wing — 331
36 Research concerning people with mental handicaps — Professor Peter Mittler — 339

PART 10 Research concerning situations in which some people seek help 351

37 Research concerning bereavement and grief reactions — Dr Colin Murray Parkes — 353
38 Research concerning family and marital therapy — Dr Michael Crowe — 361
39 Research concerning sexual dysfunction and difficulties — Dr Michael Crowe — 369
40 Research concerning homosexuality — Professor Donald West — 377
41 Research concerning people wanting to control their violence or anger — Dr Kevin Howells — 382
42 Research concerning the use and misuse of alcohol — Dr Douglas Cameron — 390
43 Research concerning the use and misuse of drugs — Dr Douglas Cameron — 400

Index 414

LIST OF FIGURES AND TABLES

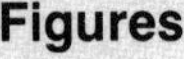

Figures

Frontispiece The ten-factor clinical formation (Herbert, 1981, adapted from Clarke, 1977)
1.1 The development of General Systems Theory (After Beishon, 1980)
1.2 A range of approaches within sociology
1.3 A range of approaches within psychology
1.4 A range of approaches within psychiatry
1.5 The process when intervening in systems (Pincus and Minahan, 1973)
2.1 A schematic overview of the research process (Beyer, 1971)
2.2 The experimental approach with one person (Sheldon, 1982)
2.3 Independent and dependent variables in a controlled experiment (Sutton, 1979)
3.1 Assertion training with a withdrawn psychiatric patient (Sheldon, 1982)
5.1 Levels of organizational conflict and its impact on effectiveness (After Stoner, 1978)
5.2 Intergroup conflict leading to intragroup cohesiveness (Stoner, 1978)
5.3 A systems formulation of negotiation/mediation (After Wall, 1981)
6.1 The two tasks and two channels of social groups (Argyle, 1972)
6.2 Styles of social behaviour (Argyle, 1972)
7.1 The distribution of participation in groups of different sizes (After Bales, Strodtbeck, Mills and Roseborough, 1951)
9.1 A feedback loop suggested by social learning theory
10.1 A five-stage plan of the initial counselling interview(s)
10.2 A treatment decision-making model of counsellor methods in relation to client needs (Nelson-Jones, 1982)
11.1 A system with sub-systems, interacting with other systems (1980)
11.2 A model of forward planning, including the critical path (After Cleland and King, 1972)
13.1 Factors affecting the experience of unemployment (Ashton, 1986)
13.2 The phase model of unemployment (Harrison, 1976)
15.1 The concepts in the World Health Organisation trial scheme (1980)
17.1 A model of intrafamily violence (Gelles, 1974)
19.1 Social conditions of British eleven-year-olds (Wedge and Prosser, 1973)
20.1 Non-attendance at school (Rutter, 1975)
21.1 General assessment guidelines in the field of children's conduct disorders, (Herbert 1981)

22.1 The frequency of bed-wetting (Morgan, 1981)
23.1 The group care field across systems (Ainsworth and Fulcher, 1981)
24.1 A social psychological model of the causes of child abuse (Gelles, 1979)
28.1 Juveniles found guilty of, or cautioned for, indictable offences per 100,000 population in set and age groups (NACRO, 1985)
28.2 Elements contributing to the occurrence of a criminal event (Clarke, 1977)
33.1 Modifying factors between stressful event and possible subsequent depressive illness (Paykel 1979)
35.1 Simplified schema for studying the origin, development and perpetuation of the schizophrenias and similar disorders (Wynne, 1977)
36.1 The causes of mental impairment and handicap (O.H.E./Mencap, 1986)
36.2 Services for disabled people in England (O.H.E./Mencap, 1986)
36.3 The 'core and cluster' principle (King's Fund centre, 1980)
38.1 An example of a geneogram (Finch and Jaques, 1985)
41.1 Determinants of anger arousal (Novaco, 1978)
42.1 An explanatory system for problem drinking (Thorley, 1985)
42.2 A tentative decision tree for those male clients wishing to control their drinking (Heather and Robertson, 1981)
43.1 A multi-variate/systems, model of opiate use and outcomes

Tables

3.1 How bad is it? How good is it? Questionnaire administered to psychiatric nurses (Oppenheim, 1976)
4.1 Community workers in the United Kingdom (Francis, Henderson and Thomas, 1984)
4.2 Organizations employing community workers, by area. Percentages (Francis, Henderson and Thomas, 1984)
4.3 A summary of community work approaches (Taylor, 1985)
8.1 Relationship between therapist dimensions of affection and activity (Bierman, 1969)
12.1 Changes in the extent of poverty 1960–81 (Britain) (Townsend, 1984)
12.2 Experience of specific problems, by number of other problems experienced (Berthoud, 1983)
13.1 Unemployment rates 1979 and 1985 – standardized to US definitions (Sinfield, 1986)
13.2 Regional unemployment 1979 and 1986 (Unemployment Unit Briefing)
13.3 Male unemployment in the previous twelve months, 1975–7 and 1983, Great Britain (*Social Trends*, 1980, 1985)
13.4 Age distribution of long-term unemployed claimants in the UK at 10 October, 1985 (Unemployment Unit Briefing, 1986)
14.1 Population of Great Britain by ethnic origin and birthplace, 1983 (*Social Trends*, 1985)
14.2 Economic status of the economically active in Great Britain, 1983 (*Social Trends*, 1985)
14.3 Tenure in major areas of black residence by ethnic group (Brown, 1984)
14.4 Amenities by ethnic group (Brown, 1984)

14.5 Victims of assault over past 16–18 months (Brown, 1984)
15.1 Persons registered as substantially and permanently handicapped (*Health and Personal Social Services Statistics for England*, 1985)
16.1 Estimated staffing of the Youth Service (*Experience and Participation*, 1982)
17.1 Victims of selected notifiable offences: by sex and age, 1984. (*Social Trends*, 1987)
17.2 Offenders found guilty at all courts or cautioned for indictable sexual offences, by offence. England and Wales (*Criminal Statistics*, 1984)
17.3 Summary of data concerning assault and wife-beating. (Dobash and Dobash, 1978)
17.4 Rape and sexual assault experienced by respondents to the Women's Safety Survey (Hall, 1985)
18.1 Households by type in Great Britain (*Social Trends*, 1984)
18.2 Marriage in Great Britain (*Social Trends*, 1984)
18.3 Divorce in England and Wales (*Social Trends*, 1984)
19.1 One-parent families: by household composition (*Social Trends*, 1985)
19.2 Circumstances of lone mothers and lone fathers (*General Household Survey*, 1984)
19.3 Family size in one-parent families (*National Council for One-Parent Families*, 1983)
19.4 Comparative incomes relative to Supplementary Benefit levels of one-parent and two-parent families (*Hansard*, 1985)
19.5 Housing: one- and two-parent families (*One-Parent Families*, 1984)
20.1 Variables differentiating diagnostic categories (Rutter, 1975)
20.2 Prevalence of psychiatric disorder among ten-year-olds in two areas (Rutter et al., 1975)
20.3 Family Adversity Index (Rutter, 1978)
23.1 Children in care of local authorities (*Health and Personal Social Services Statistics*, 1985)
23.2 Types of day services across systems (Ainsworth and Fulcher, 1981)
24.1 Deaths of children in England and Wales, 1982 and 1983 (*Mortality Statistics*, 1983, 1984)
24.2 Number of registered children by year and type and severity of abuse (Creighton, 1984, 1985)
24.3 Offenders found guilty or sentenced for indictable sexual offences by offence (*Criminal Statistics*, 1984)
24.4 Prevalence of child sexual abuse in the UK (Beezley Mrazek, Lynch and Bentovim, 1981)
24.5 Possible antecedents to child abuse (Gardner and Gray, 1982)
24.6 Child abuse: high risk rating check list (Greenland, 1986)
25.1 Accommodation of children in care (*British Agencies for Adoption and Fostering*, 1985)
26.1 Children adopted under orders registered in England and Wales, 1973–84 (Houghton Report/Office of Population Censuses)
27.1 Persons in accommodation provided by or on behalf of local authorities (*Health and Personal Social Services Statistics*, 1985)

27.2 Places and persons in voluntary and private homes for the elderly and physically handicapped (*Health and Personal Social Services Statistics*, 1985)
27.3 Homes and hostels for the mentally ill and mentally handicapped (*Health and Personal Social Services Statistics*, 1985)
28.1 14–16-year-old males found guilty 1950–78, by type of offence (Rutter and Giller, 1983)
30.1 Probation orders in England and Wales (*Social Trends*, 1985)
31.1 Sentence or order passed on offenders sentenced for indictable offences: by sex (*Annual Abstract of Statistics*, 1985)
33.1 Characteristics of depression (Dominian, 1984)
33.2 Prescriptions for preparations acting on the nervous system, England, 1975, 1980 (*Health and Personal Social Services Statistics*, 1976, 1982)
33.3 Ten models of depression (After Akiskal and McKinney, 1975)
33.4 Depression as a 'final common pathway' (After Akiskal and McKinney, 1975)
34.1 Frequency of suicide in England and Wales, by age and sex (Kreitman, 1985)
34.2 Frequency of parasuicide in Edinburgh (Kreitman, 1985)
34.3 Summary comparison of parasuicides and suicides in the UK (Kreitman, 1983)
35.1 Total admissions in England for schizophrenia, paranoia to types of hospital 1981, 1982 (*DHSS In-patient Statistics*, 1981, 1982)
35.2 Risk among relatives of schizophrenically ill people of developing the disorder (Slater, 1968)
35.3 Schizophrenic illness in the biological and adoptive families of schizophrenic index cases and controls (Wing, 1978)
36.1 The four categories of mental handicap (Quoted by Russell, 1985)
36.2 Diagnosis of underlying impairment in children with severe mental handicap (After Weatherall, 1983)
37.1 Marital condition: census figures UK
38.1 Annual interviews during the period 1981–5 (National Marriage Guidance Council, 1985)
39.1 Categories of sexual dysfunction (After Jehu, 1979)
41.1 Offenders found guilty: by offence group (*Annual Abstract of Statistics*, 1985)
42.1 Drinking habits by sex and age, 1984 (*Social Trends*, 1987)
43.1 A drugs compendium (After *Observer*, 1973)
43.2 Narcotic drugs – new addicts notified (*Social Trends*, 1986)
43.3 Offenders found guilty (*Criminal Statistics*, 1984)
43.4 Drugs used by the Cheltenham sample (Plant, 1975)

ACKNOWLEDGMENTS

A great many people have been involved directly and indirectly in the development of this book: to all of them I extend my thanks and appreciation for their contributions of time and effort.

To those who agreed to act as Consultants to the book I am personally and particularly grateful. Many of them undertook to advise me when they were already dealing with very heavy commitments, and have given me invaluable and detailed advice. Without this help, the book would not have been written.

I should like to acknowledge a particular debt to Dr Tony T. Carr, who first put to me the question, 'What is the *empirical evidence*?' That question has challenged me ever since, and has guided me in compiling this book.

Many colleagues in the School of Applied Social Sciences and Public Administration and in other Schools at Leicester Polytechnic, have been of help to me in a wide variety of ways: by drawing books and papers to my attention, by giving me detailed information and by encouraging me in times of frustration. I offer my thanks to the Head of School, Fred Bartlett, and to my colleagues: David Batchelor, Ted Cassidy, Kay Davis, Martin Davis, Peter Duke, Ray Fabes, Jean Fergus, Dorothy Hutchinson, Dick Jones, Val Marett, Pat Mounfield, Pat Osborne, Val Pleasance, Gil Pottinger, Paul Taylor, Hilary Unwin, Paul Weston, Shantu Watt and Terry Willits.

My thanks are also offered to the librarians, administrative and secretarial staff of Leicester Polytechnic, who have taken much trouble to follow up details of my inquiries, to obtain books and to prepare materials. The former include Olwyn Reynard and Elizabeth O'Neill, together with Jane Brittain, Caroline Davis, Ann Hughes, Darryl Rouse, Lesley Compton, Rhamba Khuti, Kamaljit Kaur, Mary Sullivan, Sue Holm and Dilys Hockridge; the latter include Anita Hollidge, Sue Bloy, Carole Shaw, Dorothy Astley, Margaret Austick, Lyn Boon, Sue Dewing, Janet Dickman, Barbara Geary, Janet Grundy, Gillian Lewis, Nina Kenchington, Ruth Maisey, Rachel Mayhew, Lorna Morrison, Sue Oakley and Helen Sanderson. My particular thanks are due to Dorothy Root for unfailing helpfulness.

I am also indebted to Barrie Ingham and Dennis Markillie of the Reprographic Unit of Leicester Polytechnic for their advice and practical help.

In addition I should like to acknowledge the contribution which a number of colleagues have made towards developing the plan and content of the book; these include: Brian Sheldon, Director of the School of Applied Social

Studies at Bedford New College, London University, Barbara Hudson, of the Department of Social and Administrative Studies at Oxford University, Rhoda Oppenheimer of the Academic Psychiatric Unit at the General Hospital, Leicester; Dr Roger Morgan, Deputy Director, Social Services Department, Oxfordshire County Council, together with Keith Turner, Mike Corp, Chris Cordle, Angela Holland, Joyce Scaife and Mike Hopley of Leicester District Community Psychology Team. I should also like to thank Professor Peter Warr of Sheffield University for sending me valuable material, Doug Smith of the National Youth Bureau and Christina Smakowska of the NSPCC for advice and help. Other colleagues who have given me much encouragement and aid are Dick Beak, Andrew Bunyan, Irene Dooher, Dorota Iwaniec, Robert Nisbet, Alan Pratten, Alan Sapsford, Rosemary Strange and Robert Waters.

I wish also to acknowledge my debt to a number of past and present students who brought papers or other information to my attention, and gave other forms of help. I should like to thank Wendy Bass, Steve Bettison, Penny Brown, Mike Davies, Maggie Eaton, Nick Emmet, Nigel Hinks, Pauline Hughes, Pat Oxley, Chris Shaw, Anne Walters, Lis Worsley and Gareth Wynne.

Finally, to the members of my family, Clive, Cathy, Meriel, Peter and Rowan, my gratitude for their support and encouragement over the many months it has taken to compile the book, and for putting up with it; and to Gran, to whom the book is dedicated.

For permission to reproduce material from works in copyright the author and publisher make grateful acknowledgment as follows:

The frontispiece is reprinted from *Behavioural Treatment of Problem Children*, M. Herbert, 1981, by permission of Academic Press Inc., Florida: the figure was adapted from the original in R. V. G. Clarke's 'Psychology and Crime', *Bulletin of the British Psychological Society*, reprinted by permission of the BPS and Prof. Clarke; 'Moment in Time' is from *The Psychology of Consciousness*, R. E. Ornstein, 1972, by permission of W. H. Freeman & Company, Copyright © 1972; Fig. 1.1 is reprinted from the Open University Course T243: *Systems Organisation*, Block 1, copyright © 1980 The Open University Press; Fig. 1.5 is reproduced by permission of the publisher, F. E. Peacock Publishers Inc, Itasca, Illinois, from Allen Pincus and Anne Minahan, *Social Work Practice: Model and Method*, 1973, copyright © 1973, p. 86, fig. 1; Fig. 2.1 is from *Inquiry in the Social Studies Classroom*, B. K. Beyer, 1971, published by Merrill Publishing Company; Figs 2.2 & 3.1 are from *Behaviour Modification*, B. Sheldon, 1982, published by Tavistock Publications; Table 3.1 is from *Questionnaire Design and Attitude Measurement*, A. N. Oppenheim, 1968, published by Gower Publishing Company; Tables 4.1–2 are from *A Survey of Community Workers in the UK*, D. Francis, P. Henderson and D. N. Thomas, 1984, by kind permission of the National

Institute for Social Work, London; Figs 5.1–2 are from James A. F. Stoner/Charles Wankel, *Management*, 3rd edn. © 1986, pp. 382, 390. Reprinted by permission of Prentice-Hall Inc., Englewood Cliffs, New Jersey; Fig. 5.3 is from 'Mediation. An Analysis, Review and Proposed Research', J. A. Wall Jr, in *Journal of Conflict Resolution*, Vol 23, No 1, March 1981, published by Sage Publications Inc, California; Figs 6.1–2 are by M. Argyle from the Open University course E281: *Personality, Growth and Learning*, Blocks 8/10, copyright © 1972, The Open University Press; Fig. 7.1 is by Bales, Strodtbeck, Mills and Roseborough in *American Sociological Review*, Vol. 16, reproduced from *Social Interaction*, M. Argyle, 1976, by permission of Tavistock Publications; Table 8.1 is derived from 'Dimensions of Interpersonal Facilitation in Psychotherapy and Child Development', R. Bierman, 1969, in *Psychological Bulletin*, and reproduced from *Small Groups and Personal Change*, Peter B. Smith, 1980, by permission of Methuen & Co; Figs 10.1–2 are from *The Theory and Practice of Counselling Psychology*, R. Nelson-Jones, 1982, by permission of Holt Saunders Ltd; Fig. 11.1 is from the Open University Course T243: *Systems Organisation*, 1980, Block 1, copyright © 1980 The Open University Press; Fig. 11.2 is from *Management: A Systems Approach*, D. I. Cleland and W. King, 1972, published by McGraw-Hill Publishing Co Ltd; Table 12.1 uses extracts from *The Poor and the Poorest*, B. Abel-Smith and P. Townsend, 1965, pp. 40, 44, by permission of Bell & Hyman; Table 12.2 is from R. Berthoud's 'Who Suffers Disadvantage', in *The Structure of Disadvantage*, ed. M. Brown, 1983, by permission of Gower Publishing Ltd; Figs 13.1–2 are reproduced from *Unemployment under Capitalism*, D. Ashton, 1986, by permission of Wheatsheaf Books Ltd; Tables 13.1–2, 4 are from *Unemployment Unit Briefing*, Statistical Supplement, University of Edinburgh, January 1986; Tables 14.3–5 from *Black and White Britain*, C. Brown, 1984, by permission of Gower Publishing Ltd; Fig. 15.1 is from *Children with Disabilities and their Families*, M. Philp and D. Duckworth, 1982, by permission of NFER-NELSON Publishing Co Ltd; Table 16.1 is from Cmnd 8686 *Experience and Participation: Report of the Review Group on the Youth Service in England*, A. Thompson, 1982, by permission of HMSO; Fig. 17.1 is from R. Gelles (1974), *The Violent Home*, Beverly Hills, CA: Sage Publications, used by permission of the author; Table 17.3 is from 'Man's Inhumanity to Wives', the *Sunday Times*, 9 March 1980, originally from *Violence against Wives*, R. E. and R. Dobash, 1978, Open Press, and used by permission of the authors; Table 17.4 is from *Ask Any Woman*, R. Hall, 1985, published by Falling Wall Press Ltd; Fig. 19.1 is from *Born to Fail*, P. Wedge and H. Prosser, 1973, by kind permission of the National Children's Bureau and Century Hutchinson Ltd; Fig 20.1 & Table 20.1 from *Helping Troubled Children*, Michael Rutter (Penguin Education, 1975), p. 36, 41, copyright © Michael Rutter, 1975; Table 20.2 is by Rutter *et al.* (1975), 'Attainment and adjustment in two geographical areas', from *British Journal of Psychiatry*, vol. 126; Table 20.3 by M. Rutter from *Aggression and Anti-Social Behaviour in Childhood*, eds L. Hersov, M. Berger, D. Shaffer, 1978, by permission of Pergamon Press Ltd; Fig. 21.1 is from *Behavioural Treatment of Problem Children*, M. Herbert, 1981, reproduced by permission of Academic Press, Florida, and Professor Herbert; Fig. 22.1 is from *Childhood Incontinence*, Dr R. Morgan, BA, PhD, 1981, by permission of the Disabled Living Foundation and Heinemann Medical Books Ltd; Fig. 23.1 & Table 23.2 from *Group Care for Children*, F. Ainsworth and L. Fulcher, 1981, by permission of Tavistock Publications; Fig. 24.1 is by R. J. Gelles and is reprinted, with permission, from the *American Journal of Orthopsychiatry*, copyright 1979 by the American Orthopsychiatric Association Inc; Table 24.2 is from *Trends in Child Abuse 1977–81*, S. J. Creighton, 1984, by kind permission of the NSPCC; Table 24.4 is from *Child Sexual Abuse*, by kind permission of BASPCAN; Table 24.5 is by J. Gardner and M. Gray from *Developments in the Study of Criminal Behaviour*, ed. P. Feldman, 1982, by permission of John Wiley & Sons Ltd; Table 24.6 is reproduced by kind permission of the author, Professor Cyril Greenland; Fig. 28.1 is from *Juvenile Crime*, 1985, by kind permission of NACRO; Table 28.1 from *Juvenile Delinquency*, Michael Rutter and Henri Giller, (Penguin Education 1983), p. 71, copyright © Michael Rutter & Henri Giller, 1983; Fig. 28.2 is by Professor R. G. Clarke, 'Psychology and Crime' in *Bulletin of the British Psychological Society*, 1977, Vol. 30; this article is acknowledged as being subject to Crown Copyright, and the figure is reproduced by permission of HMSO, with thanks to the BPS and Professor Clarke; Fig. 33.1 is by E. S. Paykel from *Psychobiology of Depressive Disorders*, R. Depue, 1979, by permission of Academic Press, Florida; Table 33.1 from *Depression*, J. Dominian, 1984, by permission of Collins Publishers; Table 34.3 by N. Kreitman from *Companion to Psychiatric Studies*, eds R. Kendell and A. Zealley, 3rd edn, 1983, by permission of Churchill Livingstone; Fig. 35.1 is by L. C. Wynne from *Developments in Psychiatric Research*, ed J. Tanner, 1977, published by Hodder & Stoughton; Table 35.2 is by E. Slater from *The Transmission of Schizophrenia*, eds D. Rosenthal and S. Kety, 1968, by permission of Pergamon Books Ltd; Table 35.3 from *Schizophrenia: Towards a New Synthesis*, J. Wing, 1978, by permission of Academic Press, Florida and Professor Wing; Figs 36.1–2 from *Mental Handicap: Partnership in the Community*, by permission of Office of Health Economics, London, 1978; Table 36.1 from *Mental Handicap*, D. Russell, 1985, by permission of Churchill Livingstone; Table 36.2 from *The New Genetics and Clinical Practice*, D. J. Weatherall, 1983, by permission of Oxford University Press and Professor Weatherall; Fig. 36.3 from *An Ordinary Life*, 1980, by kind permission of King Edward's Hospital Fund for London; Fig. 38.1 from *Adoption and Fostering*, R. Finch and P. Jacques, 1985, Vol. 9, No. 3, by permission of British Agencies for Adoption and Fostering; Table 39.1 from *Sexual Dysfunction: A Behavioural Approach*, D. Jehu, 1979, published by John Wiley & Sons Ltd; Fig. 41.1 is by Professor R. W. Novaco from *Cognitive Behaviour Therapy: Research and Application*, eds J. Foreyt and D. Rathjen, 1978, by permission of Plenum Publishing Corp; Fig. 42.1 from *The Misuse of Alcohol*, I. Robertson and P. Davies, 1985, by permission of Croom Helm Ltd; Fig. 42.2 from *Controlled Drinking*, N. Heather and I. Robertson, 1981, by permission of Methuen & Co; Table 43.1 from the *Observer Magazine*, 21 October, 1973, by permission of The Observer Ltd; Fig. 43.4 from *Drugtakers in an English Town*, M. Plant, 1975, published by Tavistock Publications.

Material from *Social Trends*, 1980, 1984, 1985 and 1986, and from the *Annual Abstract of Statistics* 1985 is reproduced with the kind permission of the Controller of HMSO.

Every reasonable effort has been made by the author and publishers to contact the copyright holders listed above. Where this has not been successful, as full a credit as possible has been given, and it is hoped that any omissions can be corrected in a future edition.

MOMENT IN TIME

'What is Fate?' Nasrudin was asked by a scholar.

'An endless succession of intertwined events, each influencing the other.'

'That is hardly a satisfactory answer. I believe in cause and effect.'

'Very well,' said the Mulla, 'look at that.' He pointed to a procession passing in the street.

'That man is being taken to be hanged. Is that because someone gave him a silver piece and enabled him to buy the knife with which he committed the murder; or because someone saw him do it; or because nobody stopped him?'

Quoted by Ornstein (1972)

INTRODUCTION

The main objective of this book is to bring together between one pair of covers some of the research relating to the fields of practice of a number of the helping professions. This research arises mainly from the work of sociologists, psychologists and psychiatrists. To compile the book has taken rather more than six years, and the help and advice of many colleagues, as well as that of the Consultants who agreed to peruse my drafts and offer detailed advice and comment from their specialized fields of knowledge and experience.

The idea of the book stemmed from my perception of the need for a range of sophisticated knowledge and skill on the part of the highly committed people seeking to prevent or respond to human need and misery, and the impossibility of enabling them to gain these in the time available for training.

From my own experience as a counsellor and as a social worker in a variety of fields, I knew just how varied and complex are the demands made upon such people. From my training as a psychologist, much influenced by clinical psychology, I knew how a practitioner in those fields, if confronted with an unfamiliar or difficult situation, is taught to go to the research literature and draw upon the work of sometimes hundreds of previous researchers. Such time, and training in the use of research-based approaches is, however, not available in the training of practitioners such as social workers, health visitors and probation officers, despite their heavy statutory responsibilities. It is not available for community and youth workers, or for counsellors or a range of other practitioners who encounter people's need, and sometimes desperation.

As a tutor upon courses of training in social work and youth and community development work, and as a teacher of health visitors, I have sometimes felt ethically reprehensible in colluding in the situation of working with excellent students, highly motivated and enthusiastic to learn, only to discover that one can do no more than introduce them to a handful of the issues, and a smattering of the relevant research, before their course is over and they become practising professionals.

Within my own training, and my subsequent reading and teaching, I have encountered hundreds of books, reports and papers in journals of immediate relevance to these practitioners and, hence, to the well-being of the members of the public to whom they are accountable. Yet there are enormous difficulties in disseminating such material: it seems to take decades for much of it to reach public awareness, and even longer to influence policy and practice. This book seeks to speed up the process of dissemination.

Decisions to extend the periods of training in some of the helping professions are to be welcomed, but other forms of support and training are also needed as workers incur increasing and daunting responsibilities in times of diminishing resources.

This book, then, has been written as a *source book* for members of the helping professions. The chapters seek to be summaries of the research, with all its imperfections and areas of neglect. I hope it will help readers to appreciate the range of the research which has been, and is being, conducted, both within single disciplines and in inter-disciplinary approaches, and that it will encourage them to go to the original material to peruse, appreciate and criticize it. The book attempts to be a 'snapshot' of research at this time, and as such its contents are provisional, tentative and open to challenge. Inevitably, but unintentionally, there are major omissions.

Four particular themes have constantly presented themselves to me as I undertook the reading for this book, and I wish to highlight them here. They are:

1 The importance of systems theory
2 The contribution of structural variables to people's difficulties
3 The inescapability of personal perception and subjectivity
4 The value of simple, attainable goal setting – whether with an individual, a group or family or a community.

1 The importance of systems theory

An early important discovery when compiling material for this book was the figure by Clarke (1977): Elements contributing to a criminal event. (See page 278). The way in which this figure incorporated both sociological and psychological perspectives, and explicitly acknowledged the impact of social and economic factors as well, resolved not only the inappropriate conflict which sometimes occurs between sociologists and psychologists, but placed both perspectives within a far wider context. Anything other than a multivariate analysis both of criminal events, and of many, many other situations thereafter has seemed untenable.

The value of the systems perspective was repeatedly confirmed as I read further: in almost every field wherein I examined the research the multiple nature of the variables, and their complex interactions, became apparent; the approach illustrating the occurrence of a 'criminal event' can also be applied to the schizophrenias, alcohol misuse, child abuse, and difficulties within families. All can be seen in terms of multiple influences and their interactions.

2 The contribution of structural variables to people's difficulties

It is apparent from studies in many different fields of research that structural variables, those associated with lower socio-economic class, disadvantage, and such factors as poverty and unemployment, contribute in major ways to people's difficulties. Whether we examine issues of family life, mental health, or criminology the empirical evidence is there: social inequalities are intrinsically stressful *and* make people vulnerable to additional stresses.

3 The inescapability of personal perception and subjectivity

There is no escaping personal, idiosyncratic experience and perception, and private interpretation. People really do see the same situation differently. Not only do they notice different things, but they interpret and respond to them differently, and they ascribe different meanings to them. Thus being admitted to hospital will have different meanings for different people: for many it is likely to mean distress, with no advantages of any kind; for a few it may mean relief and the 'permission to be ill', according to the perceptions and circumstances of those concerned, and the meaning it has for them. It is timely, then, that the importance of inescapable subjectivities is becoming increasingly recognized and incorporated into models of situations and practice.

4 The usefulness of agreeing simple, attainable goals

In such a situation, where the helping professions are relatively unable to change major socio-economic variables, yet are confronted repeatedly with desperate human situations, what are they to do? Whatever they decide to do, whether it is working at the level of communities, groups, families or individuals, or on several levels at once, it seems that it is helpful if they *agree simple, attainable objectives or goals with the people concerned* and work together towards them – watching meanwhile for any counter-effects which 'progress' has upon those both directly and indirectly concerned.

Such an approach, of starting where people are and involving them as fully as possible in agreeing where they hope to get to, i.e. to their goals or objectives, seems to be not only a supportively structured way of working, but an ethical one as well.

The broad convergence of the research upon the usefulness of this approach came as something of a surprise to me. Yet as I read the research in a wide variety of fields, the message came through, separately and independently, from study after study: not only from the task-centred approach of Reid and Epstein (1972), familiar to social workers, but from settings as disparate as community development and counselling. A situation may be so complex, with multiple variables from many systems interacting, that people feel overwhelmed, not knowing where to start; agreeing a few initial and *attainable* goals and working towards these with them can be an extremely positive and productive approach.

My debt to the Consultants

The immediate stimulus to the book was encountering the 'Highlights' of the National Children's Bureau. These summarize, in a single sheet, key findings concerning all children born in the United Kingdom in one week in March, 1958: as many as possible have been followed up ever since. If so much could be conveyed so succinctly, I thought, perhaps it would be possible to bring together research concerning at least some of the range of fields of practice encountered by the 'helping professions', and by the countless volunteers who do so much vital, and under-recognized work.

The list of the areas where I knew that relevant research was taking place was extensive, and it became apparent that a number of major areas, such as truancy, and important topics such as autism, would have to be omitted. Moreover, it would be improper for such a survey to be undertaken by a single person: one's knowledge is too fragmentary and one's personal biases too strong.

The publishers to whom I put this idea were interested, but requested that I should seek the help of a Consultant in each area of research to consider my summary and to make any necessary amendments. This I have done in almost all of the areas: where I have not it is because of existing personal interests of my own.

The research reported in this book has been undertaken by people from different disciplines, with different standpoints and from different ideologies. While, in my view, it is one of the strengths of the 'systems' formulation that it can accommodate differing perspectives on the same situation, it can be confusing for the reader when the standpoint of the researcher is unclear.

For researchers are human: despite attempts to maintain objectivity, they tend to be alert to data which support their hypothesis and to neglect those which do not. Hence the value of independent evaluations of research and of Consultants who come from many disciplines: sociology, psychiatry and psychology. Because it would not be possible to indicate the standpoint of every researcher quoted in these pages, I have pointed out such particular perspectives only occasionally. Happily, more and more researchers are recognizing, or discovering, evidence of the interactive nature of human experience, and are deliberately seeking the views and contributions of others from differing disciplines, professions and standpoints.

If a multi-dimensional approach to understanding the human situation is called for, then communication and co-operation between people of different viewpoints is certainly needed to reduce human misery and distress. Those whom I have invited to act as Consultants were approached because of the breadth of their vision as well as for their own contribution to empirical research. Their support and co-operation has been a source of encouragement throughout.

The structure of the book

It opens with a section on some principles of working with people in a variety of ways – with a particular emphasis upon research and evaluation within a systems framework. It continues with a closer examination of research in a number of important fields: these range from the broader areas, researched primarily by sociologists, through the more specific fields of particular interest and concern to social workers and researched largely by them, to some of the areas investigated mainly by psychologists and psychiatrists. Because of the overlap in so many of the fields and in the disciplines drawn upon to investigate them, I have found that the boundaries between both fields and disciplines are increasingly blurred. Happily this phenomenon is increasingly reflected by the establishment of multi-disciplinary teams in many fields of practice.

My hope is that some practitioners and students in the helping professions, and indeed some volunteers, will be able to use the material in the book to inform practice, and as a springboard from which further study may take place. If it serves to stimulate debate and to pose questions, that is all part of the empirical approach.

A note to readers

There exist within the English-speaking world two separate means of classifying psychiatric disorders which are in concurrent use. These have many overlapping features. They are:

1 The *International Classification of Diseases*, Ninth Revision (1977), published by the World Health Organization in Geneva. This contains a *Glossary of Mental Disorders and Guide to their Classification.*
2 The *Diagnostic and Statistical Manual of Mental Disorders* (1980) of the American Psychiatric Association, published in Washington.

Some Consultants use one form of classification: some the other. I have followed the recommendation of the Consultant concerned in each case.

References

Clarke, R. V. G. (1977), 'Psychology and crime', *Bulletin of the British Psychological Society*, vol. 30, pp. 280–3.

Ornstein, R. E. (1972), *The Psychology of Consciousness*, San Francisco: W. H. Freeman and Company.

Reid, W. and Epstein, L. (1972), *Task-Centred Casework*, New York: Columbia University Press.

PART 1

Principles and concepts of working within the human social system

1 Three disciplines within a 'systems' approach: sociology, psychology and psychiatry

1 Introducing the 'systems' approach

1.1 The need for a way of thinking of situations involving many interacting variables

It is becoming increasingly apparent that many of the difficulties which people working with people encounter are extremely complex, and are influenced by many different variables. Beishon (1980) has written that if we consider the range of problems encountered by modern society, it is difficult to see any pattern in them, and so we find a range of reactions to them. He continued,

> The truth of the matter, of course, is that there are many forces acting in society and that problems arise from complex interactions of forces, from new rates of change, and indeed from *complexity* itself. . . . We shall suggest that the search for single 'causes' of social problems is misguided and that what is needed is much greater understanding of the complex systems and their interactions which make up society. . . .

1.2 Feature of 'systems' thinking

Beishon suggested that this way of thinking directs attention to:

> the properties of 'wholes' or 'systems' rather than to the parts that make up wholes. This means that attention is focused on *complete entities* and on complexes of interlocking or interacting systems and that it is the *behaviour* of the entity that is studied. This perspective also brings out the relationship between a system and its environment, so that a system is not studied in isolation. . . .

1.3 Origins of 'systems' thinking

1. Beishon noted that the *explicit* recognition of systems thinking began with work of the biologist von Bertalanffy in the 1920s.
2. Writers, thinkers and researchers in many disciplines including mathematics, chemistry, anthropology and many others, began to formulate aspects of their work in terms of interlocking *networks of relationships*. They saw that no discipline is discrete in itself; it is essentially a *selection* from, a perspective upon the total possible field. Thus it follows that each discipline is enriched and illuminated by the insights and contributions of other disciplines.

3 By the 1950s, Beishon reported, these different strands began to converge, and a number of enthusiasts developed the Society for General Systems Theory. From this grew a productive effort to represent aspects of complexity, and to investigate whether there are features common to systems.
4 One development has been the recognition that, in many situations, it is important to understand the contribution of many variables to producing a given situation; it follows, in the world of working with people, that an inter-disciplinary approach may well be the most fruitful.

1.4 Another way of describing the systems approach: the 'ecological' perspective

Hicks and Gullett (1981) have clarified this:

> The ecological view shows that ultimately every form of life affects every other one. However, the inter-relationship may be obscure and insignificant, and may involve many links. These interrelationships have been called the 'web of life'. Persons and the organisations to which they belong are essential parts of this web. . . .

1.5 An example of a 'system': the human body

The human body can be readily understood as a 'system' in which the circulatory system, the respiratory system, the central nervous system and other sub-systems all interact in order to maintain life. Specialist disciplines have arisen which focus upon particular aspects of the whole, but the contributions of each are needed for a deeper understanding of the whole.

1.6 Three disciplines contributing to understanding the human social system

The human social system is an extremely complex affair. Since working with people takes place within this social system, a deliberate attempt has been made to consider research mainly from three among the many disciplines which investigate aspects of this system: sociology, psychology and psychiatry.

2 Sociology

2.1 Describing sociology

Cuff and Payne (1979) suggest that rather than trying to define sociology a more useful approach is to discuss the nature of *sociological perspectives*.

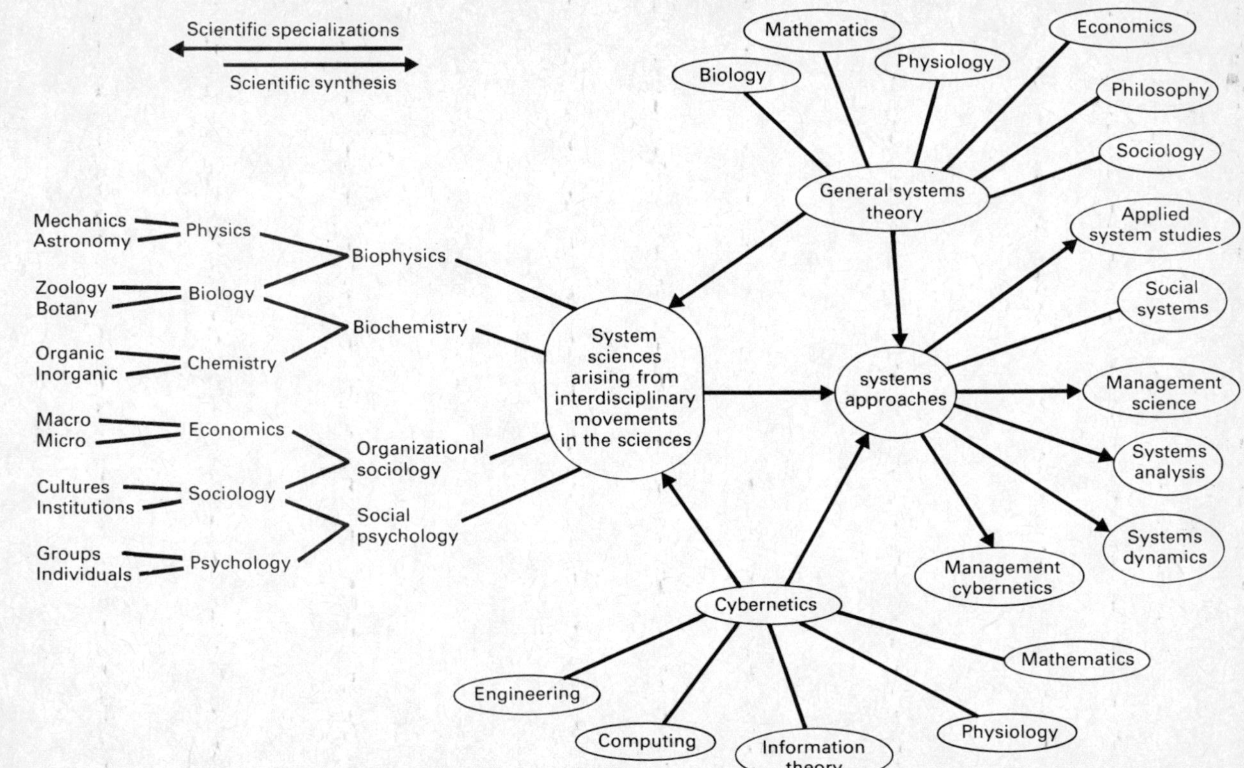

FIGURE 1.1 The development of General Systems Theory (After Beishon, 1980)

2.2 Approaches within sociology

Sociology is the analysis of the structure of social relationships. As with many disciplines, a number of different perspectives, approaches or 'models' have developed within sociology; they represent different standpoints within the total system, and they can in themselves be seen as components of the larger discipline of sociology. Some of the commonly accepted perspectives are shown below, but readers are referred to sociology texts for the detail of each.

1 Functionalism
2 Symbolic interaction
3 Exchange theory
4 Radical and neo-Marxist theory
5 Positivism
6 Phenomonology and ethnomethodology

3 Psychology

3.1 A definition

Psychology is the scientific study of behaviour. The subject matter includes processes that are observable, such as gestures, speech and

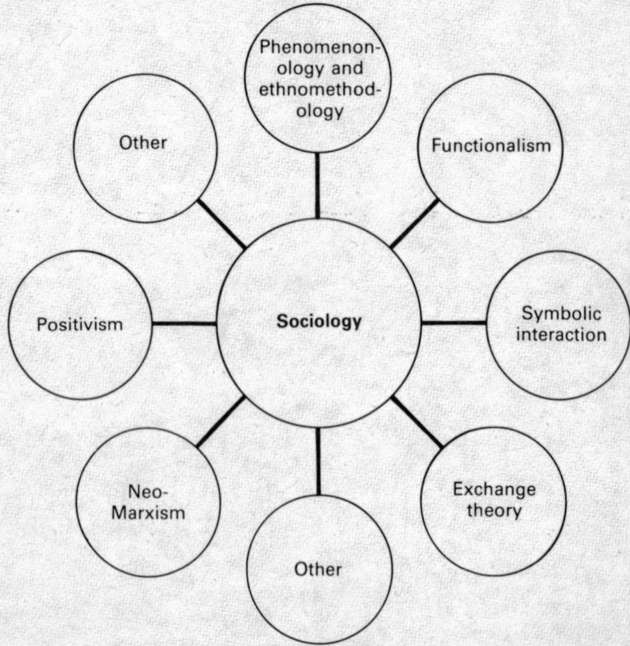

FIGURE 1.2 A range of approaches within sociology

physiological changes, as well as processes which can only be inferred, such as thoughts and dreams. (Clark and Miller, 1970)

3.2 Approaches within psychology

It is increasingly common within psychology to consider human experience, development and behaviour from a range of perspectives (cf. sociology above). These include:

1 The biological and ethological approach
2 The psychoanalytic and psychodynamic approach
3 The social learning and behavioural approach
4 The cognitive approach, which overlaps with the social learning approach
5 The humanistic or 'personal growth' approach

4 Psychiatry

4.1 A definition

Psychiatry is the branch of medicine which deals with the recognition, treatment and prevention of mental abnormalities and disorders. It

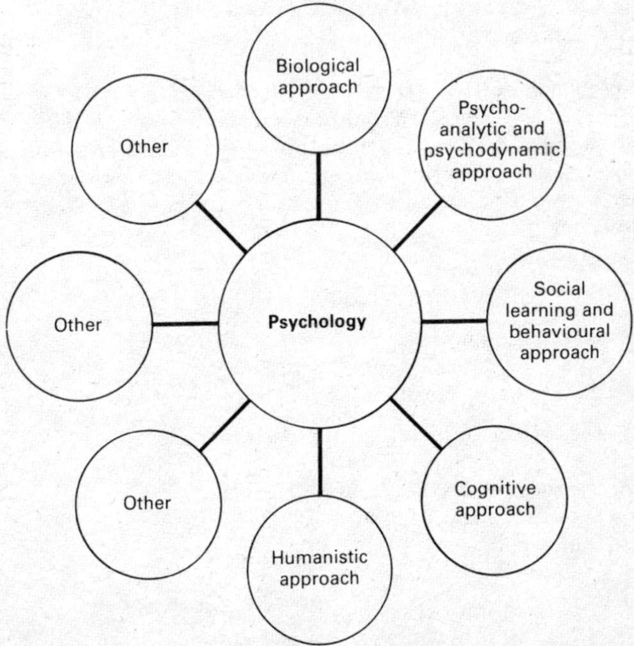

FIGURE 1.3 A range of approaches within psychology

deals with illnesses which predominantly affect a person's mental life and behaviour, i.e. his feelings, his thinking, his behaviour and social relationships. (Linford Rees, 1976)

4.2 The field of psychiatry

The section of mental disorders of the *International Classification of Diseases*, Ninth Revision, refers to three groups of disorders: psychoses, neuroses and mental retardation. In Britain the concept of mental retardation is now replaced by the concepts of 'mental impairment' and 'severe mental impairment'.

'1 **Psychoses:** Mental disorders in which impairment of mental function has developed to a degree that interferes grossly with insight, ability to meet some ordinary demands of life or to maintain contact with reality . . . (Such disorders include the schizophrenias, the severe depressions and manic-depression.)

2 **Neurotic disorders:** Neurotic disorders are mental disorders without any demonstrable organic basis in which the patient may have considerable insight . . . in that he does not confuse his morbid subjective experience and fantasies with external reality . . .
(Such disorders include excessive anxiety, hysterical symptoms, phobias, obsessional and compulsive behaviour, and the less severe depressions.)'

3 **Mental impairment:** In the UK the Mental Health Act 1983 refers to severe mental impairment as, 'a state of arrested or incomplete development of mind which includes severe impairment of intelligence or social functioning. . . .' The same Act refers to mental impairment as a lesser degree of mental handicap which 'includes significant impairment of intelligence and social functioning. . . .'

4.3 Approaches within psychiatry

Clare (1980), in his book *Psychiatry in Dissent*, a critique of the state of the discipline, noted a wide range of approaches or 'models' within psychiatry: some of these are shown in Figure 1.4.

1 The organic or biological approach
2 The psychotherapeutic approach
3 The sociotherapeutic approach
4 The behavioural approach
5 Other approaches

4.4 The growth of inter-disciplinary co-operation

1 These varying approaches, while not mutually exclusive, can seem so. This can lead to divisiveness and to practitioners' perceiving highly

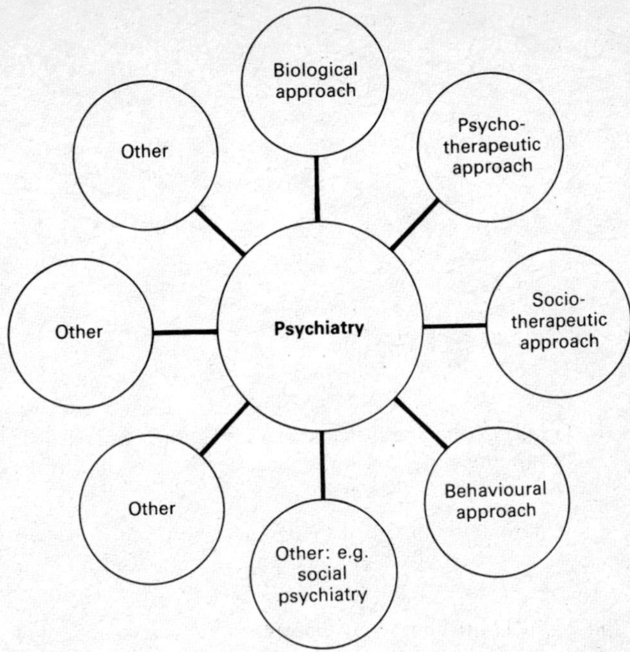

FIGURE 1.4 A range of approaches within psychiatry

complex situations in terms of a single model. Happily, as the 'systems' approach, which stresses the interaction of many variables in contributing to a given situation, gains ground, such narrow affiliations are being seen as unhelpful to people in distress.

2 For example, there has been a heartening growth of inter-disciplinary teams in which people with specialist training contribute their particular expertise towards problem-solving to help people in need. Similarly, close inter-professional co-operation is developing in many areas.

5 Some examples of thinking in terms of systems

5.1 Understanding 'problem behaviour'

The frontispiece to this book, Figure 1.1, (see page 00) shows 'problem behaviour' as precipitated by the interaction of many variables. This model, derived from evidence, can be seen as a 'systems' formulation.

5.2 Systems thinking in professional practice

1 Several researchers, including Goldstein (1973) and Pincus and Minahan (1973), have conceptualized situations, in which e.g. social workers

become involved, in terms of interacting systems. Pincus and Minahan have distinguished four such systems:

1 *Change agent system*: The change agent and the people who are part of his agency or employing organisation.
2 *Client system*: People who sanction or ask for the change agent's services, who are the expected beneficiaries of the service, and who have a working agreement or contract with the change agent.
3 *Target system*: People who need to be changed to accomplish the goals of the change agent.
4 *Action system*: The change agent and the people he works with and through to accomplish his goals and influence the target system.

2 These authors suggested that the systems framework lends itself to the analysis of any situation, and that it can be used in a variety of settings, whether the primary target be,

> an emotionally disturbed individual who needs help with personal problems, a family in conflict, absentee landlords of slum properties, or a social agency unresponsive to the needs of its consumers.

3 Pincus and Minahan urged the necessity for agreeing outcome goals with those with whom work is undertaken, and saw these as:

> a specification of the condition in which we would like to see a situation at the end of a successful planned change effort.

The process they advocated is shown in Figure 1.5.

References

Beishon, J. (1980), 'Introduction to systems thinking and organization' in *Systems Organization: the Management of Complexity*, T243, Block 1, Milton Keynes: The Open University.

Clare, A. (1980), *Psychiatry in Dissent*, London: Tavistock.

Clark, K. E. and Miller, G. A. (1970) (eds) *Psychology*, Prentice Hall.

Cuff, E. E. and Payne, G. C. F. (1979), *Perspectives in Sociology*, London: Allen & Unwin.

Goldstein, H. (1973), *Social Work Practice: A Unitary Approach*, Columbia: University of South Carolina Press.

Herbert, M. (1981), *Behavioural Treatment of Problem Children. A Practice Manual*, London: Academic Press.

Hicks, H. and Gullett, C. R. (1981), *Management*, McGraw-Hill.

International Classification of Diseases, Injuries and Causes of Death: Mental Disorders Section (1980), Geneva: World Health Organization.

Linford Rees, W. L. (1976), *A Short Textbook of Psychiatry*, London: Hodder & Stoughton.

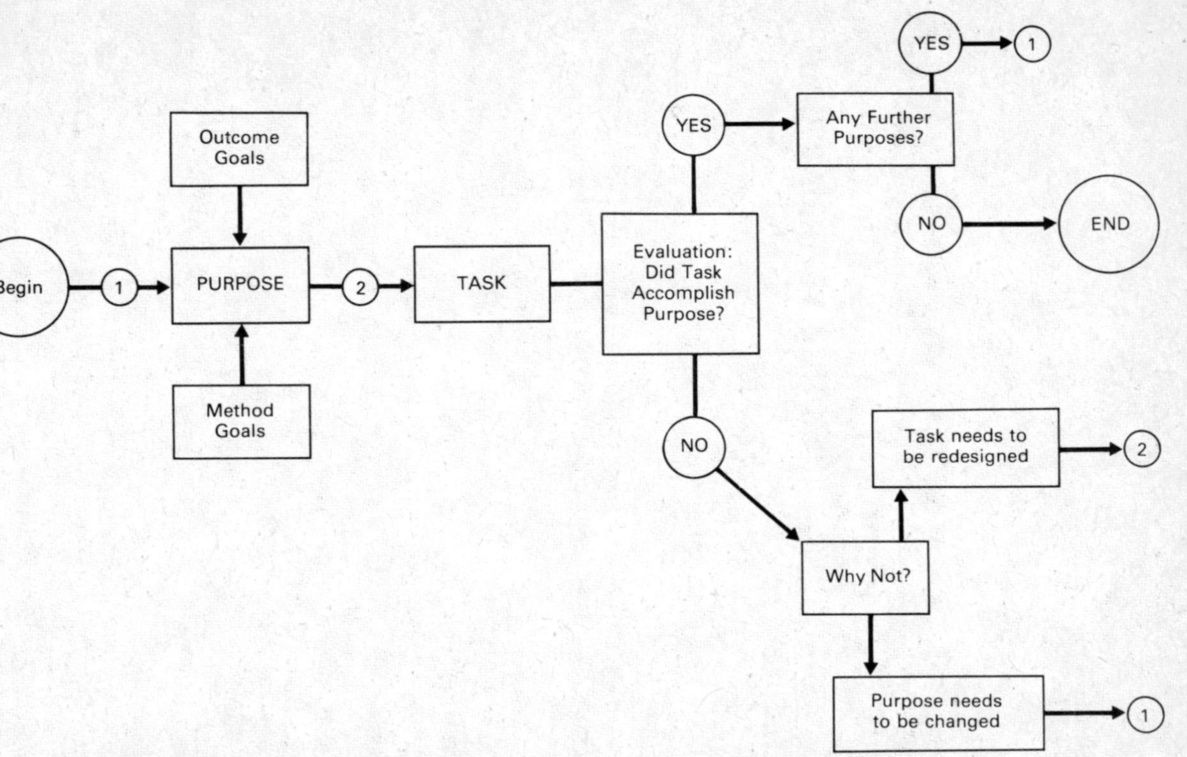

FIGURE 1.5 The process when intervening in systems (Pincus and Minahan, 1973)

Pincus, A. and Minahan, A. (1973), *Social Work Practice: Model and Method*, Itasca, Illinois: F. E. Peacock Publishers, Inc.
von Bertalanffy, L., Hempel, C. G., Bass, R. E. and Jonas, H. (1951), 'General Systems Theory: A New Approach to Unity of Science', I–VI, *Human Biology*, 23, pp. 302–61.

2 The empirical approach in the social sciences: gathering verifiable data

1 Definitions and descriptions of terms

1.1 Empirical

> Based or acting on observation or experiment, not on theory; regarding sense-data as valid information; deriving knowledge from experience alone.
>
> (Concise Oxford English Dictionary, 1976)

1.2 Social sciences

Atkinson, Atkinson and Hilgard (1983) have suggested that,

> The study of human behaviour must go beyond what happens to an isolated individual and consider the institutional arrangements in which the individuals live: the family, the community and the larger society . . . a number of fields of enquiry have developed: anthropology, economics, linguistics, political science and other specialities. Taken together, these are known as the *behavioural* and *social sciences* . . . the terms 'behavioural science' and 'social science' have come to be used interchangeably.

These authors can be seen as locating the individual within a number of *systems*: the family, the community and the larger society. They go on to suggest that the term 'social science' encompasses the study of groups of individuals in interaction, while the term 'behavioural science' emphasizes the individual and his or her specific characteristics or behaviour.

1.3 Science

The same authors wrote concerning 'science' and its aim,

> The aim of science is to provide new and useful information in the form of verifiable data: data obtained under conditions such that other qualified people can repeat the observations and obtain the same results. This task calls for orderliness and precision in investigating relationships and in communicating these to others. The scientific ideal is not always achieved, but as a science becomes better established, it rests upon an increasing number of relationships that are taken for granted because they have been validated so often.

2 Some features of the empirical approach

2.1 Asking questions, and devising hypotheses

Such questions may *seem*, at first, to be fairly simple, such as,

> Are boys more likely to become ill in childhood than girls?

or more complex, such as,

> How can people with agoraphobia be helped?

Put into the form of testable hypotheses ('hunches', the accuracy of which one can test), these might become,

> Boys are more likely to become ill in childhood than girls,

and,

> People with agoraphobia benefit from practising relaxation.

There are many difficulties, however, in reaching even approximate and provisional answers. Some of these will be discussed in 2.4.

2.2 Examining the 'literature' on the subject

1 If other people have researched the same subject, i.e. asked the same question in a systematic and organized way, then relevant reports will already exist in books and journals. Many of these will report attempts to provide data, or measurements, as the basis for their studies. Such reports, together with other bodies of information, constitute the 'research literature'.

2 This research literature may not provide any answers: it may suggest a partial answer, or it may just point to other questions. Any tentative answers which it does suggest will relate most closely to the sample of people who took part in the studies, and cannot be automatically applied to other groups of people.

2.3 Seeking answers via measurement: gathering verifiable data

1 The empirical method approaches such questions by asking, *What is the evidence?* It grounds any provisional answers upon 'observation and experiment' and upon 'verifiable data'. Typical data are often measurements of various kinds and personal reports.
2 Researchers frequently make use of questionnaires, surveys, observational studies and experimental approaches. See Section 3.

2.4 Recognizing difficulties in measuring things

Such difficulties include:

1 **Problems of sampling** No sample of a population is perfectly representative: the smaller the sample, the more unrepresentative it will be. This illustrates the need for repeating studies among different samples of people composing a particular population (group) – of, say, adolescents.

2 **Problems of gathering 'valid' information or data** There are great difficulties in being sure that the information gathered really gives a true picture. Administering even a simple questionnaire is a very complex task. People do not seem to act as naturally when they are being questioned, or when they feel under scrutiny, as when they are on their own. Researchers may also, unintentionally, encourage certain types of answers or reactions rather than others: for example, by smiling when the answers accord with their own view of an appropriate answer.

3 **Problems of gathering 'reliable' information or data** Similarly there are problems of gathering 'reliable' data: a reliable test, e.g. for depression, is one which gives broadly the same result whoever administers it, and in whatever circumstances. Such reliability in tests is very hard to attain.

4 **Problems of subjectivity of meanings** Despite a common language, people mean different things when they use the same word: e.g. 'health', 'improvement', or 'aggressiveness'. Recognizing this, many researchers will try to agree a tight or 'operational' definition of terms and meanings before starting on a given study. For example, if investigating whether one group of children was more 'aggressive' than another, it might be agreed that, in that study, aggression would be defined as:

(a) a physical blow, push, punch or bite
(b) the action of removing an object from another child who resists this action

Measuring 'aggression' between the two groups could then be carried out reasonably straightforwardly and accurately, by, for example, counting instances of the agreed behaviours by children of the two groups during a fixed period in a common setting.

3 Some methods of research and investigation

3.1 The survey method

1 **Advantages and disadvantages** Researchers in all the social sciences use this as a means of gathering a wide range of opinion, information and other data. Surveys involve large numbers of participants, and so draw upon a broad spread of opinion. Disadvantages, already mentioned, are that survey data is usually still only a sample, and that people do not always give their real views to a researcher.

2 **Stages in conducting a survey** McNeill (1985) has suggested the following key stages:

1 Choice of topic to be studied.
2 Forming of hunches and hypotheses.
3 Identification of the population to be surveyed.
4 Carrying out preparatory investigations and interviews.
5 Drafting the questionnaire or interview schedule.
6 Conducting a pilot survey.
7 Finalizing the questionnaire.
8 Selecting a sample of the population.
9 Selection and training of interviewers (if necessary).
10 Collecting the data.
11 Processing the data and analysing the results.
12 Writing the research reports.
13 Publication of the report.

Many of these stages can be readily identified in Figure 2.1.

3 **Examples of surveys**

1 The best known is the National Census, conducted every ten years, and directed towards every member of the population of the UK.
2 Another in the longitudinal study still being conducted by the National Children's Bureau upon all children, over 14,000, born in a specific week in March 1958 – or as many as can be traced. This study offers some answers to the question whether boys are more likely to become ill in childhood than girls. Most surveys are based upon much smaller samples.

3.2 The observational method

1 **Advantages and disadvantages** Advantages include the desirability of minimal interference in a natural system such as a playground or classroom. Disadvantages include 'selective perception', i.e. that observers may see what they hope to see. It is increasingly the custom to engage more than one observer to reduce this difficulty.

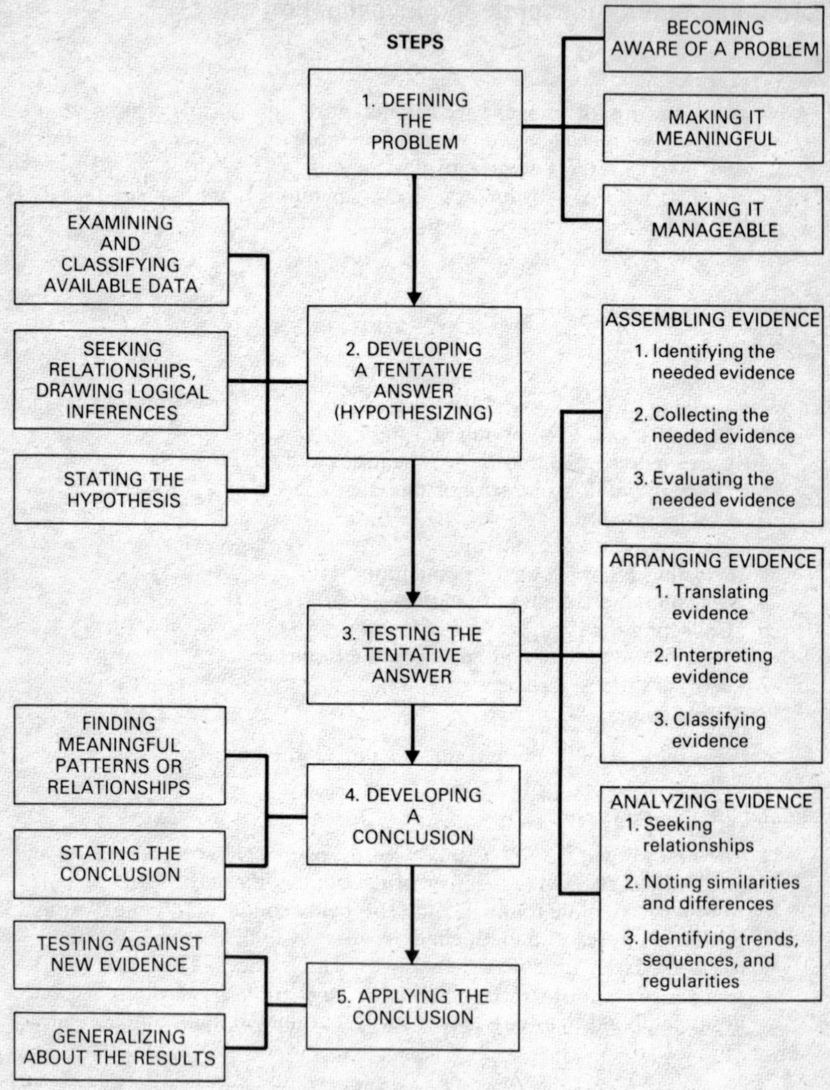

FIGURE 2.1 A schematic overview of the research process (Beyer, 1971)

2 **Examples of observational studies** Many studies have taken place, for example, of children in play settings, and differing interactions of boys and girls. (McGrew, 1972)

3.3 The experimental method

1 Features of this method

1 The aim is usually to investigate the impact of a particular variable of the total system, called the 'independent' variable, upon a situation. Such a possible effect can be measured by noting changes in one or more features of that situation: these are called the 'dependent variable(s)'.

2 Psychologists employ this method frequently: sometimes they work in laboratories, but increasingly, they, together with sociologists and psychiatrists, work in the ordinary setting (system) of the home, the playground and the shopping centre.

2 Stages in the approach There are also a number of stages in this approach: the following list is adapted from that of McNeill (1985):

1. Choice of topic to be studied.
2. Examining the literature on the topic.
3. Forming of hunches or hypotheses.
4. Identification of the population to be studied.
5. Consideration of ethical issues.
6. Planning the experimental design: e.g. 'single subject'; designs with 'experimental' and 'control' groups, etc.
7. Pinpointing a statistical analysis appropriate to the experimental design.
8. Inviting people to participate, and informing them as fully as possible about the study.
9. Conducting a pilot study.
10. Finalizing the experimental design and the materials, if necessary.
11. Selection and training of researchers, if necessary.
12. Conducting the experiment with new participants.
13. Processing the data and analysing the results.
14. Writing the research report.
15. Publication of the report.

3 An example of the experimental approach: with one individual To seek an answer to the question, How can a person be helped to overcome agoraphobia?, a possible hypothesis, devised with the research literature in mind, (see Chapter 32, page 312), might be:

Rehearsing going out each day will help a person to spend more time outdoors unaccompanied each day.

In this example, the independent variable is 'rehearsals of going out': the dependent variable is 'spending time outdoors unaccompanied'. The course of such a study is shown in Figure 2.2.

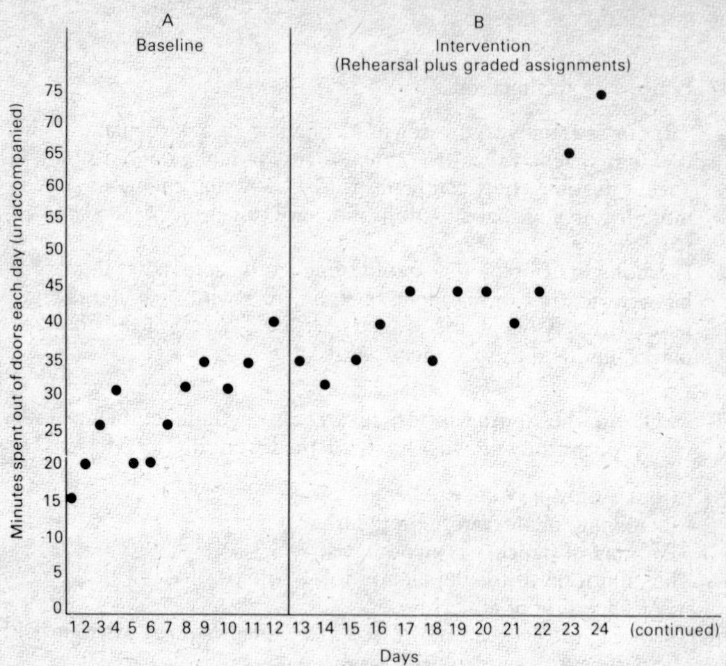

FIGURE 2.2 The experimental approach with one person (Sheldon, 1982)

4 **An example of the experimental approach with two (*or more*) groups:**

1 If there are large numbers of participants, more than say thirty or forty, allocation to the groups is made randomly: if small, then an effort is made to match each participant in one group with a participant in the other group – in terms of e.g. age, sex, social class, etc. Such an approach is called a 'controlled experiment' because there is an 'experimental group', who experience the effects of the independent variable, and a 'control group', who do not.

2 This format could be used to test the same hypothesis:

> Rehearsing going out each day will help a person to spend more time outdoors unaccompanied.

Typically, volunteers experiencing agoraphobia would be randomly allocated to the 'experimental' and 'control' groups. Pre-test measures of time currently spent outdoors would be taken. (This is called 'establishing a baseline'). Then those in the experimental group would be encouraged to practise going out unaccompanied daily for, say, one month. These in the control group would not.

3 At the end of the month the average number of minutes spent outdoors unaccompanied by members of each group would be compared. (Cf. Figure 2.3).

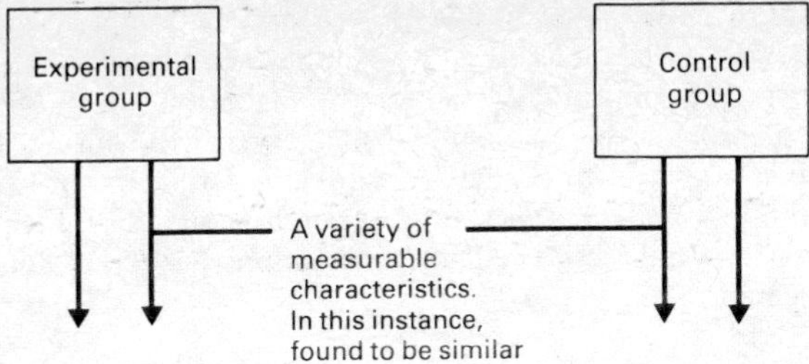

A *Pre-test situation:* two matched samples, chosed to be as similar upon as many different variables as possible: e.g. age, sex

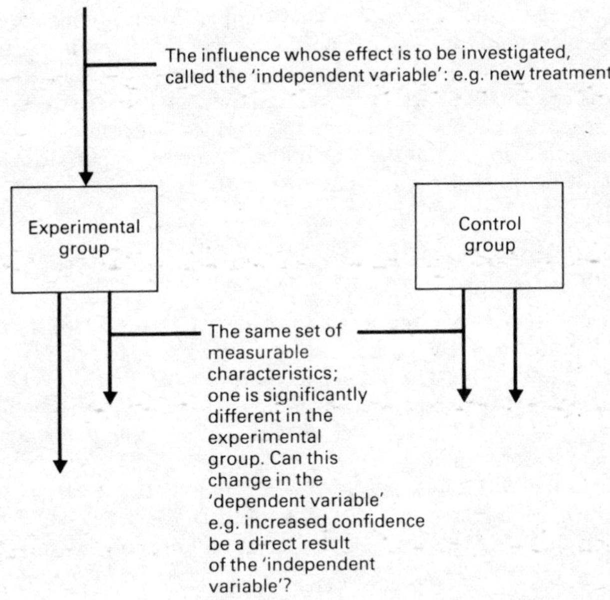

B *Test situation*: the same matched samples tested following the application of a specific influence e.g. a new drug, or a new form of treatment

FIGURE 2.3 Independent and dependent variables in a controlled experiment (Sutton, 1979)

4 Other important issues

4.1 The use of mathematical and statistical techniques

1 Because, increasingly, the behavioural and social sciences use the common currency of mathematics to report their findings

('quantitative' data) – although they may well use other verbal or written accounts as well ('qualitative' data) – they are able to employ a range of statistical techniques to examine the significance of those findings.

2 When planning a research study it is important to consider beforehand what forms of statistical analysis will be undertaken. For example, there are specific techniques appropriate to situations where the effects of several variables, and possible interactions between them, are being investigated.

4.2 Drawing provisional conclusions and acknowledging limitations

1 If the data and the statistical analyses performed thereon warrant it, it may be possible to draw some provisional and tentative conclusions as to whether the evidence does or does not support the original hypothesis. Such evidence is then compared and contrasted with other evidence found in similar fields in the literature, and implications discussed.

2 It is customary to acknowledge frankly the weaknesses and flaws of one's research, and to be open to informed criticism. Such honesty is, or should be, part of the scientific and empirical approach. The constructive criticism of one's own work and that of others is to be encouraged.

References

Atkinson, R. L., Atkinson, R. C. and Hilgard, E. R. (1983), *Introduction to Psychology*, New York: Harcourt, Brace, Jovanovich.

Beyer, B. K. (1971), 'The inquiry method', *Inquiry in the Social Studies Classroom*, Columbus: Merrill.

McGrew, W. C. (1972), *An Ethological Study of Children's Behaviour*, London: Academic Press.

McNeill, P. (1985), *Research Methods*, London: Tavistock.

Oxford English Dictionary (1976), Oxford University Press.

Sheldon, B. (1982), *Behaviour Modification*, London: Tavistock.

Sutton, C. (1979), *Psychology for Social Workers and Counsellors*, London: Routledge & Kegan Paul.

The empirical approach in the social sciences: evaluation of intervention

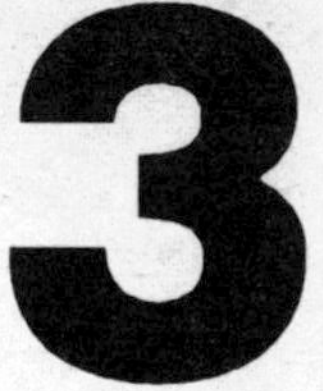

1 Definition

To evaluate an intervention means, in general terms, to assess the effects/effectiveness of an intervention: more precisely, it means to measure, using mathematically verifiable data, the effects/effectiveness of an intervention.

2 Why is it important to evaluate?

1 To arrive at the best means, within the time and resources available, for helping people with their difficulties in living.
2 To carry out ethical responsibilities towards the people in whose lives the helping professions intervene.
3 To demonstrate particular need – e.g. for resources.
4 To make an intelligent response to controversy: an examination of the *evidence* may short cut hours of debate based solely upon subjective impression or viewpoint.
5 To alert practitioners to the necessity of determining whether their efforts to help others are found to be helpful *by those others*.
6 To gather evidence concerning the usefulness or otherwise of innovations, or concerning their unintended effects upon other aspects of the total system.
7 To pinpoint key variables in settings where many variables are interacting: e.g. the importance of certain counsellor characteristics. (Truax and Carkhuff, 1967)

3 Some considerations before embarking on an evaluation

3.1 Preliminary questions

(After Herzog (1959) and Phillip, McCulloch and Smith (1975)

1 What is the purpose of the evaluation? This will often be to test the validity of research data which have been gathered, and any provisional conclusions drawn, against a hypothesis or prediction; e.g.:

Suicide increases during periods of high unemployment.
Wearing seat-belts will reduce road accident fatalities.
Volunteer counsellors are as helpful as professionals.

2 Does the researcher know the research 'literature' on the subject?
3 How representative was the sample of subjects of the larger population?
4 How were the data collected?

5 In experimental work, what were the independent and the dependent variables?
6 In experimental work, how were these variables and their possible effects measured?
7 At what point(s) were measurements made?
8 What is the evidence that any changes noted were actually due to the effect of the independent variable?
9 Is the design of the experiment repeatable?
10 Was the investigation ethically acceptable to those concerned?
11 Did all the participants understand that they were taking part in a research study, and was their agreement obtained?

3.2 The impossibility of conducting value-free research

1 No research ever takes place in a situation which is value-free. In a discussion of this, McNeill (1985) has reported the views of Halsey, Heath and Ridge (1980) concerning sociology:

> It has never, therefore, been a 'value-free' academic discipline, if such were in any event possible. Instead, it has been an attempt to marry a value-laden choice of issue with objective methods of data-collection.

2 Thus, while some steps can be taken to avoid major flaws arising from personal subjectivity, or sampling errors, it will always be important to know, as Rees and Wallace (1982) emphasized,

> who was making a judgment, from what value base, in relation to what sort of activity.

3.3 An example of rigorous criteria for evaluating outcome studies

Gurman and Kniskern (1978, 1981), in their major reviews of the field of family and marital therapy, (see Chapter 38, page 362) suggested the following vital indicators of the quality of the research, and commented thereon:

1 *Controlled assignment of clients to treatment conditions*: random assignment, matching of total groups or matching in pairs.
2 *Pre-postmeasurement of change*: it is not uncommon for family therapy research to use post-evaluations only.
3 *No contamination of major independent variables*: this includes therapists' experience level, number of therapists per treatment condition, and *relevant* therapeutic competence. . . .
4 *Appropriate statistical analysis*
5 *Follow-up*: one to three months . . . three months or more.
6 *Treatments equally valued*: tremendous biases are often engendered for both therapists and patients when this criterion is not met.
7 *Treatment carried out as prescribed or expected*: clear evidence. . . .

8 *Multiple change indices* used. . . .
9 *Multiple vantage points* used in assessing outcome.
10 *Outcome not limited to change in the 'identified patient'*: this criterion is perhaps uniquely required in marital/family therapy.
11 *Data on other concurrent treatment*. . . .
12 *Equal treatment length* in comparative studies. . . .
13 *Outcome assessment allows for both positive and negative change*
14 *Therapist–investigator nonequivalence*: earlier reviews . . . had found the two to be the same person in about 75 per cent of the studies examined.

4 Some examples of intervention which have been evaluated

1 The comparative effectiveness of paraprofessionals, such as community volunteers, and professionals, in helping some groups of people with their difficulties in living. (Durlak, 1979)
2 The usefulness or otherwise of bereavement counselling. (Parkes, 1980) (See Chapter 37, page 354)
3 The effectiveness or otherwise of electric convulsive therapy (ECT) in relieving depression. (West, 1981) (Chapter 33, page 321)
4 The effects of various kinds of sentence in reducing offending against the law. (Brody, 1976). (See Chapter 30)
5 The effectiveness of patch-based social services teams. (McGrath and Hadley, 1981)

N.B. It must be emphasized that none of the above studies is the final word upon the subjects which they address; they are, however, contributions to an on-going enquiry in each area.

5 Some of the main models of evaluation of intervention

5.1 The model based on 'the achievement of objectives'

1 **Preliminary considerations** This approach stems from management theory, (see Chapter 11, page 86), where it is discussed more fully. The approach is adaptable to many settings, including ones encountered by those working with people in difficulties. Principles include:

1 Agreeing what are the objectives of the organization, the community, the group, the family and/or the individuals concerned.
2 Agreeing *attainable* goals or objectives.
3 Agreeing what will constitute evidence that a given objective has been achieved; i.e. what will be the criteria of 'success' of, for example:
   (a) a group working to increase the take-up of welfare benefits.
   (b) a group seeking better provision for elderly people from ethnic minority groups.
   (c) a family seeking to communicate more constructively.

(d) the acceptable standard of performance of a volunteer undertaking training in counselling.

4 Deciding, *by some form of measurement*, and *for each objective*, where the participants are at the outset – in relation to their ultimate objectives; i.e. establishing a 'baseline'.

5 Following the intervention, comparing the post-intervention data with the pre-intervention data, and judging whether the agreed criteria have been met. If not, pinpointing why not, and using that feedback when planning the next effort.

2 A possible example

1 If the objective of a group is to increase the take-up of welfare benefits, the following matters, at the very least, will need to be worked out and agreed:
   (a) what is the present level of take-up in the area – in terms, for example, of numbers of claimants, or, as another example, of extent of take-up of a specific entitlement?
   (b) for how many months will the campaign last?
   (c) how will 'success' be defined? would an increased take-up by claimants of 10 per cent?, 25 per cent?, 50 per cent?, 100 per cent? count?
   (d) if not, what would?
   (e) will any unintended effects be monitored?

2 Having considered these matters, and determined both the current level of 'take-up' in an area (the baseline), and what will constitute 'success' in the campaign, the campaign runs.

3 Thereafter it would be fairly easy to calculate the extent of increased take-up of welfare benefits, and whether the post-intervention data, when compared with the pre-intervention data, met the agreed criteria or not.

5.2 The model based upon completion of a questionnaire

1 Preliminary considerations Matters to be considered will include those indicated in Chapter 2, page 18. When evaluating a study based upon a questionnaire, as distinct from another type of study, the following issues at least are important:

1 The reasons for using a questionnaire as the tool of inquiry.
2 What was the precise hypothesis under investigation?
3 If the total population, e.g. of people in receipt of a particular social service, was not approached, how was the sample thereof selected?
4 What were the key issues to which the questionnaire was addressed?
5 Did the design of questionnaire (e.g. check list, rating scale, inventory, etc.) appropriately test the hypothesis?
6 Were the kind(s) of statistical analysis used appropriate?

7 Were any conclusions drawn based clearly on data arising from the hypothesis?
8 Were ethical issues, e.g. confidentiality, addressed?

2 A possible example

1 Oppenheim (1976) reported the design of the inventory form of questionnaire shown in Table 3.1. Such a design could be used to test a hypothesis concerning the impact of training upon perceptions of 'good' and 'bad' practice among psychiatric nurses.
2 Administering the questionnaire both before and after training, and

How good or bad would it be, in your opinion, if a psychiatric nurse like yourself on your present ward did any of the following things? (Please put a check in the right column)

How bad is it if you *How good is it if you*	Very bad	Bad	Would not matter	Fairly good	Very good	It would depend
Spend a good deal of time talking to patients?						
Let some patients remain untidy?						
Sometimes show that you are in a bad mood yourself?						
Appear to the patients to be very busy and efficient?						
Forget to put on a clean uniform?						
Avoid discussion of personal problems of a patient with him because you feel that the doctor should do this?						
Take special pride in having patients who are quiet and do as they are told?						
Talk about a patient when the patient is present, acting as though the patient was not there?						
Get deeply involved with what happens to particular patients?						
Find that you have to be very firm with some patients?						

TABLE 3.1 How bad is it? How good is it? Part of a questionnaire administered to psychiatric nurses (Oppenheim, 1976)

subjecting the results to statistical analysis would offer some evidence for an evaluation of the effectiveness of the training programme.

5.3 The models based upon experimental design

1 Evaluation of intervention with a single individual

(a) A common model is the design

A B . . . . . follow-up

where A represents a baseline
where B represents an intervention
where follow-up takes place, typically, some weeks later

(b) A possible example Figure 3.1 shows a study reported by Sheldon (1982), illustrating the effectiveness of a programme of modelling, rehearsal and graded assignments, plus a back-up reinforcement scheme, for a withdrawn psychiatric patient. The evaluation, occurring at the follow-ups at fourteen and twenty-eight weeks, suggests that the effect of the training programme had been maintained.

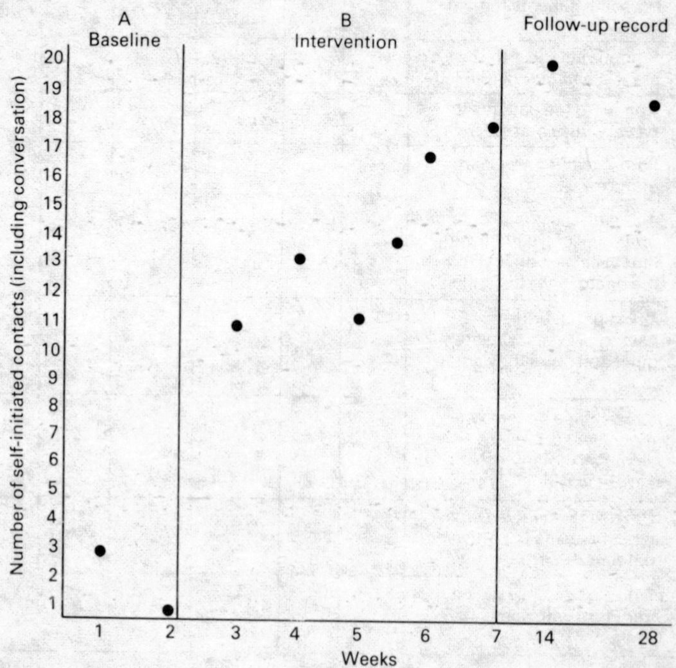

FIGURE 3.1 Assertion training with a withdrawn psychiatric patient (Sheldon, 1982)

2 **Evaluation of intervention with an experimental group and a control group**

(a) Here, the design below is commonly followed

Experimental group:	A B	......	follow-up
Control group:	A	......	follow-up

where A represents a baseline
where B represents an intervention
where follow-up takes place, typically, some weeks later

Thus the experimental group experiences a specific intervention: the control group does not.

(b) An example of this design is a study by Kassebaum et al (1967) with two groups of offenders, each with 484 prisoners. Counselling (the independent variable) was offered to one group, the experimental group: it was not offered to the second, control, group. At follow-up, after discharge from prison, the prevalence of re-offending (the dependent variable) was the same for both groups. The evaluation thus offered no evidence that the provision of counselling for prisoners had an effect upon the probability of their re-offending – though it may have had other beneficial effects.

(c) It is now professional practice among most sociologists, psychologists and psychiatrists to evaluate the effects/effectiveness of their interventions. All groups who intervene in the lives of others carry ethical responsibility for evaluating the effects of their work.

6 Difficulties with these 'classical' models of evaluation

1 It is being increasingly recognized that the models of evaluation described above, the so-called 'classical' models, do not lend themselves readily to the complexity of many situations where intervention is requested (e.g. in family work), or implicit (e.g. in community development).

2 There is also increasing recognition that events occur within a context or system, and that 'it is impossible just to do one thing'; that is, there are always side effects, unforeseen implications or unintended consequences.

3 In these circumstances, there are moves towards trying to develop systems models of evaluation. These are at an early stage, however, and until they become practicable many writers, e.g. Weiss (1972), suggest the 'objectives model' has advantages for evaluating outcomes in complex situations. Other possible approaches have been suggested by the London Voluntary Service Council (1981) and by Hedley (1985).

References

Brody, S. (1976), *The Effectiveness of Sentencing: a Review of the Literature*, London: HMSO.

Durlak, J. (1979), 'Comparative effectiveness of paraprofessional and professional helpers', *Psychological Bulletin*, vol. 86, pp. 80–2.

Gurman, A. S. and Kniskern, D. P. (1978), 'Research on marital and family therapy: progress, perspective and prospect' in Garfield, S. and Bergin, A. E., (eds), *Handbook of Psychotherapy and Behaviour Change*, New York: Wiley.

Halsey, A. H., Heath, A. F. and Ridge, J. M. (1980), *Origins and Destinations. Family, Class and Education in Modern Britain*, Oxford: The Clarendon Press.

Hedley, R. (1985), *Measuring Success. A Guide to Evaluation by Voluntary and Community Groups*, London: Advance.

Herzog, E. (1959). *Some Guidelines for Evaluative Research*. Washington, D.C.: Department of Health Education and Welfare.

Kassebaum, G., Ward, D. and Wilner, D. (1971), *Prison Treatment and Parole Survival*, New York: Wiley.

London Voluntary Service Council (1981), *Evolution of Community Work*. London: London Council of Social Service.

McGrath, M. and Hadley, R. (1981), Evaluating patch-based social services teams: a pilot study. In E. M. Goldberg and N. Connelly (eds), *Evaluative Research in Social Care*. (Policy Studies Institute Series), London: Heinemann Educational Books.

McNeill, P. (1985), *Research Methods*, London: Tavistock Publications.

Oppenheim, A. N. (1976), *Questionnaire Design and Attitude Measurement*, London: Heinemann Educational Books.

Parkes, C. M. (1980). 'Bereavement counselling: does it work?', *British Medical Journal*, 5 July, 1980.

Philip, A. E., McCulloch, J. W. and Smith, N. J. (1975), *Social Work Research and the Analysis of Social Data*, Oxford: Pergamon.

Rees, S. and Wallace, A. (1982), *Verdicts on Social Work*, London: Edward Arnold.

Sheldon, B. (1982), *Behaviour Modification*, London: Tavistock Publications.

Truax, C. and Carkhuff, R. (1967), *Towards Effective Counselling and Psychotherapy*, Chicago: Aldine.

West, E. (1981), 'Electric convulsion therapy in depression: a double blind controlled trial', *British Medical Journal*, vol. 282, 31 January 1981.

Weiss, C. (1972), *Evaluation Research*, Englewood Cliffs, New Jersey: Prentice-Hall.

Community work and community development

4

Consultant: Paul Taylor, Senior Lecturer, Youth and Community Development Course, Leicester Polytechnic.

1 Definition

There is no one accepted definition of community work. It may therefore be helpful to give a definition of *community workers* and a description of their work.

1.1 Community workers and their work

Francis, Henderson and Thomas (1984) have defined community workers as:

> paid staff whose *primary responsibility* is to develop groups in the community, whose members experience (and wish to tackle) needs, disadvantage or inequality.

1.2 A description of the work

These same writers have suggested:

> Community workers
>
> - help people to identify needs, to come together in a group and support them in their action.
> - help groups to achieve their goals.
> - seek to improve the skills, confidence and awareness of group members, and their understanding of problems and issues.
>
> They do not usually deal with problems on a one-to-one basis but encourage people to work on problems collectively, enabling them to acquire resources and influence. They enable groups to deal with issues in a number of fields including health, education, social services, employment, the environment, housing, planning, recreation, youth work and the arts.
>
> The groups may be based on a neighbourhood or on common interests, and will include a variety of action groups, care and self-help groups, committees, co-operatives and federations.
>
> Community work sometimes involves making services more flexible

and relevant, developing community resources and influencing statutory, voluntary and private organisations to make them more responsive and open to people's needs and demands.

This description echoes many of the stated aims and objectives of the Association of Community Workers (1982).

2 Statistics

Francis, Henderson and Thomas (1984) give the following data upon the numbers of community workers (as defined above):

Statutory sector	2,201
Voluntary sector	3,164
	5,365

Of those in the statutory sector, 27 per cent were employed by Social Services Departments and 47 per cent by Local Education Authorities.

TABLE 4.1 Community workers in the United Kingdom. (Francis, Henderson and Thomas, 1984). Reprinted with permission.

2.1 The employment of community workers

	UK overall	London	Metro England	Shire England	Wales	Scotland	Northern Ireland
Social Services	11	10	13	11	13	12	9
Education	19	4	10	7	7	63	2
Leisure services	5	2	2	11	4	1	24
Housing	2	2	2	2	5	1	—
Chief Executives	1	2	1	*	2	1	2
Planning	1	1	1	1	1	*	—
Other or unspecified local authority	1	1	2	1	2	*	—
Probation	*	—	*	*	1	n/a	—
Development corporations	1	*	*	3	—	1	—
Health authorities and CHCs	1	1	*	1	1	—	—
Councils of Voluntary Service/RCCs	7	3	5	14	7	4	5
Community Relations Councils	4	7	6	3	1	1	—
Other voluntary organisations	49	67	58	45	58	15	58
Total %	102	100	100	99	102	99	100
n =	5365	1138	1104	1255	186	1230	192

TABLE 4.2 Organizations employing community workers, by area. Percentages. Figures are rounded (Francis, Henderson and Thomas, 1984). (Reprinted with permission)

3 Some approaches to, or models of, community work

3.1 A well-recognized classification

The work described in 1.2, above, is commonly identified in practice as three interrelated models:

1 Community organization
2 Community development
3 Community action

3.2 One possible set of definitions/descriptions

Stevens (1978), building on the work of Armstrong and colleagues (1974), gave a brief summary of each approach:

'1 **Community organization** This is the most traditional strategy of community work. The aim of those employing this strategy is usually to maintain or improve levels of social welfare provision either by:

(a) Maximizing the utilization of resources which exist *within* communities, for example, by establishing 'Good Neighbour' Schemes . . .
and/or
(b) Co-ordinating and improving the efficiency of service provision, especially of voluntary services
and/or
(c) Securing higher levels of provision from government agencies.'

2 **Community development** Taylor (1985) has suggested that community development is more a community-based *process* based on a wide range of issues. Stevens (1978) sees theory here as more wide-ranging and more overtly political than community organization. While the latter mainly addresses aspects of social service provision, community development:

1 encourages analysis of issues, such as health, housing, education and unemployment.
2 allows for the input of governmental intervention and resources
3 makes processes of participation and self-help more central.

3 **Community action** Stevens (1978) suggested that community action theorists propound a conflict analysis, and that the view of most such theorists is that given the nature of capitalism, working-class communities will inevitably be exploited by élite groups. . . . This analysis is likely to lead to the employment of a number of strategies by community workers, including encouraging groups to engage in 'direct action' (such as harassing officials, rent strikes and squatting) to educational programmes based on Marxist theory, and attempts to unite local groups with more powerful organizations, such as Trades Unions.

Taylor (1985) has pointed out that community action is not exclusively a left-wing response or strategy, but can equally be used by right-wing activists: e.g. responding with a conflict approach to social issues.

4 Further explorations of the philosophy, practice and types of activity within the three models

4.1 Explorations of the philosophy

Lovett (1983) has described how educational processes are forming the essential underpinning of the three models, and describes these as follows:

1 **The Community organization/education model** Lovett saw this as akin to the work already undertaken by many community colleges, involving community education tutors and out-reach workers; these often attempt both to respond to consumer demand for conventional educational opportunities and to generate popular, particularly working-class, efforts to influence the response of the system to people's needs. Lovett comments that this approach, however, 'does nothing for problems of poverty and inequality which community development strategies seek to eliminate. . . .'

2 **The Community development/education model** Lovett described this as an approach in which educators work in community projects giving help, advice, resources and taking opportunities for teaching specific skills for more actively co-operative community development approaches to those who hold power and make policies: e.g. councillors, clergy, social workers, police and planners. A major weakness however is its 'assumption that the problems found in deprived areas can be solved by such co-operation, co-ordination and improved understanding'.

3 **The Community action/education model** Lovett described this model as placing greater stress

> on combining community education and community action, on the role of conflict in resolving local problems and the importance of creating alternative institutions and organisations. It emphasises the need for adult educators to identify with, and commit themselves to, local working class communities. . . .

Lovett has drawn the parallel with the work of Freire (1978) who seeks, via his approach of dialogue and discussion with people in oppressed and powerless communities, to increase their awareness of political and economic factors which maintain their condition.

4.2 Some examples of practice associated with the three models

1 **The Community organization/education model** Examples are the Law Centre movement or Claimants' Unions, which have concerned themselves with

resources and the provision of social welfare, but which have used these consciously to educate the community concerning rights and benefits, planning policies and environmental controls.

2 **The Community development/education model** An example is a project such as Second Chance to Learn, which originated in the early 1970s in Liverpool's dockland. This course consists of a day-a-week social studies course for twenty weeks, with priority given to activists.

Yarnit (1980) has described how the educators linked with this work seek to convey an understanding of the position of the working class, but that this has to develop from the starting points of the participants.

3 **The Community action/education model** Lovett described two different forms of this:

> In the first model the role of adult education in community action is seen as one of providing the working class with an effective educational service so that they can take full advantage of the educational system *and* make the best use of their individual talents and abilities . . .

Within the second model,

> there is a consistent emphasis on the need to engage the residents in relevant education of a high standard. . . . Working class activists are to 'be given the chance to come to terms with a subject, skill or field of knowledge so that they can understand its internal rules, and become expert as far as possible'.

He stressed the links with earlier movements for radical change with an adult education base, such as the Antigonish movement in Nova Scotia and the Highlander Folk School in Tennessee, USA.

4.3 Some characteristic activities associated with the three models

Below are shown some typical activities in which community workers might be engaged within the three models:

1 The Community organization/education model

(a) Surveying local provision for particular groups, e.g. the elderly, and organizing the efforts to meet this need.
(b) Supporting and promoting self-help groups.
(c) Encouraging the active involvement of people in plans to improve their circumstances by fostering participation.
(d) Liaising between community groups and local government officials.
(e) Working for community provision for particular groups: e.g. the recovering mentally ill.
(f) Encouraging adult participation in education.

2 The Community development/education model

(a) Longer-term work than in community organization.
(b) Attempting to educate people concerning their rights and entitlements.
(c) The active taking up of issues by those affected by them: e.g. those with inadequate housing or warmth.
(d) Educating people to a political perspective on issues.
(e) The empowerment of under-privileged people.

3 Within the Community action/education model

(a) Gallacher, Ohri and Roberts (1983) suggest that responses, e.g. within the field of unemployment, include:

helping to establish welfare rights services
helping to establish claimants' unions
providing organizational support for campaigns
building alliances with trade unions
interpreting situations as political, not personal

(b) supporting local activists within a range of social, political, economic and environmental issues: e.g. housing, peace campaigns, anti-racism, drug-related issues and public inquiries.

4.4 A summary of community work approaches

Taylor (1985), drawing upon a number of other models, has proposed the following summary overview:

	Community organisation	*Community development*	*Community action*
1 Related educational provision	Compensatory education	Community education	Alternative education
2 Main processes	Coordinating, planning, convergence seeking	Education, control, consensus seeking	Confrontation, conflict seeking
3 Key role of the worker	Organiser, enabler	Multiplier, animator	Activator, challenger

TABLE 4.3 A summary of community work approaches (Taylor, 1985)

5 The range of research and evaluation initiatives within community work and community development

5.1 One way of categorizing research efforts

In an effort to 'order and codify' what has been written about research and community work, Thomas (1980) distinguished between three main forms, and confirmed the three groupings made by Specht (1976): service research (sometimes called 'action research'), evaluation research and knowledge-development research.

1 *Service research*: This concerns inquiries directly related to furthering the aims of community work initiatives, and may include gathering information about organizations, documentation of the extent of social problems and issues in the community, and the '. . . simultaneous involvement of the research activity in both studying the community work intervention and contributing to its development'.
2 *Evaluation research*: This seeks to monitor the activities of a community work intervention, and to assess outcomes. 'Hard-line' evaluation, using classical research designs, is exceedingly difficult; 'softline' evaluation is less difficult, but yields less reliable information.
3 *Knowledge-development research*: Such research, intended to generate general statements about the nature of community work intervention, would examine this in the (a) pre-planning and planning stages; (b) the phases of the implemention and action; and (c) the stage of termination.

5.2 Limitations of the traditional models of evaluation – and an alternative model

1 As Harris and colleagues (1978) have recognized, community work is not a field which lends itself to the conventional research designs. It is not even a field which lends itself very easily to the objectives model, whereby 'measurable indicators of goal achievement' can be pinpointed and attained: e.g. the impact of a Take Up (of welfare rights) campaign.
2 Harris *et al.* thus favour an ecological or systems approach – an attempt at evaluation which takes account of multiple variables, one which asks, in effect: 'When such a community programme is introduced what then happens?'

   They argue that such evaluation will not be concerned with detached assessment, 'but rather with being a dynamic part of the whole situation'.

5.3 The contribution of the ecological/systems approach

A number of positive aspects of this approach are highlighted in the work of Fordham, Poulton and Randle (1979), in their evaluation of learning networks in adult education on a Southampton estate. They recommended a number of 'working principles':

1 The growth of adult education within an area should be ecological. It begins where people are and assists their intellectual, social, psychological, cultural and political growth. . . .
2 It is necessary to establish a belief in the abilities, a respect for the values and a reinforcement of the potential of people. . . .

3 Control over the setting and carrying out of tasks in a neighbourhood forms a vital learning process. It should be passed to the people involved. . . .
4 A flexible support system should be available for groups to use as required. . . .
5 Neighbourhood organizations should also play an active part in conveying their particular message to audiences through media most fitted for the occasion. It is extremely important that people in local organizations are encouraged to present their ideas to others, irrespective of the outsider's status.

References

Armstrong, R., Davies, C., Doyle, M. and Powell, A. (1974), *Case Studies in Community Work*, vol. 1. Manchester Monographs.

Association of Community Workers (1982), *A.C.W. Definition of Community Work*.

Calouste Gulbenkian Foundation (1973), *Current Issues in Community Work*, London: Routledge & Kegan Paul.

Fordham, P., Poulton, G. and Randle, L. (1979), *Learning Networks in Adult Education*, London: Routledge & Kegan Paul.

Francis, D., Henderson, P. and Thomas, D. N. (1984), *A Survey of Community Workers in the United Kingdom*, London: National Institute for Social Work.

Freire, P. (1978), *Pedagogy in Process: the letters to Guinea-Bissau*, translated by Carmen St John Hunter, New York: Continuum.

Freire, P. (1985), Education, liberation and the Church. In D. Macedo (ed.), *The Politics of Education, Culture, Power and Liberation*, London: Macmillan.

Gallacher, J., Ohri, A. and Roberts, L. (1983), 'Unemployment and community action', *Community Development Journal*, vol. 18, pp. 2–9.

Harris, P., Blackmore, M., Blackmore, E., Davis, A., Robinson, D., Smith, J., Taylor, B. and Williams, G. (1978), *Evaluation of Community Work*, London Voluntary Service Council.

Lovett, T. (1983), 'Community education and community action'. In J. Campling (ed.), *Adult Education and Community Action*, London: Croom Helm.

Specht, H. (1976), *The community development project*. London: National Institute of Social Work.

Stevens, B. (1978), 'A fourth model of community work?' *Community Development Journal*, vol. 13, pp. 86–94.

Taylor, P. (1985), Personal communication.

Thomas, D. (1980), 'Research and community work', *Community Development Journal*, vol. 15, pp. 30–40.

Yarnit, M. (1980), 'Second chance to learn'. In J. Thompson (ed.), *Adult Education for a Change*, New York: Anchor Press.

Managing organizational or intergroup conflict

5

1 Definitions

1.1 Organizational conflict

A disagreement between two or more organization members or groups arising from the fact that they must share scarce resources or work activities and/or from the fact that they have different status, goals, values or perceptions. Organization members or subunits in disagreement attempt to have their own cause or point of view prevail over others. (Stoner, 1978)

1.2 Intergroup conflict

Disruptive disagreement arising between two or more groups within a larger system.

2 Fields of research in this area

1. The contribution of the systems approach to understanding intergroup conflict, negotiation and mediation.
2. Concepts of organizational or intergroup conflict within a systems framework.
3. Characteristics of intergroup conflict.
4. The reduction of intergroup conflict.
5. Models of the negotiation/mediation system.

3 The contribution of the systems approach to understanding intergroup conflict

1. Just as it is helpful to consider an organization such as a hospital or school as an interdependent grouping of units and sub-units (see Chapter 11, page 86), which functions within the context of the larger community, so this systems approach can contribute to understanding conflict.
2. From his research, Mintzberg (1979) concluded that at different times people or groups within an organization bid for influence therein. Similarly, outside organizations and pressures bring influence to bear upon the organization, and it is the totality of these internal and external pressures, held in tension, which constitute the system. Conflict, as well as co-operation, are thus integral parts of a system.
3. Stoner (1978), writing from the standpoint of business management,

suggested that conflict within an organization can be either functional or dysfunctional and has potential for improving or impairing organizational performance, depending upon how it is managed. He illustrated the potential of constructive conflict in Figure 5.1. The same principles appear to be relevant when applied to intergroup conflict within the wider community.

4 It is generally accepted however that much intergroup and organizational conflict is counter-productive and dysfunctional; negotiation and mediation skills are important for such situations.

4 Concepts of intergroup or organizational conflict within a systems framework

4.1 The social identity/social comparison theory of intergroup conflict

1 **The in-group/out-group phenomenon** From their own and many other researchers' studies of this phenomenon, Tajfel and Turner (1979) concluded:

> that the mere perception of belonging to two distinct groups – that is, social categorization per se – is sufficient to trigger intergroup discrimination favouring the in-group. In other words, the mere awareness of the presence of an out-group is sufficient to provoke intergroup competitive or discriminatory responses on the part of the in-group.

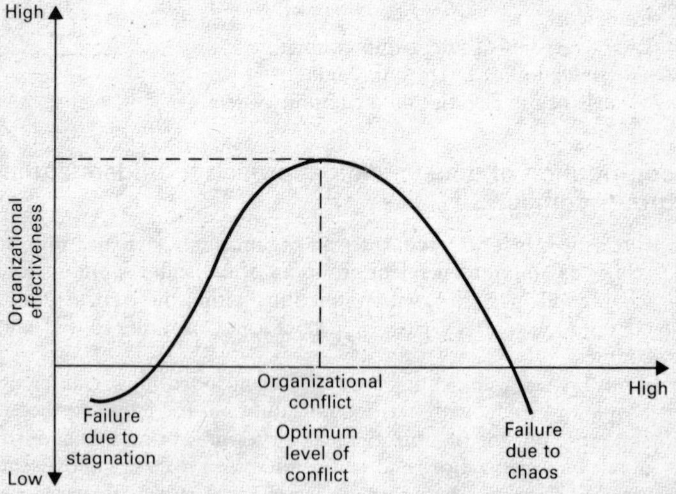

FIGURE 5.1 Levels of organizational conflict and its impact on effectiveness (After Stoner, 1978)

2 **Principles from Tajfel's social-identity theory** Tajfel and Turner proposed the following theoretical principles:

1 Individuals strive to achieve or to maintain positive social identity.
2 Positive social identity is based to a large extent on favourable comparisons that can be made between the in-group and some relevant out-groups: the in-group must be perceived as positively differentiated or distinct from the relevant out-groups.
3 When social identity is unsatisfactory, individuals will strive either to leave their existing group and join some positively distinct group and/or to make their existing group more positively distinct.

N.B. It is noteworthy, however, that many of the studies from which the above statements are drawn were conducted almost entirely with males: studies with females might give different results.

4.2 Characteristics of intergroup conflict

Experimental studies by Sherif and colleagues (1954) have been confirmed by other researchers, and there is broad consensus that the following phenomena, described by Stoner (1978), and shown in schematic form in Figure 5.2, are features of conflict between groups:

1 *A rise in internal cohesion.* Group members tend to set aside former disagreements and to close ranks in the case of a real or perceived threat from another group.
2 *The rise of leaders.* As intergroup conflict increases, those people who are more aggressive, able or articulate are given power by the group – in the expectation that they will lead the group to victory.
3 *Distortion of perception.* Group members' perceptions of their own in-group, and of the out-group, become distorted. Each in-group tends

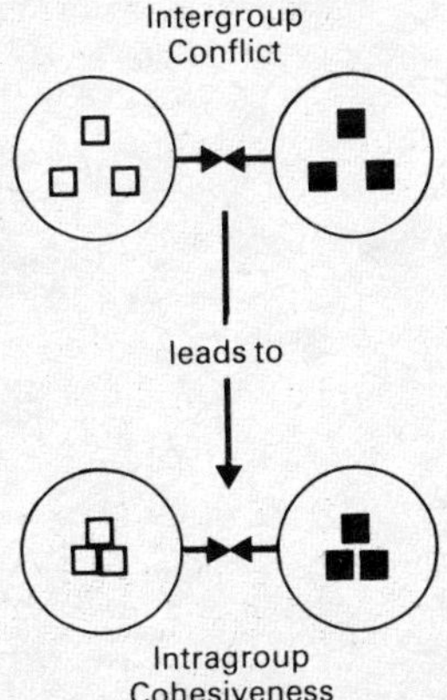

FIGURE 5.2 Intergroup conflict leading to intragroup cohesiveness (Stoner, 1978)

to regard the skills and characteristics of their group as superior to those of the out-group.

4 *Rise of negative stereotypes.* As each group belittles the other's ideas, the differences between the groups are seen as *greater* than they actually are, while the differences within each group are seen as *less* than they actually are.
5 *Selection of strong representatives.* Each group selects representatives who, it believes, will not capitulate under pressure from the other side. Each group tends to view its own leaders positively and the opposing leaders negatively.
6 *Development of 'blind spots'.* Strong identification with the in-group develops, and this tends to obscure clear thinking and the resolution of differences.

5 The reduction of intergroup conflict

There are several relevant fields of research, but they mainly concern situations where power is broadly equal.

5.1 Circumstances in which promoting co-operation between opposing groups may be effective – or not

Worchel's (1979) review of the evidence suggests:

1 *The effects of intergroup contact are unpredictable.* Such contact is as likely to heighten conflict as to reduce it. While some intergroup contact is probably a necessary condition for the reduction of conflict, it does not reliably reduce it.
2 *Negotiation by representatives is also hazardous.* Blake and Mouton (1961) found that not only did representatives have great difficulty in reaching agreement, but when an agreement was reached, their groups often rejected it. There is broad consensus among researchers that representatives who reach agreements which the group regard as unsatisfactory, are often ridiculed and rejected by the group.
3 *The importance of working together towards shared goals.* There is substantial agreement among researchers, e.g. Sherif (1966), that bringing groups together in a *series* of situations to work towards goals *which both groups separately want, but which they cannot achieve alone* does reduce intergroup conflict.

5.2 'Graduated reciprocation in tension reduction'

Osgood (1962), from his research, advocated a model of conflict reduction whereby one group unilaterally demonstrates a reduction of threat. After each reduction, the other side can be invited to demonstrate good faith by making a similar reduction in its threat capacity.

5.3 'Negotiating agreement without giving in'

Fisher, Ury and Patton (1983) distinguished a number of key principles in the field of negotiation:

1 Separate the people from the problem: i.e. treat opponents with personal respect.
2 Focus on interests, not positions: i.e. look forward to what both parties have to gain from a negotiated agreement, not at present entrenched positions.
3 Invent options for mutual gain: i.e. think divergently and creatively about possible solutions.
4 Insist on objective criteria: i.e. once agreement is arrived at, work out precisely how it shall be implemented, and what will constitute the evidence thereof.

5.4 The effects of facilitating intergroup co-operation

Worchel (1979) found that intergroup co-operation resulting in success produced increased intergroup attraction; intergroup co-operation resulting in failure produced decreased intergroup attraction.

5.5 The contribution of social exchange theory

1 The exchanges between groups can be thought of in terms of 'social exchange theory' (Thibaut and Kelley, 1959). This suggests that people and groups try to maximize their rewards, and minimize their costs, *as they perceive both*. (There are close parallels here with the concept of the cost-benefit analysis in economic theory, but individual perceptions, expectancies and values are explicitly included as part of the total equation.)
2 This way of looking at human interactions seems to be similar to the concept of the 'subjectively expected utility' framework of Walton and McKersie (1965) for understanding negotiation, and to the 'maximization theory' of Rachlin, Battalio, Kagel and Green (1981). These suggest that an organism behaves in such a way as to maximize a set of properties or advantages in its environment. Groups often seem to behave in the same way.

5.6 The value of open and consistent conciliation

Lindskold (1979) reported in his survey of both real-world and laboratory evidence 'that: the evidence seems to give consistent support to the proposition that open and consistent conciliation can make for more trusting and cooperative relations.'

5.7 Managing perceived threat

Blake and Mouton (1961) found that strong, active and dominant people were chosen in preference to people seen as constructive and helpful to represent a group in negotiation situations. This seems to suggest that such situations are perceived as implicitly threatening. Several studies have shown how perceived threat may best be managed; the following points seem to be important:

1 *The enhancement of trust*: Deutsch (1973) has suggested that trust can be increased by each side's rehearsing the other's case in order to demonstrate that the case of each has been 'heard and understood'.
2 *The avoidance of insult*: Tjosvold and Huston (1978) found in negotiation settings that those who deliberately or unwittingly affronted *as people* those with whom they were bargaining, obtained less favourable outcomes; i.e. attack should be at the case presented, not at the person presenting it.

6 A model of the negotiation/mediation system

6.1 Negotiation/mediation within a systems framework

1 Negotiation/mediation can be understood in terms of systems theory. In negotiation representatives of the parties in dispute exchange views and opinions, while in mediation a third party attempts actively to conciliate between two parties who alone have been unable to arrive at a mutually acceptable solution.
2 Wall (1981) has represented this negotiation/mediation system schematically. (see Figure 5.3). He conceptualizes the relationships in terms of social exchange theory, suggesting that each participant, negotiator, mediator and group member, can be understood as trying to maximize his perceived rewards at least cost to himself, in terms of his group responsibilities, his aspirations and his personal values.

References

Austin, W. G. and Worchel, S. (eds), (1979), *The Social Psychology of Intergroup Relations*. California, Brooks Cole.

Blake, R. R. and Mouton, J. S. (1961), 'Perceived characteristics of elected representatives', *Journal of Abnormal and Social Psychology*, vol. 62, pp. 693–5.

Blake, R. R. and Mouton, J. S. (1961), 'Reactions to intergroup competition under win–lose conditions', *Management Science*, vol. 7, pp. 420–35.

Deutsch, H. (1973), *The Resolution of Conflict*, New Haven: Yale University Press.

Fisher, R., Ury, W. with Patton, B. (ed.), (1983), *Getting to Yes*, London: Hutchinson.

Lindskold, S. (1979), 'Managing conflict through announced conciliatory

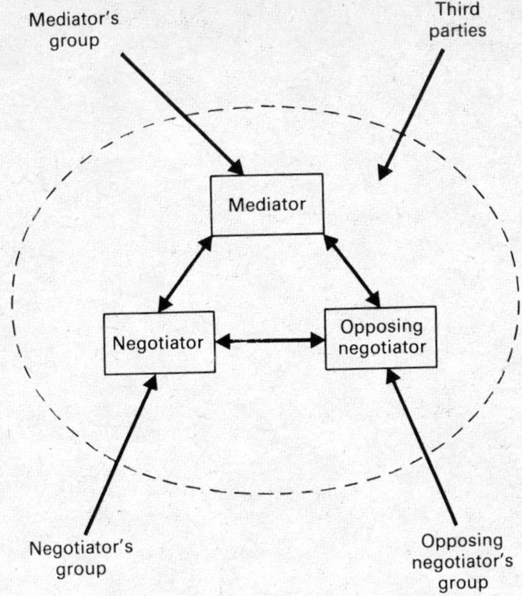

FIGURE 5.3 A systems formulation of negotiation/mediation (After Wall, 1981)

initiatives backed by retaliatory capacity' in W. G. Austin and S. Worchel (eds), *The Social Psychology of Intergroup Relations.*

Mintzberg, H. (1979), *The Structuring of Organizations*, Englewood Cliffs, New Jersey: Prentice Hall.

Osgood, C. E. (1962), *An Alternative to War or Surrender*, Urbana: University of Illinois Press.

Rabbie, R. R. and Mouton, J. S. (1961), 'Reactions to intergroup competition under win–lose conditions', *Management Science*, vol. 7, pp. 420–35.

Rachlin, H., Battalio, R., Kagel, J. and Green, L. (1981), 'Maximization theory in behavioural psychology'. *The Behavioural and Brain Sciences*, vol. 4, pp. 371–417.

Sherif, M. (1958), 'Superordinate goals in the reduction of intergroup conflict', *American Journal of Sociology*, vol. 43, pp. 349–65.

Sherif, M. (1966), *Group Conflict and Cooperation: Their Social Psychology*, London: Routledge & Kegan Paul.

Sherif, M. (1979), 'Superordinate goals in the reduction of intergroup conflict: An experimental evaluation', in W. Austin and S. Worchel (eds), *The Social Psychology of Intergroup Relations.*

Sherif, M., Harvey, O. J., White, B., Hood, W. R. and Sherif, C. (1954), *Experimental Study of Positive and Negative Intergroup Attitudes between Experimentally Produced Groups: Robbers' Cave Study.* Norman, University of Oklahoma.

Sherif, M. and Sherif, C. W. (1969), *Social Psychology*, New York: Harper & Row.

Sherif, M. and Sherif, C. W. (1979), 'Research on intergroup relations', in W. G. Austin and S. Worchel (eds), *The Social Psychology of Intergroup Relations*.

Stephenson, G. (1976), 'How to strike the right bargain', *Psychology Today*, vol. 2, pp. 25–9.

Stoner, J. A. (1978), *Management*, London: Prentice Hall International.

Tajfel, H. and Turner, J. (1979), 'An integrative theory of intergroup conflict', in W. Austin and S. Worchel (eds), *The Social Psychology of Intergroup Relations*.

Thibaut, J. and Kelley, H. (1959), *The Social Psychology of Groups*, New York: Wiley.

Tjosvold, D. and Huston, T. (1978), 'Social face and resistance to compromise in bargaining', *Journal of Social Psychology*, vol. 104, pp. 57–68.

Wall, J. A. (1981), 'Mediation: An analysis, review and proposed research', *Journal of Conflict Resolution*, vol. 25, pp. 157–80.

Walton, R. E. and McKersie, R. B. (1965), *A Behavioural Theory of Neighbour Negotiations*, New York: McGraw Hill.

Worchel, S. (1979), 'Cooperation and the reduction of intergroup conflict: some determining factors', in Austin, W. G. and Worchel, S. (eds), *The Social Psychology of Intergroup Relations*.

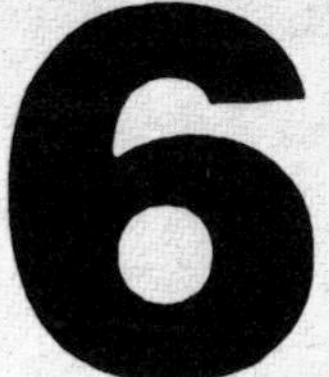

Small group work

Consultant: Dr Michael Argyle, Reader in Social Psychology, Department of Experimental Psychology, University of Oxford.

1 Definition

For the purposes of this chapter, a 'small group' is one which contains between three and fifteen members.

2 Research concerning features common to all groups

Certain characteristic features have consistently been noted; they may be grouped under the following headings.

1 Dimensions of groups.
2 The contribution of verbal and non-verbal communication within the group.
3 The composition of the group.
4 Aspects of group formation and development.

These will be considered separately below.

3 Dimensions of groups

3.1 Task behaviour and sociable behaviour

Argyle (1972) has described the two types of activity which occur in *any* group: task-related behaviour and sociable behaviour: he illustrated these in Figure 6.1

	task	sociable
verbal	e.g., committee discussion	e.g., gossip, discussion of personal problems
non-verbal	e.g., helping another	e.g., pouring coffee, practical joke

FIGURE 3.1 The two tasks and two channels of social groups. Reprinted from Argyle, M. (1972). The nature of social relationships. In *Social Relationships*, The Open University.

3.2 Interaction between task-related and sociable behaviour

It is generally agreed that a group of whatever kind is likely to feature both task-related and sociable behaviour; at any time one or the other may predominate, but both feature and should not be ignored. (Argyle, 1972)

3.3 A leader for each type of behaviour?

It was noted by Slater (1955) and endorsed by Argyle (1972), that two complementary leaders often emerge within a group: a task leader who takes business forward, and a socio-emotional leader who seeks to soothe interpersonal tension. In some groups a single leader may have to play both roles.

4 The contribution of verbal and non-verbal communication

4.1 Interacting channels of communication

There is now a strong body of empirical evidence (Eibl-Eibesfeldt, 1975; Exline, Ellyson and Long, 1975) that there are two parallel and interacting channels of communication: the verbal and the non-verbal.

4.2 Aspects of non-verbal communication

Argyle (1978) has reported the major channels of non-verbal communication: these include:

1. *Bodily contact*: . . . In Britain it is used for greetings and farewells; elsewhere it signals friendship and intimacy.
2. *Bodily proximity*: . . . there are wide cross-cultural differences.
3. *Bodily orientation*: Co-operating pairs sit side by side; competing or hostile pairs sit facing; those in discussion or conversation prefer 90°.
4. *Bodily posture*: indicates whether a person is tense or relaxed; the person of highest status sits least formally.
5. *Gestures* . . . communicate general emotional arousal, as well as specific emotions, e.g., fist-clenching for aggression . . .
6. *Head nods* act as reinforcers to encourage others to talk more, etc. . . .
7. *Facial expression* communicates emotions and attitudes to others – though it is heavily controlled and hence hard to interpret. It also provides immediate feedback on what others are saying. . . .
8. *Eye movements* . . . are used to collect feedback on the other's reactions. . . .
9. *Appearance* of clothes, face, hair, etc., is used to send messages about the self – occupation and social status. . . .
10. *Emotional tone of speech* is a more reliable indicator of emotions than facial expression, since it is not so well controlled. . . .

4.3 Aspects of verbal communication

A well-known way of categorizing verbal communication is that of Bales (1950), who distinguished twelve categories; these can be further grouped as follows: the participant

1 agrees or supports
2 gives a suggestion
3 asks for a suggestion
4 disagrees or challenges

Argyle (1972) also noted such major variables as,

1 the content or information value of speech
2 the degree of rewardingness of the communication
3 the degree of self-revealingness of the communication.

4.4 Interaction between verbal and non-verbal channels

A classic study by Argyle and colleagues (1970) examined which channel, the verbal or non-verbal, carried more weight in an encounter. They reported,

> the non-verbal style had more effect than the verbal contents, in fact about five times as much; when the verbal and non-verbal messages were in conflict, the verbal contents were virtually disregarded.

The researchers suggested an innate biological basis to the non-verbal signals, evoking powerful emotion.

5 The composition of the group

5.1 The size of the group

Several researchers have examined the effects of different numbers of people in groups. Krech, Crutchfield and Ballachey (1962) pointed out that the optimum size varies according to the type of task, but Argyle (1972) reported that many people would *prefer* to work with four or five other members.

5.2 Styles of social behaviour

Several researchers, including Schaefer (1959), Foa (1961) and Brown (1965), on the basis of work with a wide range of groups, have arrived at a model which shows the key dimensions of styles of social behaviour. This is shown in Figure 6.2 and summarizes the work of these researchers.

Argyle suggests that a person's position in this chart indicates his or her preferred style of social behaviour.

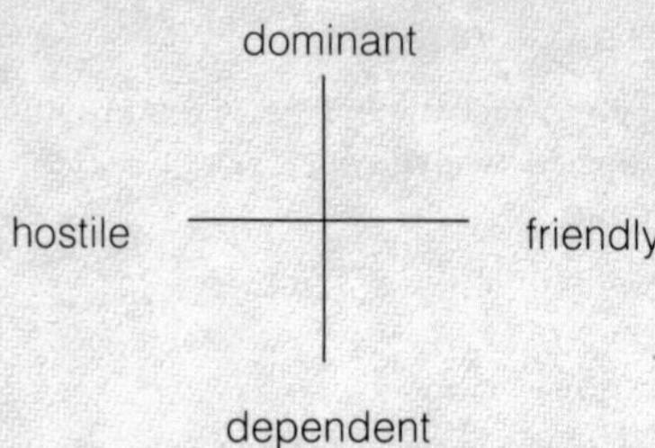

FIGURE 6.2 Styles of social behaviour. Re-printed from M. Argyle (1972), The nature of social relationships. In *Social Relationships*, Open University.

5.3 Behaviour of dominant personalities

Argyle (1972) suggests that those who prefer a dominant social style seek to exercise that style – although this will be affected by the situation. Similarly, it has been found that those higher in dominance motivation, extraversion or intelligence do come to dominate in groups; they also talk more. If a group contains two or more people high in dominance, they are likely to compete.

5.4 Conflicting personalities within the group

Schutz (1953) found some groups contained members so incompatible that they could not achieve a solution to tasks which required co-operation: such groups were those:

1 in which two or more people vied for dominance
2 in which members had very different levels of affiliation motivation.

6 Aspects of group formation and development

6.1 The sequence of stages

Tuckman (1965) found that many newly-formed groups such as T-groups pass through a broad sequence of stages:

1 *Forming*: characterized by anxiety, looking for a leader, uncertainty about the task and the situation.
2 *Storming*: marked by conflict between individuals and sub-groups, challenge to the leadership and resistance to both the rules and the task.
3 *Norming*: marked by greater stability, with the development of a group structure, leading to the recognition of norms, and the growth of cohesiveness.
4 *Performing*: marked by increased attention to the task, and the constructive solution of problems.

6.2 Distinctive features of any group and its development

Argyle (1969) suggested these fall into three categories:

1 The norms of behaviour particular to the group.
2 The hierarchical structure of leadership, power and social influence.
3 The networks of liking and disliking between members of the group.

Each of these will be considered separately below.

6.3 The norms of behaviour particular to the group

1 **The kinds of norm that prevail** Argyle (1972) summarized these as follows:

1 Norms about the task: e.g. methods of work.
2 Norms about interaction in the group.
3 Norms about attitudes: these tend to be those of the dominant members of the group.
4 Norms about appearance and style of dress.

2 **Pressure to conform to norms** Argyle has suggested,

> All small social groups develop 'norms', i.e. shared patterns of perceiving and thinking, shared kinds of communication, interaction and appearance, common attitudes and beliefs, and shared ways of doing whatever the group does. . . . Anyone who fails to conform is placed under pressure to do so, and if he does not he is rejected. Numerous experiments show that a deviate becomes the object of considerable attention, and of efforts to persuade him to change his behaviour.

3 **Attempts to change norms** Muscovici (1976) reported from his research that it *is* possible for a persistent minority to change norms, but generally *two* people are needed, acting in support of each other. Any given individual seeking to change majority opinion needs the support of someone of high status in the group, or of someone who is an expert in that particular field.

4 **Challenging group norms** Considerable disarray can be produced by deliberately setting out to challenge group norms: e.g. by introducing conflict into a group accustomed to operate by consensus. Dominance contests are likely to occur, with the winner either re-establishing or modifying the prevailing norms.

6.4 The hierarchical structure of leadership and power

1 **The spontaneous emergence of hierarchical structure** Many researchers, including Knipe and Maclay (1972), Barkov (1975) and Argyle (1983) agree in seeing the human species as one in which hierarchical patterns of organization are constantly and spontaneously emerging. Argyle (1983) has written:

'All groups of animals and men form hierarchies and there are advantages in having leaders who are able to direct activities and prevent conflict in the group. During the early meetings of the group there is a struggle for status among those individuals strong in dominance motivation. When the order has settled down a characteristic pattern of interaction is found. The low status members at the bottom of the hierarchy talk little, they address the senior members politely and deferentially, and little notice is taken of what they have to say.'

2 **Fluctuations within the hierarchy**

1 Campbell and Singer (1979) noted that in many groups individuals with particular skills, or with particular goals, emerged into more central positions in the course of the life of the group. If their skills were of great importance to achieving the group task, then they might retain such a position, and move up the hierarchy.

2 Moreover, personality variables such as dominance motivation are often found to interact with situational variables: thus a person who is talkative and influential in one type of group setting may sit silent in another, seeking to exert no influence. It depends on his or her knowledge or expertise.

6.5 The networks of liking and dislike between group members

1 **The importance of cohesiveness and interpersonal needs** Of these, Argyle (1969) has written:

> Members will be drawn towards the group if they are valued, popular and prestigeful in the group – those who are lowest in these respects are the most likely to leave it. Certain kinds of group behaviour are more satisfying and produce cohesion – democratic leadership, and cooperation rather than competition. External threat can lead to an increase of group cohesiveness. . . . (Lott and Lott, 1965).

2 **The importance of cohesiveness and task-related needs** Of these, Argyle (1969) has written:

> Satisfaction of needs related to the task also generates group cohesiveness. Shared success in group tasks, especially if this leads to an increase of status or other rewards, acts in this way, as a number of experiments show. Attraction to the group may be based on the prestige of belonging to it, the economic benefits incurred, the opportunities for work or play, together with attraction to other members. (e.g. Ross and Zander, 1957)

6.6 Other ways of making groups more cohesive

It was noted by Thibaut and Kelley (1969) that groups are often in a state of mixed co-operation and competition, but in addition to cohesiveness increasing under circumstances of external threat (see above) it has also been found to increase when the goals of the group are set out in a democratic way, i.e. with the participation of the membership, and as a result of skilled leadership. (Argyle, 1957)

References

Argyle, M. (1957), *The Scientific Study of Social Behaviour*, London: Methuen.

Argyle, M. (1969), *Social Interaction*, London: Methuen.

Argyle, M. (1972), 'The nature of social relationships I', in *Social Relationships*, Milton Keynes: Open University Press.

Argyle, M. (1972), 'The nature of social relationships II', in *Social Relationships*, Milton Keynes: Open University Press.

Argyle, M. (1983), *The Psychology of Interpersonal Behaviour*, 4th edn, Harmondsworth: Penguin Books.

Argyle, M., Salter, V., Nicholson, H., Williams, M. and Burgess, P. (1970), 'The communication of inferior and superior attitudes by verbal and non-verbal signals', *British Journal of Social and Clinical Psychology*, vol. 9, pp. 221–31.

Bales, R. F. (1950), *Interaction Process Analysis*, Cambridge, Mass.: Addison-Wesley.

Barkov, J. (1975), 'Prestige and culture: a biosocial interpretation', *Current Anthropology*, vol. 16, pp. 553–72.

Becker, W. C. and Krug, R. S. (1964), 'A complex model for social behaviour in children', *Child Development*, vol. 35, pp. 371–96.

Brown, R. (1965), *Social Psychology*, London: Collier Macmillan.

Campbell, F. and Singer, G. (1979), *Brain and Behaviour: Psychology of Everyday Life*, Australia: Pergamon Press.

Eibl-Eibesfeldt, I. (1975), *Ethology: The Biology of Behaviour*, Holt, Rinehart & Winston, Inc.

Exline, R. V., Ellyson, S. L. and Long, B. (1975), 'Visual behaviour as an aspect of power role relationships', in P. Pliner, L. Kramer, and T. Alloway (eds), *Nonverbal Communication of Aggression*, New York: Plenum.

Foa, U. G. (1961), 'Convergences in the analysis of the structure of interpersonal behaviour', *Psychology Review*, vol. 68, pp. 341–53.

Hall, J. (1971), 'Decisions, Decisions, Decisions', *Psychology Today*, November, p. 54.

Hare, A. P. (1976), *Handbook of Small Group Research*, Glencoe, Illinois: The Free Press.

Knipe, H. and Maclay, G. (1972), *The Dominant Man*, London: Souvenir Press.

Kogan, N. and Wallach, M. A. (1967), 'Risk taking as a function of the situation, the person and the group', in *New Dimensions in Psychology 3*, New York: Holt, Rinehart & Winston.

Krech, D., Crutchfield, R. S., and Ballachey, E. L. (1962), *Individual in Society*, New York: McGraw Hill.
Lott, A. J. and Lott, B. E. (1965), 'Group cohesiveness as interpersonal attraction: a review of relationships with antecedent and consequent variables', *Psychological Bulletin*, vol. 64, pp. 259–309.
Muscovici, S. (1976), *Social Influence and Social Change*, London: Academic Press.
Ross, I. and Zander, A. (1957), 'Need satisfaction and employee turnover', *Personnel Psychology*, vol. 10, pp. 327–38.
Schaefer, E. S. (1959), 'A circumflex model for maternal behaviour', *Journal of Abnormal and Social Psychology*, vol. 59, pp. 226–35.
Schutz, W. C. (1953), 'Construction of high productivity groups', Tufts College Department of Systems Analysis.
Slater, P. E. (1955), 'Role differentiation in small groups', in A. P. Hare (ed.), *Small Groups*, New York: Knopf.
Thibaut, J. W. and Kelley, H. H. (1959), *The Social Psychology of Groups*, New York: Wiley.
Tuckman, B. W. (1965), 'Developmental sequences in small groups', *Psychological Bulletin*, vol. 63, pp. 384–99.

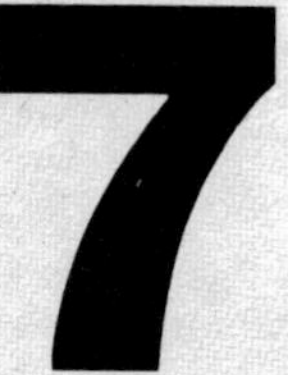

7 Problem solving and decision-making group work

Consultant: Dr Michael Argyle, Reader in Social Psychology, Department of Experimental Psychology, University of Oxford.

1 Definition

Problem-solving, decision-making and task-focused groups come together with prior objectives in mind: these are related to the achievement of appropriate goals.

2 Research concerning features of problem-solving, decision-making and self-help groups

These can be grouped under the following headings:

1 Aspects of leadership.

2 Research into problem-solving groups.
3 Research into decision-making groups.
4 Research into self-help groups.

These will be considered separately below.

3 Research into aspects of leadership of such groups

3.1 The emergence of a leader

Argyle (1969), reviewing the research, suggested that:

1 The emergence of a hierarchy, headed by a leader, seems to be a universal feature of human groups.
2 Informal groups may be led by the person accepted as leader. This depends on his or her expertise, past conformity, social skills and other such factors.
3 Formal groups tend to have formally appointed leaders who take the chair; if not formally appointed, the leader may be the person of highest status in the organization.

3.2 The relationship between rank position and participation

Much work has been conducted by Bales (1951, 1953) into patterns of participation in problem-solving groups. The graphs on page 60 represent the relationships which he found, in groups of differing sizes, between the rank position of the participants and the percentage of the total acts of communication engaged in by the members.

3.3 Leadership skills in problem-solving and decision-making groups

Maier (1967), after extensive research, has pinpointed the following skills of effective leadership:

1 Identifying the problem, calling for factual information and for members' views about key factors.
2 Acknowledging disagreements within the group, and trying to arrive at creative solutions.
3 Asking questions to stimulate creative solutions.
4 Evaluating different solutions against constraints.
5 Dividing problems into component parts, so that each may be considered in turn.

3.4 Leadership skills in the socio-emotional sphere

Argyle (1972) has reported that many studies of successful leadership point to the following skills:

1 Planning work, showing people how to do it, and checking that it is done; this is done with 'a very light touch'.

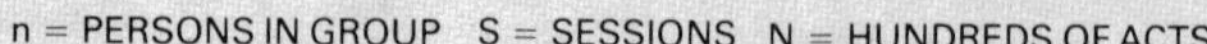

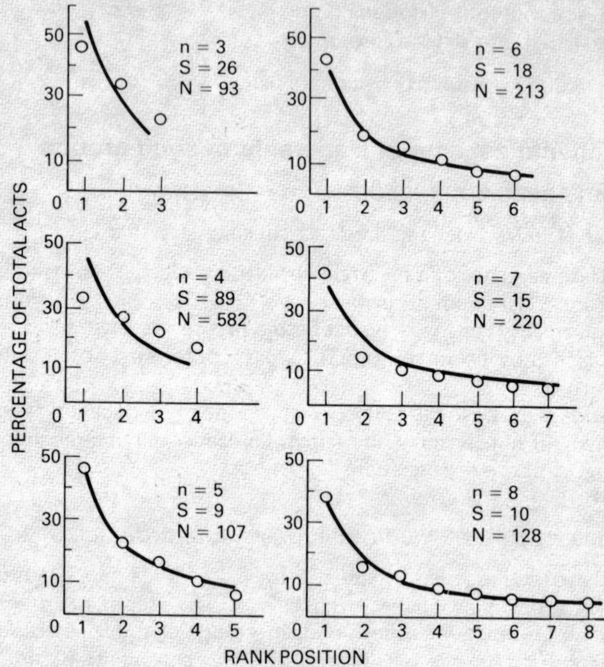

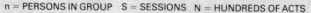

FIGURE 7.1 The distribution of participation in groups of different sizes (After Bales, Strodtbeck, Mills and Roseborough, 1951)

2 Establishing a friendly relationship with members, and taking a personal interest in them as people.
3 Using democratic methods and group decision-making.

3.5 Leadership skills for committee work

Argyle (1972) suggested that particular skills here include,

1 Restraining the working of the status hierarchy.
2 Encouraging the expression of minority opinions.

4 Research into aspects of problem-solving groups

4.1 Advantages of group problem-solving

Argyle (1969), and Stoner (1978), separately reviewing the research, suggested the following advantages:

1 The problem can be divided up and each part dealt with by the persons best able to do it.

2 The group has greater knowledge than a single person working alone.
3 If a solution has been worked out among members of the group there is likely to be better understanding and increased acceptance thereof.

4.2 Disadvantages of group problem-solving

Stoner (1978), drawing upon Maier (1969) suggested these:

1 Premature decisions: in some settings, consensus is so rare that the first suggestion to win approval may be accepted.
2 Domination by one or more individuals; such people may not be the most able.
3 Bi-polarisation may occur, so that 'winning the battle' may become more important than finding the best solution.

4.3 Conditions under which problem-solving is most effective

Argyle (1972) has summarized these as follows:

1 There should be members with the necessary skills: if there are not, the necessary people should be co-opted.
2 Cooperative groups are more effective than competitive ones, as they elicit greater commitment from members.
3 All members should be listened to, regardless of status, although the leaders may well have the greatest relevant knowledge.
4 The chairperson needs actively to control the hierarchy and to check inappropriate dominance behaviour of members.
5 The chairperson needs to monitor time constraints.

5 Research into aspects of decision-making groups and committees

5.1 The danger of making 'risky' decisions

There is considerable evidence, since the phenomenon was first noted by Kogan and Wallach (1967), that groups tend to come to riskier decisions than do individuals: i.e. they take chances, neglect implications and make assumptions. This may be because of some of the following processes:

1 'Diffusion of responsibility' takes place, with each person assuming another will implement a decision.
2 The value attached to being 'risky' by some participants.
3 In the balancing of arguments from one side and the other, group bi-polarisation can readily occur.

5.2 Emerging guidelines for committee members

The group decision process was seen by Hall (1971) as having a single aim: the creative resolution of conflicts by reaching consensus. He sees consensus not as unanimity, but as a condition in which each member accepts the group's decisions because they seem both logical and feasible. He suggested the evidence supports the following guidelines:

1 A clear statement of one's own position, avoiding a 'pushing' of one's own view.
2 The basing of one's views upon sound logic and evidence, which can be demonstrated.
3 The holding to one's own position if the logic supports it, even at the cost of harmony.
4 Seeking to avoid bi-polarisation, and win or lose positions.
5 Avoiding techniques that bypass logic for the sake of reducing conflict, such as bargaining.
6 Accepting that differences of opinion are inevitable.

6 Research into aspects of self-help groups

6.1 Common features of many self-help groups

The authors of *Guide to Self-Help Groups* considered,

> the essential characteristics of what may be described as self help would be governed by the presence of the following factors:
>
> 1 A membership or group consisting of people who share a common condition, common situation, experience, cause or concern.
> 2 The group is mainly self-governing and self-regulating, each member being involved and equal to another; there is no distinction between helpers and helped.
> 3 The group usually advocates self-reliance, giving support to others and receiving support as well . . .
> 4 Groups tend to be self-supporting financially and professionally . . .

6.2 The importance of the helper principle

There appear to be many advantages derived by the helper from the experience of helping others. Caplan and Killilea (1976) have reported the conclusions of Skovholt (1974), whose views, although arising from the field of therapy, seem to be relevant to a wide range of self-help group situations:

> (1) the effective helper often feels an increased level of interpersonal competence as a result of making an impact on another's life, (2) the effective helper often feels a sense of equality in giving and taking between himself or herself and others, (3) the effective helper is often the recipient of valuable personalized learning acquired while working with a helpee, and (4) the effective helper often receives social approval from the people he or she helps.

6.3 The importance of clear objectives

The authors of *Guide to Self Help Groups* also stated,

> The objectives of a self help group should be clear and easily understood. If they are not clearly stated confusion and dissent will inevitably arise with disputes between members. It would also be advisable for groups to define in writing the difference between a primary objective (goal) and secondary objective.

6.4 The effects of increased size and success

Stares (1984) has noted the challengers brought by the very success of some enterprises. These seem to apply to all self-help groups, and include the following:

1. Changes in scale and complexity can require the recruitment of additional (often specialist) staff.
2. Such changes may call in question established priorities.
3. The changes may involve a loss of control by the originators of the group or by the central committee, and one which may not always be appreciated by them.

References

Argyle, M. (1969), *The Scientific Study of Social Behaviour*, London: Methuen.

Argyle, M. (1972), 'The nature of social relationships I', in *Social Relationships*, Milton Keynes: Open University Press.

Argyle, M. (1972), 'The nature of social relationships II', in *Social Relationships*, Milton Keynes: Open University Press.

Argyle, M. (1976), *Social Interaction*. London; Tavistock.

Argyle, M. (1983), *The Psychology of Interpersonal Behaviour*, Harmondsworth: Penguin Books.

Bales, R. F. (1953), 'The equilibrium problem in small groups', in T. Parsons, R. F. Bales and E. A. Shils (eds), *Working Papers in the Theory of Action*, Glencoe, Illinois: Free Press.

Bales, R. F., Strodtbeck, F., Mills, T. and Roseborough, M. (1951), 'Channels of communication in small groups', *American Sociological Review*, vol. 16, pp. 461–8.

Caplan, G. and Killilea, K. (1976), *Support Systems and Mutual Help*, New York: Grune and Stratton.

Hall, J. (1971), 'Decisions, decisions, decisions', *Psychology Today*, November 1971.

Killilea, M. (1976), 'Mutual help organizations: interpretations in the literature', in G. Caplan and K. Killilea (eds), *Support Systems and Mutual Help*, New York: Grune & Stratton, Inc.

Kogan, N. and Wallach, M. A. (1967), 'Risk taking as a function of the

situation, the person and the group', in *New Dimensions in Psychology 3*. New York: Holt, Rinehart & Winston.
Maier, N. R. (1967), 'Assets and liabilities in group problem solving', *Psychological Review*, vol. 74, pp. 239–49.
Share Publications. *Guide to Self-Help Groups*, London: Share Community Ltd.
Skovholt, T. M. (1974), 'The client as helper: A means to promote psychological growth', *Counseling Psychologist*, vol. 4, pp. 58–64.
Stares, R. (1984), *Insights into Black Self-Help*, London: Commission for Racial Equality.
Stoner, J. A. F. (1978), *Management*, London: Prentice-Hall International.

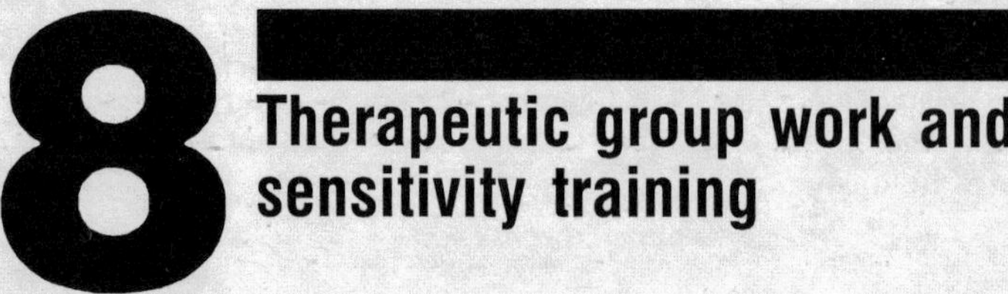

8 Therapeutic group work and sensitivity training

Consultant: Dr Peter B. Smith, Reader in Social Psychology, University of Sussex.

This chapter draws substantially upon *Small Groups and Personal Change* (1980a), edited by Peter B. Smith and published by Methuen.

1 Definition

Group-work is a finite activity whereby a small group seeks to create change within their own behaviour and feelings. (Smith, 1980a)

2 Generally accepted features of therapeutic group work

Therapeutic groups, which include sensitivity groups, encounter groups, 'T' (Training) groups, and groups in clinical settings, often have the following characteristics:

1 The intention of creating some change in members' behaviour and feelings.
2 The group has a leader or facilitator, with skills relevant to the facilitation of change.

3 The group's procedure is based on an examination of its own behaviour, past, present or future.
4 The group is usually of limited duration and consists of between seven and fifteen members, meeting on a face-to-face basis.

3 Research concerning effects of sensitivity training and encounter

Smith (1980a) reviewed reports of sensitivity training among groups which met for at least twenty hours, and which included a 'pre' and 'post' training measure; he noted the small proportion which included a 'follow-up' measure. His account is summarized below:

3.1 Studies using global measures of the self-concept as indicators of effectiveness

1 Among fifteen studies employing a control group, twelve groups of participants saw themselves more positively after training, while controls reported no change. Of those six studies carrying out follow ups, however, only three found the effects persisted for six months or more.
2 In a group of twenty studies using psychometric tests, only seven reported change after sensitivity training: of these, three found persisting effects at follow up.
3 Summarizing these, and other studies, Smith concluded that:

> Of forty-four studies which included some type of global self-concept measure, twenty-one detected change. Nine of these included follow-up measures among which six found persistence of change.

3.2 Studies using specific measures of the self-concept as indicators of effectiveness

1 Smith (1980a) reports that of twenty-four studies using an enhanced sense of personal effectiveness to measure the usefulness of training, ten found increases not found in controls. Only two out of seven found this increase persisted at follow up.
2 Similarly of fifteen studies which employed broad measures of openness and reduced prejudice, seven found a positive effect following sensitivity training, by comparison with controls. Four of these included follow-up measures but only one of these found the effects to have persisted two months later.
3 Of twenty-four further studies which focused on measures of increased participation, sixteen found favourable effects. Of these, seven had follow-up measures, but only one showed a persisting effect.

3.3 Studies using tests of specific skills or of everyday work behaviour

1 Smith examined the information on tests of specific skills, such as communication or empathy. Eight out of eleven studies found positive effects. Only one, however, included follow-up data, and this reported no effect.
2 Similarly, of fourteen studies which examined the effects of sensitivity training upon everyday performance, eight reported a positive effect, but six did not. Of the five studies which included follow-up data, three showed persistence of effects.
3 It thus appears that a good deal of measurable change does occur after groups which is not found among controls. However, these effects quite frequently fade out and we must turn to studies of group processes to determine why this might be.

4 Research concerning processes in therapeutic groups

Several aspects of group processes have been studied which may be important in producing positive or negative changes in participants.

4.1 Characteristics of participants

1 Epps and Sikes (1977) surveyed 757 volunteers who took part in 'personal growth' groups in America. They reported that:
   1 Participants usually became interested in the group because someone told them about it.
   2 The 'higher' one's education, occupation and income, the greater the probability of participation.
   3 The 35–44 age group was the most likely to participate in a 'personal growth' group.
   4 Divorced and separated persons participated in proportionately larger numbers than others.
   5 Females were more likely to participate than males.
   6 Persons whose stated goal was learning about themselves were somewhat more likely to have a negative experience than those who stressed other goals.
2 Mitchell (1975) found that persons who changed most as a result of sensitivity training had a high degree of achievement, responsibility, vigour, dominance and endurance. This could be because work-oriented persons have more to learn from groups than person-oriented individuals, who are often more at home in such settings.
3 Reddy and Lippert (1980) summarize these and a number of other studies of participants in such groups thus:

> In general, small group participants are 'people' rather than 'task' oriented. They attend primarily for psychotherapeutic or remedial purposes. . . . Many participants enrol with the intention to deal with what they perceive as personal deficits and want to do so in a relatively

painless and speedy manner. The probability, of course, is that neither of these goals is realistic. The research on personal change is clear – it is painful and lengthy.

4.2 Structure and design

Experiential groups are often described as unstructured. Reddy and Lippert examined a number of studies concerning the degree of structure within the group which is found to be helpful by participants. They concluded that structure is not always anathema to effective learning. Structured groups seem more satisfying to some participants and can also contribute to positive change.

4.3 Composition of the group

1 Reddy (1975) concluded from a series of studies that when groups consist of some people high in a particular need and others low on that need, then the probability of positive change is increased.
2 Bertcher and Maple (1977) showed that effective groups require some similarity and some diversity. They proposed that groups should be homogeneous on demographic qualities, but heterogeneous on behavioural qualities.

4.4 Phases of group development

1 Tuckman (1965) has proposed four stages in the development of groups: see Chapter 6, page 54.

   1 Forming
   2 Storming
   3 Norming
   4 Performing

2 More recent studies indicate broadly similar sequences: e.g. Lundgren and Knight (1978), in an investigation of twenty 'T' groups, noted three general stages:

   1 The initial encounter, characterised by restraint.
   2 Interpersonal criticism and confrontation.
   3 Mutual acceptance, marked by the resolution of conflict and a renewal of more positive interactions.

3 Brown (1981) pointed out the importance of a terminal or 'mourning' phase. No research exists which links phase progression to outcome.

4.5 Leader behaviour

1 Reddy and Lippert (1980) reported the findings of Bierman (1969) of the effects of different therapist behaviour upon outcomes. These are reproduced in Table 8.1.
2 Lieberman and colleagues (1973) found that the outcome was most favourable when leaders were high on 'caring' and 'meaning

		Affection: High	Affection: Low
Activity	High	Produces strong positive results	Produces strong negative results
	Low	Produces mild positive results	Produces mild negative results

TABLE 8.1 Relationship between therapist dimensions of affection and activity (Derived from Bierman, 1969)

attribution' (i.e. explaining to group members what was going on) and moderate on 'emotional stimulation' (i.e. confronting members' emotions) and 'executive function' (i.e. structuring the group). Later studies have also supported the importance of these dimensions, particularly the first three.

3 Reddy and Lippert (1980) pointed out the finding that trainers are seldom accurate in their judgments of participants, which supports the view that learning in groups does not necessarily all derive from the leader.

4.6 Learning mechanisms in groups

1 The term 'feedback' refers to mutual sharing of perceptions on one another's behaviour.

2 Lieberman *et al.* (1973) found that in their groups neither the amount of feedback, nor of self-disclosure, was directly linked to positive outcome.

3 Reddy and Lippert (1980) reviewed experimental studies showing that superior outcomes can be more readily attained when feedback situations are provided by the trainers rather than left to develop by chance. They reported that positive feedback was rated as more accurate than negative feedback, as well as being more desirable, more influential and productive of greater intention to change. Positive feedback, followed by negative feedback, was found to be more effective than the reverse order.

4 Smith (1980b) proposed that learning occurs in groups when a member experiences both support and confrontation from others. However, the effective mechanism of change may be not the receipt of feedback but how it is experienced by the recipient.

5 Lieberman *et al.* (1973) showed that those for whom the effects of

groups did *not* fade out were those who made plans as to how they wished to sustain change.

5 The usefulness of groups in clinical settings

5.1 Group psychotherapy with children

Abramowitz (1976) reviewed forty-two empirical studies of group therapy with children; of these only nineteen met such criteria as having a control group. These nineteen employed twenty-six types of treatment:

eight of the twenty-six were behaviourally based, with six (75 per cent) effective.
nine of the twenty-six were counselling based, with five (56 per cent) effective.
nine of the twenty-six were activity/play based, with four (45 per cent) effective.

These studies provided little follow-up data.

5.2 Group psychotherapy with neurotically ill people

Smith, Wood and Smale (1980) found that an encouraging number of studies report more favourable outcomes for patients than controls. They reported that the issue is increasingly not whether group therapy can be effective, but for which conditions it can be as quickly effective as some forms of behaviour therapy. Groups based on psychoanalytic theory have less often shown positive outcomes.

5.3 Group psychotherapy with psychotically ill people

Hospital discharge policies and the development of drug treatments mean that group therapy for schizophrenically ill people is now largely restricted to post-discharge support groups. Smith, Wood and Smale (1980) concluded that while such groups have been shown to create some positive effects, these do not directly affect relapse rates.

5.4 Therapeutic communities

1. Smith, Wood and Smale (1980) found that these compared well with traditional psychiatric treatment, at least for people able to participate in social living and interaction. They found that people who improved were those who took part actively in the community and made close relationships.
2. They commented that therapeutic communities may not be appropriate for severely withdrawn or disturbed people who are unable to participate in this way; they also pointed out that patients have eventually to leave the community for the outside world, and some are unable to maintain

the benefit they have derived, and to generalize the effects of therapy to other relationships.

5.5 Parent counselling and training

Tavormina (1974), in a review of studies using two models of parent counselling, the reflective (client centred) and the behavioural, concluded that there was research evidence that both models resulted in improved behaviour by the child, but that there was inadequate evidence of the comparative usefulness of the two approaches.

References

Abramowitz, C. C. (1976), 'The effectiveness of group psycho-therapy with children', *Archives of General Psychiatry*, vol. 33, pp. 320–6.

Bertcher, H. and Maple, F. (1977), *Creating Groups*, London: Sage.

Bierman, R. (1969), 'Dimensions of interpersonal facilitation in psychotherapy and child development', *Psychological Bulletin*, vol. 72, pp. 338–53.

Brown, A. (1981), *Groupwork*, London: Heinemann.

Epps, J. and Sikes, W. W. (1977), 'Personal growth groups: who joins and who benefits?', *Groups and Organizational Studies*, vol. 2, pp. 88–100.

Lieberman, M. A., Yalom, I. D. and Miles, M. B. (1973), *Encounter Groups: First Facts*, New York: Basic Books.

Lundgren, D. C. and Knight, D. J. (1978), 'Trainer style and member attitudes towards trainer and group in T-groups', *Journal of Applied Behavioural Science*, vol. 14, pp. 204–22.

Mitchell, R. R. (1975), 'Relationship between personal characteristics and change in sensitivity training groups', *Small Group Behaviour*, vol. 6, pp. 414–20.

Reddy, W. B. (1975), 'Interpersonal affection and change in sensitivity training: a composition model' in C. L. Cooper (ed.), *Theories of Group Processes*, London: Wiley.

Reddy, W. B. and Lippert, K. M. (1980), 'Studies of the processes and dynamics within experiental groups' in P. B. Smith (ed.) (1980a), *Small Groups and Personal Change*, London: Methuen.

Smith, P. B. (1980a), *Small Groups and Personal Change*, London: Methuen.

Smith, P. B. (1980b), *Group Processes and Personal Change*, London: Harper & Row.

Smith, P. B., Wood, H. and Smale, G. G. (1980), 'The usefulness of small groups in clinical settings' in Smith, P. B., *Small Groups and Personal Change*.

Tavormina, J. B. (1974), 'Basic models of parental counseling: A critical review', *Psychological Bulletin*, vol. 81, pp. 827–35.

Tuckman, B. W. (1965), 'Developmental sequences in small groups', *Psychological Bulletin*, vol. 63, pp. 384–99.

Social learning theory and goal-setting approaches

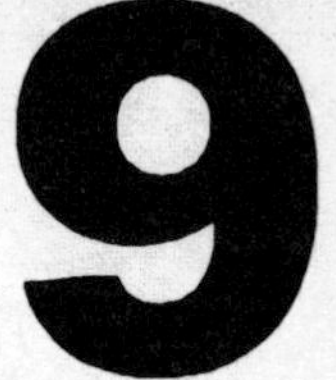

***Consultant:* Professor Martin Herbert, Professor of Clinical Psychology, Department of Psychology, University of Leicester.**

1 Definitions and descriptions of relevant terms

1.1 Social learning theory

This is a body of theory concerning the patterns of behaviour which an individual *learns* in coping with the environment; it focuses upon the interaction between the individual and the system of which he or she is part. Particular features which have been researched include:

1. The social context in which learning takes place.
2. The antecedents to learning.
3. The effects of reinforcement and feedback.
4. How principles of reinforcement work.
5. Cognitive, perceptual and thinking processes.
6. Learning by the observation of other people.
7. Interaction between the individual and the system.

1.2 Goal-setting approaches

These methods of intervention are grounded in social learning theory, and take account both of how the above processes affect behaviour and how they can be drawn upon to enable people to change, or to try to change, their behaviour in ways which have been agreed with them. Clarifying very precise but attainable goals, as a focus for effort, has been found to be particularly helpful.

2 Research leading to the formulation of social learning theory

As indicated in 1.1, several fields of research are accommodated within social learning theory; these are considered separately below:

2.1 The social context in which learning takes place

Herbert (1981) has emphasized that learning occurs in a social context. Thus a young child, for example, learns skills and gains abilities within the larger system of his or her relationships with parents or other caretakers, of the setting for the learning and of the wider environment.

2.2 Research about antecedents or previous circumstances

1 The system shown in the Frontispiece, (page vi) illustrates the interacting variables which may lead to a problem behaviour.
2 At the sociological level, these can include the broad predisposing variables, shown in Boxes VII and VIII, and known to contribute to stress: poverty, overcrowding, unemployment. Research concerning these variables is considered in e.g. Chapter 12.
3 At the psychological level, there may be events or cues which act as specific triggers to problem behaviour – shown in Box X: particular persons, places, times and circumstances.

2.3 Research about reinforcement and feedback

Much learning seems to occur via a series of feedback loops. For example, learning the language of one's community, while underpinned by innate (genetically-based) factors, is clearly influenced by the feedback a child receives. Similarly, aspects of other behaviour, such as problem behaviour, are likely to be acquired in comparable ways. (See Figure 9.1) Some of the variables involved include:

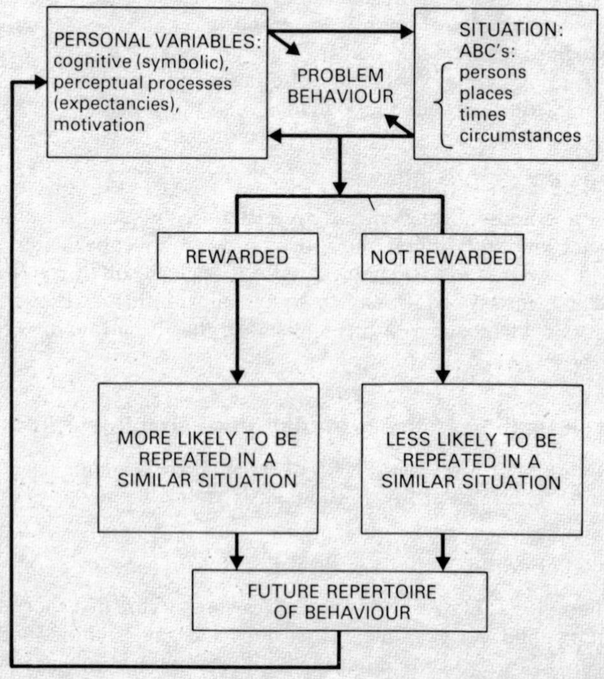

FIGURE 9.1 A feedback loop suggested by social learning theory (Emmet 1986)

1 **Positive reinforcement (reward)** This is any event which has the effect of increasing the probability of the behaviour which preceded it occurring again: e.g. thanks, praise, attention, or wages or salary for work. A child commended for effort at school is likely to go on trying hard; a person who is paid for his or her work is likely to continue in employment.

2 **Negative reinforcement** This is, technically, any happening which, because it is unpleasant, such as loud noise, has a rewarding effect when it stops. In popular usage, however, negative reinforcement often means penalty.

3 **Penalty (punishment)** Any event which has the effect of decreasing the probability of the behaviour which preceded it occurring again: e.g. criticism, blame, being ignored. Thus a person whose contribution to a discussion group is ridiculed is less likely to contribute again. For many children, however, any attention, even punishment, is better than none.

2.4 Research about how principles of reinforcement work

These principles are apparently operating whether we are aware of it or not, and whether we intend it or not. Some ways in which this happens are shown below:

1 **Continuous positive reinforcement** The rewarding of a behaviour *every time* it occurs: e.g.

(a) the praising by parents of every instance of speech by a child with almost none, in order to encourage further speech.
(b) laughing each time a small child swears is likely to increase instances of swearing.

2 **Intermittent positive reinforcement** The rewarding of a behaviour *occasionally*: this schedule of reinforcement has the effect of maintaining a behaviour in existence for a long time. For example,

(a) the paying of a wage or salary is a reward offered on an occasional, though regular, basis for work completed. It has the effect of contributing to maintaining the behaviour of 'going to work' for years on end.
(b) the occasional thanking of volunteers by those who benefit from their work. This is likely to contribute to maintaining the voluntary work of the volunteer.

3 **Extinction of a behaviour** The dying away of a behaviour because it is not reinforced. For example,

(a) A child whose whining is ignored is likely to stop whining. However, the efforts of a child to please parents or teacher, if not attended to and rewarded, are also likely to stop.

(b) Similarly, the efforts of the volunteer whose efforts are not recognized by thanks or appreciation are likely to extinguish.

4 **Generalization of a behaviour** It has been found that many behaviours, especially well-learned ones, tend to carry over from their original settings into new situations. For example,

(a) childhood patterns of friendliness, reserve, dominance or submissiveness are likely to carry over into adult life.
(b) the skill of relating with empathy to people, learned in ordinary day-to-day life, generalizes into the specialized situation of counselling among effective counsellors. (Truax and Carkhuff, 1967)

5 **The effect of immediate, versus delayed, reward** Reward offered immediately following a behaviour, rather than after a delay, makes it more likely that the behaviour will recur. Thus children learning to read do so most easily when the feedback (i.e. teacher's comments) on their achievements is immediate and specific rather than delayed. This stimulates motivation. Similarly, penalty administered immediately after a behaviour makes a recurrence less likely.

6 **The impact of large, versus small, reward** Large rewards, such as generous praise, have been found to increase or maintain a behaviour more than small ones – provided the reward is seen as sincere, and is offered in a way which the receiver finds acceptable.

7 **The impact of 'differential reward of other behaviour'** It has been found that the penalizing of one behaviour and the rewarding of its opposite is a very potent way of teaching new patterns of behaviour. For example,

(a) the systematic checking of every instance of hitting, biting or pushing by an aggressive child, together with the warm commendation of every act of kindness by that child has been found to bring about marked behaviour change in the child.
(b) the careful withholding of attention by teachers from disruptive pupils, and the appreciation by them of those pupils' constructive activity, has been found markedly to improve the academic and social skills of those pupils.

2.5 Cognitive, perceptual or thinking processes

1 Mischel (1981) has considered some of the individual differences in thinking, judging and valuing which contribute to the very personal ways in which we perceive and behave in day-to-day living. These will arise from an interaction between our personal tendencies to behave in certain ways, e.g. in a dominant manner, and the features of the particular situation or system, e.g. the location, who else is present, people's levels of arousal, and how we perceive these. Some of these

variables have been summarized by Atkinson, Atkinson and Hilgard (1983):

1 Competencies
2 Cognitive strategies: ways of dealing with situations
3 Expectancies
4 Personal values.

2 An example: contributing in a discussion group

a) *Competencies* People differ in their skills: e.g. a request at the meeting for someone to take the Minutes will be perceived very differently by a former secretary and by someone who doesn't know what the request means.
b) *Cognitive strategies* People differ in what they attend to: e.g. a person may feel strongly upon an issue but have adopted a 'never get involved' approach to participation.
c) *Expectancies* People differ in how they anticipate the outcome of different actions; some people have learned that their views and actions can influence change: others have learned helplessness.
d) *Personal values* People differ in their values; e.g. what is acceptable to one person in a meeting, as a 'necessary political strategy', may be unacceptable to another.

3 If the contribution of one participant is well received and he or she is rewarded by the interest and attention of the audience, that person is more likely to speak again: if the contribution is ignored, or publicly ridiculed, so that the speaker feels embarrassed or 'put down', that person is less likely to repeat the behaviour of speaking in the discussion.
4 As Atkinson, Atkinson and Hilgard (1983) have written,

> All of these person variables interact with the conditions of a particular situation to determine what an individual will do in that situation.

2.6 Learning by observing other people

Social learning theory also takes account of the phenomenon of 'modelling' – i.e. the way in which people imitate certain others. Bandura (1973) has carried out particular studies of the effects of aggressive models, particularly upon children. Why some possible models are chosen, and not others, is still being investigated, but it is suggested that those imitated include:

1 Friendly and kind people, particularly by children.
2 People whose behaviour is seen to be rewarded.
3 People who have power and status in the same social system as both model and imitator.

2.7 Interaction between the individual and the system

1 Bandura (1973) emphasized the multi-dimensional interactions which are implicit in human affairs, and builds this idea into social learning theory. For example, while people are much influenced by their upbringing and the socialization experiences they have had, they can also react against these, and actively choose to follow, or not to follow, similar patterns in bringing up their own children.

2 Many investigators would go further, and point out the multi-directional interactions between individuals and the total system, social and economic, which they inhabit. Such complex interaction can perhaps only be teased out via sophisticated statistical tools, but acknowledgment of the complexity is implicit in social learning theory.

3 Research arising from social learning theory

3.1 Social learning theory as a partial explanatory framework

While social learning theory is far from being an all-inclusive theory, it can often provide people with a preliminary explanatory framework to enable them to make sense of at least some aspects of their circumstances.

1 From a sociological perspective, for example, a young person may come to see that arising from early disadvantage, the lack of opportunities and the want of active encouragement at school, he was socialized into thinking of himself as a 'failure'.

2 From a psychological perspective, a person may realize that her difficulties in making friends are linked with intense shyness arising from never having played with other children before the age of five.

3.2 Research into applied aspects of social learning theory

A great deal of research has been devoted to three particular areas of investigation, which are themselves linked: behavioural approaches, goal-setting approaches and the use of contracts.

1 Behavioural approaches

(a) These are methods of intervention which have been found to be of great value in helping to resolve a wide variety of difficulties. Such approaches are grounded on very precise and detailed assessment, intervention and evaluation.

(b) Herbert (1981) has shown the various components of assessment of a child showing very difficult behaviour: see Figure 21.1. It will be noted that this focuses upon the *behaviour* in question, and the variety of the contributory factors which may be involved.

(c) Following initial assessment, an analysis in terms of the following concepts is usually helpful:

A: Antecedent: what occurs just before a given behaviour, or what are the *cues* to a behaviour.

B: Behaviour: what the behaviour itself consist of: what someone *does*.

C: Consequence: what happens immediately after the behaviour: i.e. is the behaviour rewarded or penalized?

(d) After such an analysis, it is then possible to agree with those concerned how both the antecedents and the consequences of a given behaviour could be altered, with a view to bringing about the desired behavioural change. Thus a parent, asking for help in managing the sleeping difficulties of a young child, can, following the above analysis, be encouraged *not* to hurry to the child's bedside each time he stirs.

(e) Behavioural approaches have made important contributions to helping people who are experiencing a wide range of difficulties. These take account of cognitive factors, i.e. people's perceptions and expectancies, and there is ample evidence of their use in:

Anxiety and stress management: phobias and obsessions.
Management of depression.
Managing children's difficult behaviour.
Sexual difficulties.
Alcohol misuse.
Precision learning for the mentally handicapped.

2 Goal-setting approaches

1 Several fields of research (Locke, Shaw, Saari and Latham (1981), Seligman, Klein and Miller, (1976)) have converged upon the finding that the setting of clear, attainable goals is helpful in enabling people to bring about change in the direction that they want. The attainment of each goal is likely to be rewarding, and thus to motivate people to aspire to the next. It is very important that such goals should be attainable, as success, and particularly early success, is very important indeed.

2 There are also indications that when goals to be attained are thought of terms of a hierarchy, with simple, easily achieved tasks at the bottom, and the final, culminating objectives at the top, this can be extremely helpful in stimulating motivation.

3 The use of contracts These are formal written agreements, carefully devised between at least two parties. They often specify goals, written in terms of behaviour, which each party has agreed to work towards: e.g. that John will return home by 10.30 p.m. each evining and in return his parents will refrain from criticizing John's friends. When negotiated, written down and monitored with care, such contracts have been found to be very helpful. (Goldberg and Connolly, 1981; Sheldon, 1982)

3.3 Convergence of research findings

There appears to be a general convergence of the research findings in the fields of social learning theory, behavioural approaches and management research. These findings seem to point to the importance of the following considerations when planning an intervention or an undertaking:

1 Agreeing the goals or objectives of the undertaking.
2 Involving as many people as possible in agreeing the goals.
3 Specifying what will constitute 'success', either against agreed criteria, or in terms of precise evidence.
4 Monitoring progress towards the goals with a range of methods: charts, data sheets, diaries, verbal accounts. (i.e. both quantitative and qualitative methods).
5 Giving feedback and active encouragement.
6 Negotiating fresh goals in the light of experience.

3.4 A note upon ethical issues

Principles of reinforcement, reward and penalty, seem to be operating in ordinary life, with or without our awareness. People who work with people have a responsibility to be aware of what they are rewarding or penalizing – often unwittingly. Since, however, the principles can be employed in a planned, conscious, way, by teachers, counsellors, nurses and by people who wish to change *their own* behaviour, many groups have devised Codes of Practice or Ethical Guidelines. These usually involve agreeing the goals of intervention with those concerned, or their guardians or care-takers, and monitoring such interventions closely in order to evaluate their effectiveness.

References

Atkinson, R. L., Atkinson, R. and Hilgard, E. L. (1983), *Introduction to Psychology* (8th edn), New York: Harcourt, Brace, Jovanovich.

Bandura, A. (1973), *Aggression. A social learning analysis*, Englewood Cliffs, N.J.: Prentice Hall.

Bandura, A. (1977), *Social Learning Theory*, Englewood Cliffs, N.J.: Prentice Hall.

Goldberg, M. and Connolly, J. (eds) (1981), *Evaluative Research and Social Care*, London: Heinemann Educational.

Herbert, M. (1981), *Behavioural Treatment of Problem Children*, London: Academic Press.

Locke, A. E., Shaw, K., Saari, L. and Latham, G. P. (1981), 'Goal setting and task performance', *Psychological Bulletin*, vol. 90, pp. 125–52.

Mischel, W. (1981), *Introduction to Personality* (3rd edn), New York: Holt, Rinehart & Winston.

Seligman, M. E., Klein, D. C. and Miller, R. W. (1976), 'Depression' in H.

Leitenberg (ed.), *Handbook of Behaviour Therapy*, New York: Appleton-Century-Crofts.

Sheldon, B. (1982), *Behaviour Modification*, London: Tavistock Publications.

Truax, C. and Carkhuff, R. (1967), *Toward Effective Counselling and Psychotherapy*, New York: Aldine.

Counselling and brief psychotherapy

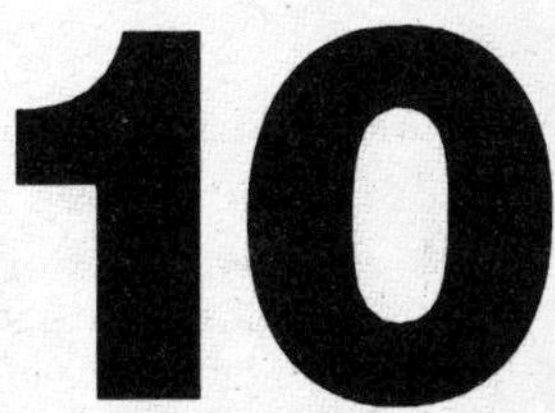

1 Some definitions

1 The British Association for Counselling suggested in 1985,

> People become engaged in counselling when a person, occupying regularly or temporarily the role of counsellor offers or agrees explicitly to offer time, attention and respect to another person or persons temporarily in the role of client.
>
> The task of counselling is to give the client an opportunity to explore, discover and clarify ways of living more resourcefully and toward greater well-being.

2 Writing of counselling psychology, Nelson-Jones (1982) has suggested,

> Counselling psychology is an applied area of psychology which has the objective of helping people to live more effective and fulfilled lives. Its clientele tend to be not very disturbed people in non-medical settings. Its concerns are those of the whole person in all areas of human psychological functioning, such as feeling and thinking, personal, marital and sexual relations, and work and recreational activity.

2 Research in counselling and brief psychotherapy

2.1 Research into effective counselling and psychotherapy

1 **The contribution of Truax and Carkhuff (1967)** Their major review of the research literature, *Toward Effective Counselling and Psychotherapy*, concluded that:

> *average* counseling and psychotherapy as it is currently practiced does not result in average client improvement greater than that observed in clients who receive no special counseling or psychotherapeutic treatment. . . .

and they drew the obvious inference that:

> if psychotherapy has no overall average effect, but that there are valid specific instances where it is indeed effective, then there must also be specific instances in which it is harmful. That is, to achieve this average, if some clients have been helped, then other clients must have been harmed.

2 **Characteristics of effective counsellors** Truax and Carkhuff then distinguished three characteristics of counsellors who *were* able to benefit their clients:

1 *Genuineness*: the capacity to respond to another person naturally, spontaneously and openly.
2 *Non-possessive warmth*: the attitude of positive caring demonstrated to clients by friendliness, a non-critical manner and active encouragement.
3 *Accurate empathy*: the ability to give the person seeking help a deep sense of being 'understood'.

2.2 Three main counselling traditions

Nelson-Jones (1982) suggested that while many sub-schools of counselling may exist, three main traditions stand out:

1 *Humanistic approaches*: associated with the 'client-centred' approach of Rogers (1951) and the ideas of Maslow (1954).
2 *Psychoanalytic approaches*: associated with the ideas of e.g. Freud (1949) and his successors.
3 *Behavioural approaches*: associated with the ideas of e.g. Wolpe (1973).

While there is not space to develop the particular contributions of these three traditions here, there is evidence that each has a contribution to make.

2.3 The move to an integrated/eclectic approach

1 In the light of the evidence offered by Truax and Carkhuff above, and several studies (e.g. Thorne, 1969) indicating that counselling or therapy based on any single theoretical system was inadequate, there has been a trend towards a more integrated approach.
2 Thus, while training in counselling tends to be grounded in the humanistic and client-centred approach, which emphasizes the counsellor characteristics distinguished by Truax and Carkhuff (1967), attention is increasingly being given to training counsellors in particular skills, such as that of teaching clients behavioural relaxation, which extends their repertoire of knowledge and resources.

4 Stages of counselling and brief psychotherapy

Commonly recognized stages in counselling often include:

1 **Gaining an overview** This often takes place in the first or first two meetings, although further matters needing consideration may well arise subsequently. An accepting and positive relationship is crucial, and so is establishing confidentiality or its limitations.

2 **Agreeing goals** Counsellor and client work out and agree how often they will meet and what will constitute the goals of their meetings. These may be put in the form of a 'contract' or agreement.

3 **Intervention** In which the counsellor draws upon a wide repertoire of relationship and other skills and offers a supportive structure so that both counsellor and client move towards attaining agreed goals.

4 **Evaluation** In which the client and counsellor consider the extent to which the agreed goals have been achieved, and arrange the follow-up.

4.1 Gaining an overview: aspects of the initial interview(s)

Nelson-Jones (1982) has summarized these in Figure 10.1.

Stage	Illustrative counsellor tasks
Introductions	• Meeting, greeting, seating • If necessary, establishing confidentiality or its limitations • Starting the development of rapport and trust • Basic data collection (?)
Presenting concerns	• Facilitating client self-disclosure and self-talk • Exploration of presenting concerns assisting client amplification and specification engaging in clarification
Reconnaissance	• Structuring • Facilitating client self-disclosure and self-talk • Broader exploration of client's mode of living, background, current stresses, self-concept, coping abilities, motivation, expectancies, etc. • Assisting exploration • Engaging in clarification
Contracting	• Summarizing • Formulating and discussing goals • Presenting a treatment method or methods • Handling questions • Establishing a treatment 'contract'
Termination	• Clarifying administrative details • Arranging next appointment • Parting

FIGURE 10.1 A five-stage plan of the initial counselling interview(s) Nelson-Jones (1982).

4.2 Agreeing goals

1 These serve to provide a structure to the series of meetings between counsellor and client. They are thus of particular value in time-limited counselling. Often counsellors can help clients distinguish some of the different areas of difficulty they are experiencing, rather in the manner of the 'task-centred' approach advocated by Reid and Epstein (1972), and then to agree how to move towards resolving these difficulties.

2 Such goals will be highly individual and selected primarily by the client, but negotiated with the therapist in the light of time available and reality factors.
e.g. That by the end of the counselling sequence the client,
1 shall feel more positive about himself;
2 shall feel clearer about a decision facing him;
3 shall have widened his circle of friends and acquaintances.

4.3 Intervention: using a range of methods towards agreed goals

1 This is likely to involve the counsellor's drawing upon the repertoire of his or her knowledge and skill in a shared endeavour to attain previously agreed goals. Such counsellor methods have been set out by Nelson-Jones (1982) in Table 10.2.

2 For example, this may involve considering the past, and how relationships or events then are still having damaging effects in the present; sometimes it may involve talking through a decision to be made, or events such as a bereavement or a broken relationship; sometimes it may be fitting for the counsellor to act as educator, and teach the client new skills such as relaxation or making positive statements about himself.

3 The counselling 'contract', mentioned above, can be very useful. Rosenhan and Seligman (1984) write concerning the broad field of counselling and psychotherapy,

> Many therapists arrive at an agreement with clients, not only regarding the goals of treatment, but also how long treatment will last. That agreement is put in the form of a contract and serves to remind each party of their aims and obligations.

Such agreements are often written down and initialled by those concerned; they can then be readily referred to as appropriate.

4.4 Evaluation – against the goals agreed at the outset

1 Having an agreed set of goals, which can be renegotiated if necessary, makes the task of evaluation much easier. It is then possible for *the client* to say to what extent he or she feels that these goals have been attained: fully, partially, or not at all. If necessary, fresh goals can be agreed or a referral made elsewhere.

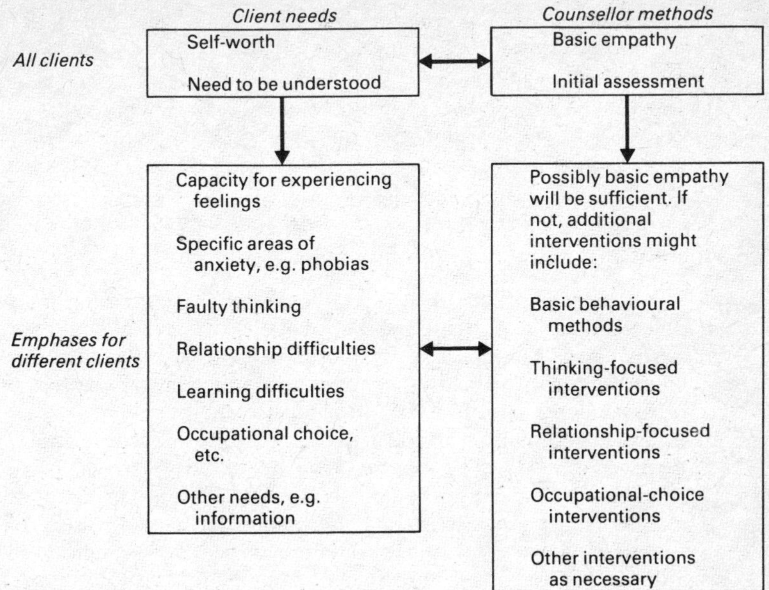

FIGURE 10.2 A treatment decision-making model of counsellor methods in relation to client needs (Nelson-Jones, 1982)

2 Similarly, clients can be invited to say at e.g. a three months' follow-up, how far they feel that any progress made has been maintained.

5 Further research upon counselling

Sutton (1979) summarized these thus:

5.1 Ideas having a measure of empirical support

1 It can be helpful if the counsellor speaks now and then of his or her own experience
Studies, e.g. by Jourard (1971), suggest that brief reference in appropriate circumstances to his or her personal experience by the counsellor can be very beneficial to those seeking help. This reduces 'distance' and makes the exchange less unequal.

2 Certain client characteristics are associated with a positive outcome
Truax and Carkhuff (1967) reported general indications from the literature that people with the greatest sense of emotional distress, and with the least behavioural disorder, e.g. an inclination to violence, were most likely to show improvement.

3 Counsellors high in persuasiveness have beneficial effects
Studies such as Bednar (1970) indicate that counsellors who encourage

an optimistic frame of mind in those with whom they work, and who subsequently foster that optimism are likely to prove helpful.

4 Those clients who most need help receive the least
Goldstein (1973) and others report that counsellors and others in the helping professions spend more time with and feel more committed to helping those in the higher, rather than the lower, socio-economic groups.

5.2 Ideas having considerable empirical support

1 The importance of clarifying clients' expectations concerning counselling
Several studies, e.g. Heine and Trosman (1960), have shown that clarifying expectations is very important. The evidence indicated that when counsellor and client do not agree on the aims or methods of help, the latter tends to break off contact early.

2 Counsellor 'commitment' to clients is a predictor of outcome
Lerner and Fiske (1973) reported that the attitude of conviction of the counsellor that he or she could help, even in unpromising circumstances, was very important. Swensen (1972) confirmed that a counsellor characteristic which he called 'commitment' was very significant in influencing positively the outcome of counselling.

3 Counselling, even when non-directive, is a social-influence process
Egan (1975) and others have pointed out that the inherent status of the counsellor and her or his perceived trustworthiness and expertise are clear, if subtle, factors in influencing clients, their thinking and behaviour.

4 Lay counsellors can be as effective as professionals
Several studies, particularly those of Carkhuff and Truax (1965) and of Durlak (1979), have shown that appropriate training of the order of 100 hours can enable lay counsellors to be as effective as professionals.

References

Argyle, M. (1972), *The Psychology of Interpersonal Behaviour*, Harmondsworth: Penguin.

Bednar, R. L. (1970), 'Persuasability and the power of belief', *Personality and Guidance Journal*, 1970, vol. 48, pp. 647–52.

British Association for Counselling (1985), *Counselling: Definition of Terms in use with expansion and rationale*, Rugby: B.A.C.

Carkhuff, R. and Truax, C. B. (1965), 'Lay mental health counselling: the effects of lay group counselling', *Journal of Consulting Psychology*, vol. 29, pp. 426–31.

Durlak, J. (1979), 'Comparative effectiveness of paraprofessional and professional helpers', *Psychological Bulletin*, vol. 86, pp. 80–92.

Egan, G. (1975), *The Skilled Helper: A Model for Systematic Helping and Interpersonal Relating*, Monterey, California: Brooks Cole.

Freud, S. (1949), *An Outline of Psychoanalysis*, New York: W. W. Norton.

Goldstein, A. P. (1973), *Structured Learning Therapy: Toward a Psychotherapy for the Poor*, New York: Academic Press.
Heine, R. W. and Trosman, H. (1960), 'Initial expectancies of the doctor-patient interaction as a factor in continuance in psychotherapy', *Psychiatry*, vol. 20, pp. 275–8.
Jourard, S. M. (1971), *The Transparent Self*, New York: Van Nostrand, Reinhold.
Lerner, B. and Fiske, D. (1973), 'Client attributes and the eye of the beholder', *Journal of Consulting and Clinical Psychology*, vol. 40, pp. 272–7.
Maslow, A. (1954), *Motivation and Personality*, New York: Harper & Row.
Nelson-Jones, R. (1982), *The Theory and Practice of Counselling Psychology*, London: Holt Rinehart & Winston.
Reid, W. and Epstein, L. (1972), *Task-Centred Casework*, New York: Columbia.
Rogers, C. (1951), *Client-Centred Therapy*, Boston: Houghton Mifflin.
Rosenhan, J. and Seligman, M. (1984), *Abnormal Psychology*, Guilford Press.
Sutton, C. (1979), *Psychology for Social Workers and Counsellors: An Introduction*, London: Routledge & Kegan Paul.
Swensen, C. H. (1972), 'Commitment and the personality of the successful therapist', *Psychological Bulletin*, vol. 77, pp. 400–4.
Thorne, F. C. (1969), 'Editorial opinion: Toward a better understanding of the eclectic method', *Journal of Clinical Psychology*, vol. 25, pp. 463–4.
Truax, C. and Carkhuff, R. (1967), *Toward Effective Counselling and Psychotherapy*, Chicago: Aldine.
Wolpe, J. (1973), *The Practice of Behaviour Therapy*, Oxford: Pergamon Press.

11 Some research concerning general management skills

Consultant: Hilary Unwin, Senior Lecturer, Certificate of Qualification in Social Work Course, Leicester Polytechnic.

1 Some fundamental concepts

1.1 A possible definition

The following is suggested by Stoner (1978),

> Management is the process of planning, organizing, leading and controlling the efforts of organizational members and the use of other organizational resources in order to achieve organizational goals.

It is noteworthy, however, that concepts of management have traditionally been drawn from experience in industry, and tend to emphasize features of a hierarchical model. By contrast, many groups who work with people seek to minimize and even eliminate hierarchical features.

1.2 Some essential components of management knowledge and skill

1 The importance of understanding the place of one's unit within the larger system.
2 The importance of being clear about the objectives of the group or unit, and of the larger organization, in precise and measurable ways.
3 The importance of rational decision-making.
4 The need for careful planning of the use of time.
5 The importance of building on the motivation of those involved.
6 The need for the constructive management of conflict.

Each of these will be considered separately below.

2 The importance of understanding the place of one's unit within the larger system

2.1 One possible model of organizations: the systems approach

The systems formulation is one useful way of thinking of relationships within and between organizations. Thus an organization can be seen as an interdependent group of units and sub-units, where the activities of each affect others, and all are affected by the influences of outside organizations, policies and resources.

1 **A hospital as an example** This engages the services of nurses, porters, administrators, catering staff, doctors, pharmacists, laboratory technicians, domestics, physiotherapists and many others, all of whom need to co-operate to provide care for sick people. A hospital, however, is itself affected by outside political influences and decisions, by the influences brought to bear by groups such as unions of medical, nursing or clerical staff, and by pressure groups such as those concerned about ethical issues and patient welfare.

2 **The relevance of the model to many organizations** No organization is free of such internal and external pressures. It is thus important for members of any organization to understand the location of their particular group within the larger context, and how decisions made elsewhere in the system, upon for example, funding policy, impinge directly and indirectly upon the work of the organization.

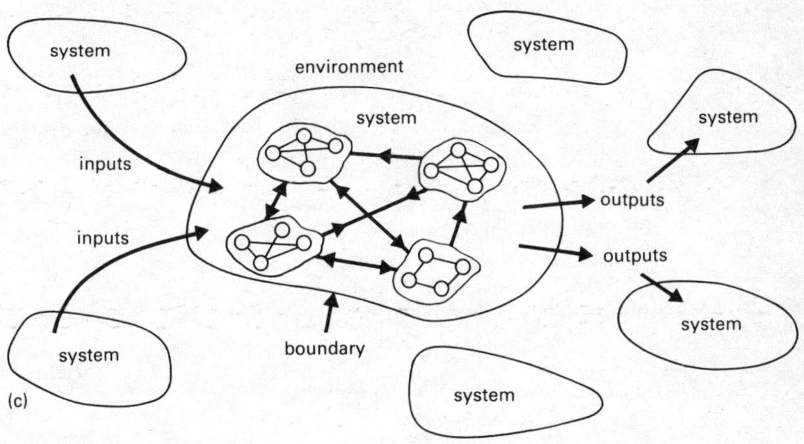

FIGURE 11.1 A system with sub-systems, interacting with other systems. From *Systems Organization: The Management of Complexity.*

2.2 The structure of activities within an organization

1 **The tendency to form hierarchies** Within the general systems approach, many organizations seem to develop a structure broadly resembling a hierarchy. In some, such as the armed forces, the structure may be formal and rigid: in others, such as some women's groups, there is a deliberate practice of rotating the offices of chairperson, secretary and others to minimize hierarchical tendencies.

2 **Competing bids for influence** Mintzberg (1979), on the basis of his studies, concluded that at different times, different groups bid for influence within the structure of the organization; it is the way in which these tensions are resolved that, at any given time, produces the form of the organization.

2.3 Typical groupings in tension within an organization

Mintzberg (1979) has suggested that within many organizations members fall into five broad categories:

1 Those who determine goals and policies.
2 Those with the responsibility for ensuring that policies are implemented and objectives attained: 'middle managers'.
3 Those who work most directly to provide the product or service of the organization.
4 Those who facilitate the work of others by offering particular skills.
5 Those who, while not carrying out the main task of the organization, are nevertheless indispensable to that task.

2.4 An example: a hospital

1 Those who determine policies have traditionally been the senior members of various hierarchies: doctors, nursing officers and others. Sometimes people are appointed to this group from outside the organization.
2 This responsibility is carried by the medical, nursing and other officers who seek to implement policies agreed at senior level.
3 This responsibility falls to the nurses, doctors, radio-therapists and others whose work most directly affects patients.
4 This group includes technicians, analysts and others with special relevant skills.
5 These staff include domestic workers, secretaries, orderlies, porters and many others.

3 The importance of being clear about the objectives of the group or unit, and of the larger organization

3.1 The objectives-setting approach

This expression was developed within American industry in the 1950s and 1960s. It emphasizes the importance of agreeing goals or objectives for given areas of activity which are co-ordinated with those of other areas and of the larger organization.

3.2 Features of an objectives-setting approach

Stoner (1978), on the basis of his studies, has suggested that these include the following:

1 Effective objective/goal setting and planning.
2 Setting of individual goals by group/unit leaders – in relation to the broader goals of the organization.
3 Considerable freedom in reaching these goals.
4 Frequent review of performance as it relates to objectives.
5 Commitment to the approach at all levels of the organization.

There is also, in many settings, a clear effort made to *measure* the extent to which goals have been met, either using quantitative (e.g. numerically-based) methods, or qualitative (e.g. opinion-based) methods.

3.3 Research from industry: relevance for human services work

Carroll and Tosi (1973) reviewed the research on some principles of the objectives approach. Despite their industrial context, and origins, their findings have relevance for working with people in human services settings.

1 **Concerning specifying goals** People who are involved in setting their own goals tend to aim to improve on past performance. If they achieve this, they set themselves even higher goals: if they do not, they set less ambitious goals. Locke, Shaw, Saari and Latham (1981) endorsed this finding.

2 **Concerning inviting participation from junior staff** People who are involved in setting their own goals are likely to show higher levels of performance than those whose goals are set for them.

3 **Concerning giving feedback on performance** Giving feedback, if it is specific and immediate, tends to lead to improvement in performance. Feedback should be given in a tactful manner, particularly if it is critical: otherwise hostility and reduced performance may follow.

3.4 An example: working with volunteers

In a voluntary agency, depending heavily upon volunteers for its work to support mentally ill people in the community, it might be valuable for staff to meet with volunteers to agree objectives. For example:

1 To put volunteers in touch with mentally ill people in the community.
2 To provide training for volunteers in aspects of mental illness.
3 To provide regular supervision and support for volunteers.
4 To develop agreements with volunteers concerning the range and extent of their commitment.

Such working out of priorities with all concerned, and *how the extent to which they have been achieved can be evaluated*, can contribute towards enlisting volunteers in the first place and towards retaining them thereafter.

3.5 Advantages of the objectives approach

A survey by Tosi and Carroll (1968) of managers on their experience of objectives found that its major advantages were that it:

1 Lets individuals know what is expected of them.
2 Aids planning by clarifying goals and target dates.
3 Improves communication between management and other staff.
4 Makes people more aware of the organization's goals.
5 Makes evaluation more effective by focusing upon specific and positive achievements.

3.6 Disadvantages of the objectives approach

Jamieson (1973), however, has noted a number of difficulties which recur among those seeking to use management-based objectives. These include:

1 Difficulties in enlisting full organizational support.
2 Difficulties in making the changes in structure, patterns of authority and procedure required.
3 Deficiencies of interpersonal skill in those responsible for judging performance and giving feedback.
4 Difficulties of devising specific objectives for individuals and shortage of time for monitoring these.
5 Difficulties of measuring output in service provision settings.

3.7 General relevance of the principles to working with people

While much of the research reported above took place in the context of industry, nevertheless, some of the principles seem to have more general relevance. These include:

1 Clear goal/objective setting for the organization/group.
2 Consultation with staff upon the nature of these goals, and upon priority tasks for the individuals and the group.
3 A clear agreement as to priorities on a regular basis.
4 Some independence for each unit in how goals shall be met.
5 Frequent review of the team's performance against goals.
6 Giving supportive and tactful feedback to team members.
7 Agreement upon how the extent to which goals have been met shall be measured/evaluated.

4 The importance of rational decision-making

4.1 Stages in the process of rational decision-making

Many researchers suggest the following stages:

1 Asking relevant questions: e.g. do we know enough about the situation?

2 If not, where do we get the information from? e.g.:
   (a) those personally affected.
   (b) others affected by the situation.
   (c) others who have encountered and solved the same problem.
3 The generation of a range of solutions.
4 The evaluation of each possibility using actual data so that the decision is made on the basis of *evidence*.
5 Assigning responsibility for implementing the decision and agreeing means for monitoring outcome.
6 Monitoring effects of the decision upon others in the larger system.

4.2 An example

People thinking it would be a good idea to open accommodation for homeless young people, might find it useful to bear the following questions in mind:

1 *Starting from grassroots* Is there really a need? Have we talked to enough homeless young people? What *particular* provision are they asking for? Short-term? Long-term? Hostel? What is the existing provision and where is it?
2 *Gathering and analysing relevant information* This might include information from:
   (a) Potential users of any provision: i.e. homeless young people.
   (b) Information from social workers, community workers, youth workers upon the need for provision.
   (c) People elsewhere who have recognized and responded to the need, and what their experience has taught them.
3 *Thinking of a range of solutions* What is *desirable*?
4 *Evaluating a range of solutions* What is *possible* in the light of information about need, others' experience, funding, etc? Adopting one plan rather than others.
5 *Who will take action to put the decision into practice*? i.e. who will write the letters, sit on committees, make the applications for funding? Basically, who will do the work?
6 *Monitoring effects* Who will report progress – to whom? Who will liaise with other groups, report reactions from those affected, and co-ordinate developments?

5 The need for careful planning of the use of time

5.1 The concept of the 'critical path'

1 This is another concept developed within industry, but with relevance for working with people generally. It is particularly important in the area of planning. (See Figure 11.2)

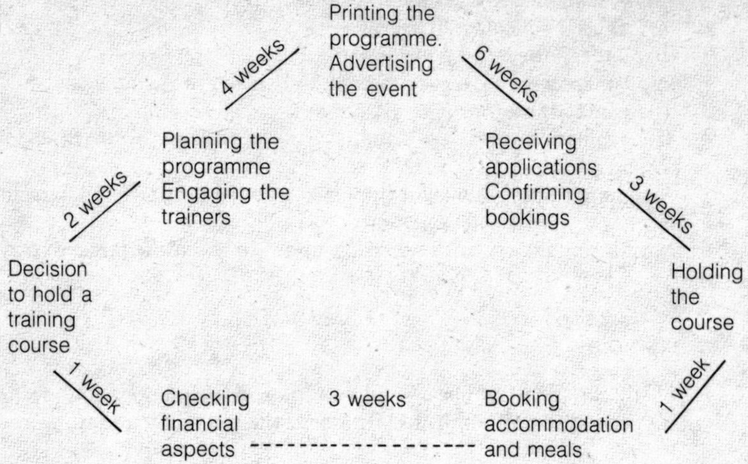

FIGURE 11.2 A model of forward planning, including the critical path (After Cleland and King, 1972)

2 Cleland and King (1972) have pointed out,

> the final event cannot be reached until all preceding activities are completed, and this cannot take place any sooner than the time required for the longest path through the network – the critical path.

3 In the above example, the upper path is the most time-consuming path, so it is the critical path.

5.2 Some further examples

1 **Forward planning, without a fixed date for completion** If a public meeting is to be convened upon the issue of, say, the provision of heating for the elderly, then a planned programme is needed which takes into account time for the completion of tasks essential to holding the meeting. These will include:

1 Agreeing objectives
2 Agreeing who will do what
3 Raising funds
4 Booking accommodation
5 Engaging speakers
6 Devising publicity
7 Distributing publicity

2 **Forward planning, where a fixed deadline has to be met** If a report upon a student placement has to be submitted by a fixed date, the following stages are likely to feature on the critical path:

1 Noting the deadline date by all concerned.
2 Agreeing the prior date by which all those with contributions to make to the final report should submit these to the practice teacher or supervisor.
3 Devising a draft report by the practice teacher.
4 Discussion of the draft with the student; making any amendments or alterations.
5 Sending the final draft for typing.
6 Signing and posting the report.

5.3 Some additional useful practices

1 Devising written lists of objectives: for the year, the month, the week or the day.
2 Listing all tasks to be completed concerning a given objective.
3 In relation to 1 and 2, pinpointing priorities.
4 Writing down priority tasks to be completed on every single day: five or six seems to be the most useful number.
5 Writing down checklists for important procedures.

6 Enlisting the motivation of all those involved

6.1 People as maximizing their satisfactions

Lorsch (1974) and Sutton (1979) have written of the implicit cost-benefit analysis in which individuals seem constantly to be engaged. Considerations seem to include:

1 Perceptions and expectations of what is involved
2 Anticipated outcomes and expectations of benefit and cost
3 Considerations based on past personal experiences
4 Personal values
5 Personal factors concerning who else is involved, demands upon time and energy, etc.
6 Availability of support networks, etc.
7 Other competing activities

These are all highly individual, interact according to situation and others involved, and for some people involve factors such as the possibility of financial, status and power rewards: for others, their personal values are crucial considerations.

6.2 A possible example

Thus it is often possible to find people to chair local committees and interest groups, because these roles are fairly prestigious, carry some status, are not onerous and allow the exercise of some power and authority. It is much less easy to find people to act as secretary, because such a role is time-consuming, personally demanding, less prestigious and fairly thankless.

6.3 The importance of consultation

Many researchers agree that people appreciate being consulted upon decisions that affect them, and feel angry when such decisions are taken without consultation.

7 The constructive management of conflict

7.1 Some primary sources of conflict

Walton and Dutton (1969), among others, suggested the following main sources of conflict:

1 The need to share resources, and competition for them.
2 Differences in values or perceptions.
3 Differences in goals or objectives.
4 Dominance tendencies of individuals.
5 Ambiguities within the organization.

7.2 The constructive potential of conflict

Stoner (1978) suggested that while it used to be thought that all conflict was undesirable, the view that some level of conflict may be constructive or even desirable is gaining ground. He reported that the research suggests that suppressing or avoiding conflict has been found to be less effective in the long run than recognizing and dealing with it. Thus constructive handling of conflict is one of the manager's skills.

7.3 The resolution of conflict

While some means of resolving inter-group conflict have already been discussed in Chapter 5, page 43, Hicks and Gullett (1981) have suggested several strategies characteristically adopted towards conflict. These include:

1 Avoidance: stemming from the hope that if a problem is ignored it will go away.
2 Competition: sometimes a straight head-on confrontation occurs; this, however, can have far-reaching and long-lasting reverberations throughout the larger system.
3 Compromise: wherein both parties give up some demands while obtaining others.
4 Collaboration: where parties concerned *actively work together* to resolve a difficulty. (This tends to assume that a 'felt power equality' exists: i.e. that both parties feel they have equal power.)

Hicks and Gullett go on to illustrate examples of these different strategies, and favour the collaborative approach as the most constructive for all concerned.

References

Carroll, S. J. and Tosi, H. (1973), *Management by Objectives – Applications and Viewpoints*, New York: Macmillan.

Cleland, D. I. and King, W. (1972), *Management: A Systems Approach*, New York: McGraw-Hill.

Hicks, H. and Gullett (1981), *Management*, New York: McGraw-Hill International Book Company.

Jamieson, B. D. (1973), 'Behavioural problems with management by objectives', *Academy of Management Journal*, vol. 16, pp. 495–505.

Locke, A. E., Shaw, K., Saari, L. and Latham, G. P. (1981), 'Goal setting and task performance', *Psychological Bulletin*, vol. 90, pp. 125–52.

Lorsch, J. W. (1974), *Managing Change*, Note prepared for class discussion at the Harvard Business School, and distributed by the Intercollegiate Clearing House, Soldiers Field, Boston, Mass. 02163.

Mintzberg, H. (1979), *The Structuring of Organizations*. Englewood Cliffs, New Jersey: Prentice-Hall.

Open University (1980), *Systems Organization. The Management of Complexity*. T 243, Block 1. *Introduction to System Thinking and Organization*, Milton Keynes: Open University Press.

Stoner, J. (1978), *Management*, Englewood Cliffs, New Jersey: Prentice-Hall.

Sutton, C. (1979), *Psychology for Social Workers and Counsellors*, London: Routledge & Kegan Paul.

Tosi, H. and Carroll, S. (1968), 'Managerial reaction to management by objectives', *Academy of Management Journal*, vol. 11, pp. 415–26.

Walton, E. and Dutton, J. (1969), 'The management of inter-departmental conflict', *Administrative Science Quarterly*, vol. 14, pp. 73–84.

PART 2

Research concerning people experiencing particular stress and disadvantage

Research concerning people in poverty and at social disadvantage

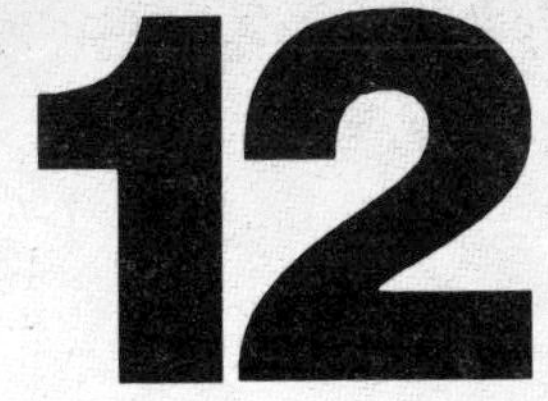

1 Some definitions and indicators

The concept of 'poverty' is controversial: there is no consensus upon a definition.

1.1 Society's definition of poverty

Townsend (1979) in his major survey, *Poverty in the United Kingdom*, reported that he viewed *society's* definition of poverty as, 'the basic rates paid by the Supplementary Benefits Commission to families of different composition.'

1.2 Poverty as a relative and dynamic concept

1 Sinfield (1975), and Townsend (1979) have, however, criticized this apparently 'scientific and value-free measure of subsistence' and highlighted instead, 'the social nature of the concept of poverty'.
2 Sinfield and Townsend thus view poverty as a *relative and dynamic* concept closely linked to issues of structural inequality. In the light of this, Townsend (1979) has suggested,

> Individuals, families and groups in the population can be said to be in poverty when they lack the resources to obtain the types of diet, participate in the activities and have the living conditions and amenities which are customary, or at least are widely encouraged or approved, in the societies to which they belong. Their resources are so seriously below those commanded by the average individual or family that they are, in effect, excluded from ordinary living patterns, customs and activities.

1.3 Indicators of social disadvantage: the DHSS/SSRC inquiry

Berthoud (1983) has reported the twenty indicators of social disadvantage used by the joint Department of Health and Social Security and Social Science Research Council inquiry (Brown and Madge, 1982) into transmitted deprivation and disadvantage:

N.B. I am much indebted to Professor Adrian Sinfield, of the Department of Social Policy and Social Work, University of Edinburgh, for advice and help with this chapter.

Indicators of social disadvantage

Resources	low income (lack of assets)
Employment	low occupational status low earnings unemployment (poor conditions of work)
Housing	lack of standard amenities overcrowding poor conditions of dwellings (homelessness)
Education	lack of qualifications
Health	general ill-health mortality mental disorder
Family	marital breakdown lone parenthood large families juvenile delinquency children in care

Multiple disadvantage

N.B. Brackets indicated that these indicators were only partially considered through shortage of data.

Each of these areas will be considered separately below.

2 Resources: the extent of poverty

2.1 Changes in extent of poverty

Income in relation to supplementary benefit scales	Numbers in thousands			
	1960	1975	1979	1981
Below supplementary benefit level	1,260	1,840	2,100	2,810
Receiving supplementary benefit	2,670	3,710	3,980	4,840
At or up to 40 per cent above supplementary benefit level	3,510	6,990	5,210	7,350
Total	7,440	12,540	11,290	15,000
	Percentage			
Below supplementary benefit level	2.3	3.5	4.0	5.3
Receiving supplementary benefit	4.9	7.0	7.6	9.1
At or up to 40 per cent above supplementary benefit level	6.4	13.2	9.9	13.8
Total	14.2	23.7	21.4	28.2

Notes

a. The data are for the UK and are on a household rather than an income unit basis. It should be noted that the estimates are based on national assistance scales, not supplementary benefit scales.
b. Drawn separately from supplementary benefit sample inquiry with people drawing benefit for less than 3 months excluded. . . .

TABLE 12.1 Changes in the extent of poverty 1960–81 (Britain). (Abel Smith and Townsend, 1965; Townsend 1984)

2.2 A major survey: 'Poverty in the United Kingdom'

This survey, reported by Townsend (1979), is based mainly on a representative national stratified sample carried out in 1968–9 with over 6,000 people from 2,050 households. It gathered data upon wealth, income, work and use of social services. A summary of the conclusions included the following:

1 **Numbers in poverty** The data confirmed the figures shown in Table 12.1, and suggested that

> *the Government's standard of poverty is pitched too low, especially for families with children . . .*

2 **The 'structure' of poverty** The risks of poverty are highly correlated with occupational class, and also with employment status, dependency and age.

> The highest risks are to be found among those of advanced age, especially if they are disabled, but are also high among children.

3 **The rich and the control of resources** The survey indicated that:

> even on a wide definition of wealth 5 per cent were found to own 45 per cent of net assets. . . . *Wealth is highly correlated with occupational class and people of the professional class account for the majority of the rich.*

4 **Social class** The summary of the survey reported,

> On both subjective and objective indicators class is strongly and uniformly correlated with poverty. Class consciousness is rooted in economic circumstances. . . .

3 Employment: unemployment and low paid employment

1 **The inadequacy of benefits** Many studies, e.g. Townsend (1979), have shown that benefits are inadequate to meet day-to-day costs. This has not only directly harmful effects, such as poor diet, upon recipients and their families, but also indirect effects, such as demoralization, depression and increased

social isolation. The impact of unemployment is considered further in Chapter 13, page 107.

2 **The impact of low income** Burghes (1984) reported the extent of low paid employment,

> By 1981, two-thirds of a million people (680,000) were living on an income below the supplementary benefit level even though they were in families with at least one full-time wage earner.

3 **Children living in poverty** Concerning the impact of these circumstances upon children, Burghes reported,

> of a total of more than 13 million children in Great Britain, well over 3½ million were living in or on the margins of poverty – well over a quarter of all the children in the country. Of this total number of children, half a million were actually living below the poverty line (supplementary benefit), another million plus on supplementary benefit and a further two million within 40 per cent of the supplementary benefit line.

4 **Employment and class status** Brown (1983), considering evidence from a number of studies, stated that although age, gender and race were all important,

> The importance of employment as a determinant of class status, and hence of disadvantage, is well known and documented (e.g. Rutter and Madge, 1976). . . .

4 Housing and housing deprivation

In the survey, *Poverty in the United Kingdom*, Townsend (1979) reported the extent of housing deprivation in his own and other official studies. Part of his summary noted:

> Twenty-two per cent of households experienced structural defects, 21 per cent inadequate housing facilities, and 11 per cent insufficient bedrooms, by conventional social standards. Another 44 per cent had only one of their rooms (or none) heated in winter, and 5 per cent had insufficient internal play-space for children. According to these five measures, 13 million, 11 million, 10 million, 22 million and 4 million people respectively in the United Kingdom were deprived. . . .
>
> By most criteria, households consisting of a man and woman and four or more children experienced the worst housing. Single-person households were more likely than households with all numbers of children to have inadequate facilities and only one room heated in winter. . . .
>
> Much the most important structural factor found to be associated with

housing deprivation was occupational class. By nearly all criteria, we found a consistent relationship between lower incidence of deprivation and higher class. . . .

More households living in poverty or on the margins of poverty also experienced poor housing than did other households. . . .

5 Education

1 **Evidence from the National Child Development Study**

1 An early study by Wedge and Prosser (1973), using data from the Child Development Study, which traced the progress of as many as possible of the 16,000 or so children born in one week in March, 1958, made a particular study of disadvantaged children. According to their criteria, at age eleven, one child in every sixteen (6 per cent) was disadvantaged.

2 Wedge and Prosser then compared the progress of these children against that of children who experienced none of their criteria of disadvantage. In terms of educational progress, they concluded,

> one in four of the disadvantaged children was 'maladjusted' but only one in eleven of the ordinary children . . .
>
> one in six of them was receiving special help within the normal school for 'educational backwardness' compared with one in sixteen of the ordinary group . . .
>
> on average, disadvantaged children were some three-and-a-half years behind ordinary children in their reading scores . . .

3 In a commentary on later surveys of the children's school attainment and on performances of children disadvantaged at eleven, those disadvantaged at sixteen, and non-disadvantaged, or 'ordinary', children, Wedge and Essen (1982) reported,

> the attainment of all the pupils in our study was tested at the age of 11 as well as at the age of 16 and hence it was possible to examine the scores at 16 of various groups of children who began secondary schooling with the same range of test scores at 11. The results made it clear that the differences in attainment between disadvantaged and ordinary children accumulate during adolescence. The differences that exist at 11 increase during the secondary school period.

2 **The micro and the macro level** There is a great body of additional evidence, e.g. that leading to the setting up of Educational Priority Areas, and the publication of the Halsey Report (1972), which links social disadvantage with educational under-achievement. Robinson (1976) has written,

> Education is related to poverty at both the micro and the macro level. At the micro level is the under-achievement of an individual coming

> from a home which might be insecure, lacking in material resources and possessing a wealth of society's disadvantages. . . .
>
> The response to the macro challenge of poverty must be a broad framework of *policy* . . . (my italics).

6 Health

1 Townsend and Davidson (1982) have edited the Report of the Working Group on Inequalities in Health (the Black Report). This Report considered the evidence of, and some of the reasons for, the major disparities which exist in health between various groups, and in summarizing the data on the pattern of present health inequalities, they concluded:

> There are marked inequalities in health between social classes in Britain. . . . Mortality tends to rise inversely with falling occupational rank or status, for both sexes and at all ages. At birth and in the first month of life twice as many babies of unskilled manual parents as of professional parents die. . . .
>
> A class 'gradient' can be observed for most causes of death and is particularly steep for both sexes in the case of diseases of the respiratory system and of infective and parasitic diseases. . . .

2 In their general Summary they reported:

> Inequalities exist also in the utilization of health services, particularly and most worryingly of the preventive services. Here, severe under-utilization by the working classes is a complex result of under-provision in working-class areas and of costs (financial and psychological) of attendance. . . .

3 And they continued:

> *In our view much of the evidence on social inequalities in health can be adequately understood in terms of specific features of the socio-economic environment*: features (such as work accidents, overcrowding, cigarette smoking) which are strongly class-related in Britain. . . .
>
> there is undoubtedly much which cannot be understood in terms of the impact of such specific factors, but only in terms of the more diffuse consequences of the class structure: poverty, working conditions and deprivation in its various forms.

7 Families and social disadvantage

1 There seems to be increasing agreement among researchers, e.g. Rutter (1978) and Madge (1983) that families undergoing many forms of social disadvantage can be understood as experiencing multiple and

measurable *stresses*. Rutter, for example, was able to devise a table of stress factors (see Family Adversity Index, Chapter 20, page 185) which were associated with childhood psychiatric and behavioural disorders.

2 Many studies have examined the implications of the difficulties of disadvantaged families. Burghes (1984), for example, reported the study by the Child Poverty Action Group and Family Service Units of sixty-five families living on supplementary benefit. Concerning the children, it was found,

> parents protected their children as well as they could from the effects of family poverty. . . . In 4 out of 10 families, children would have to go without meals from lack of money. . . . Fuel was a particular problem for these families and there was no way of protecting their children against the cold when they could not afford heating. . . .
>
> In 4 out of 10 families, second hand clothes were the norm, a cause of distress to some children, especially those in their teens.

3 Further, Burghes (1984) noted that more than 700,000 families living below or on the margin of poverty were experiencing illness and disability and that, 'by 1981 there were almost 200 thousand children in families suffering sickness and disability.'

8 Multiple disadvantage

8.1 An analysis of multiple disadvantage

Berthoud (1983) has reported an attempt to pinpoint many interacting stresses, and used the General Household Survey to yield the following index of multiple disadvantage:

Education	head of family left school at minimum age, *and* has no qualifications
Family	lone parent, *or* divorced/separated *or* four or more children
Housing	more than one person per room *or* lacks sole use of kitchen, bath/shower or inside WC
Income	roughly the bottom fifth in the income distribution: i.e., below 140 per cent of the SB entitlement
Sickness	head of family long-term ill *or* currently not working through sickness
Work	head of family semi- or unskilled manual worker, *or* unemployed *or* earns less than £30 per week, full-time (in 1975).

Berthoud (1983) commented that Table 12.2 shows that,

> the more of the other problems a family has, the greater the probability of experiencing any problem.

8.2 Experience of specific problems and other problems

Experience of specific problem	*Number of OTHER problems*					
	None %	*One* %	*Two* %	*Three* %	*Four or five* %	*Correlation (r)*
Income	4	13	24	39	65	0.36
Work	24	38	53	69	84	0.32
Education	30	43	54	63	71	0.23
Family	4	6	9	18	31	0.22
Housing	14	17	22	25	36	0.14
Sickness	21	23	25	30	36	0.09

Source: Special tabulations from the General Household Survey 1975

TABLE 12.2 Experience of specific problems, by number of other problems experienced: families whose heads were of working age. (Berthoud, 1983)

References

Abel-Smith, B. and Townsend, P. (1965), *The Poor and the Poorest.* LSE Occasional Papers. London: Bell and Hyman.

Berthoud, R. (1983), 'Who suffers disadvantage?' in M. Brown (1983) (ed.), *The Structure of Disadvantage.* (DHSS/SSRC Studies in Deprivation and Disadvantage: 12), London: Heinemann Educational Books.

Brown, M. (1983) (ed.), *The Structure of Disadvantage.* (DHSS/SSRC Studies in Deprivation and Disadvantage: 12), London: Heinemann Educational Books.

Brown, M. (1983), 'Deprivation and social disadvantage', in M. Brown (ed.) (1983), *The Structure of Disadvantage.*

Brown, M. and Madge, N. (1982), *Despite the Welfare State; A Report on the SSRC/DHSS Programme of Research into Transmitted Deprivation,* London: Heinemann Educational Books.

Burghes, L. (1980), *Living from Hand to Mouth: a Study of 65 Families Living on Supplementary Benefit,* Family Service Unit/Child Poverty Action Group.

Burghes, L. (1984), 'Children in poverty', *Concern,* National Children's Bureau, No. 50, pp. 7–10.

Halsey, A. H. (1972), *Educational Priority. Vol. 1. E.P.A. Problems and Policies,* (The Halsey Report), London: HMSO.

Madge, N. (1983), 'Identifying families at risk', in N. Madge (ed.), *Families at Risk.* (SSRC/DHSS studies in Deprivation and Disadvantage: 8), London: Heinemann Educational Books.

Robinson, P. (1976), *Education and Poverty,* London: Methuen.

Rutter, M. and Madge, N. (1976), *Cycles of Disadvantage: A Review of Research,* London: Heinemann Educational Books.

Rutter, M. (1978), 'Family, area and school influences in the genesis of conduct disorders' in L. A. Hersov, M. Berger and D. Shaffer (eds), *Aggression and Anti-social Behaviour in Childhood and Adolescence*, Oxford: Pergamon Press.

Sinfield, A. (1975), 'We the people and they the poor', *Social Studies* (Irish Journal of Sociology) vol. 4, pp. 3–25.

Townsend, P. (1979), *Poverty in the United Kingdom*, Harmondsworth: Penguin.

Townsend, P. (1979), *Poverty in the United Kingdom*, London: Allen Lane.

Townsend, P. (1984), 'The reaction of mass poverty in Britain', in P. Townsend, *Why are the Many Poor?*, London: Fabian Society, Tract no. 500.

Townsend, P. and Davidson, N. (eds) (1982), *Inequalities in Health*. (The Black Report), Harmondsworth: Penguin.

Wedge, P. and Prosser, H. (1973), *Born to Fail*. London: Arrow Books/ National Children's Bureau.

Wedge, P. and Essen, J. (1982), *Children in Adversity*. London: Pan Books in association with Heinemann Educational Books.

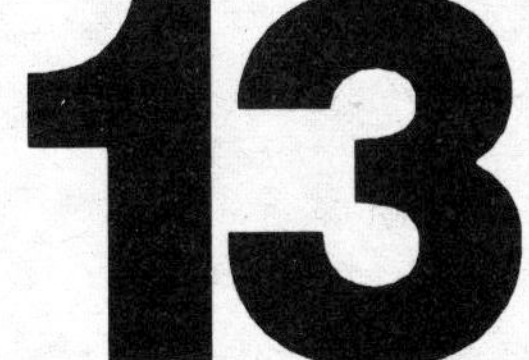

13 Research concerning unemployed people

1 Some definitions

There is controversy over a definition of 'unemployment'; two different ones, giving rise to different statistics, are:

1.1 A definition by the Department of Employment

Since October, 1982, the UK Department of Employment has defined the unemployed as,

> people claiming benefit at Unemployment Benefit Offices on the day of the monthly count who on that day were unemployed and able and willing to do any suitable work.

Footnote: I am much indebted to Professor Adrian Sinfield, of the Department of Social Policy and Social Work, University of Edinburgh, for advice and help with this chapter.

It is made clear, however, that students claiming benefit between terms are excluded.

1.2 A definition by the International Labour Organisation

Sorrentino (1981) summarized this,

> the I.L.O. definitions include as unemployed all persons who during a specified time period, were without a job, available for work and seeking work.

2 Statistics concerning unemployment

2.1 Some official statistics

1 Unemployment rates: Great Britain and other countries

	G.B.	U.S.A.	Canada	France	West Germany	Japan	Sweden
April 1979	5.7	5.7	7.6	6.2	3.3	2.1	2.2
Dec. 1985	13.0	6.8	10.0	9.8	7.7	2.9	2.7
change 79–85	+128%	+19%	+32%	+58%	+133%	+38%	+23%

TABLE 13.1 Unemployment rates 1979 and 1985 – standardized to US definitions. Percentages. (Figures calculated by Sinfield (1986) from US Sources).

N.B. An attempt has been made to allow for the different ways in which countries define employment and unemployment.

2 Regional unemployment

	May, 1979 %	January, 1986 %
South East	3.6	9.8
East Anglia	4.2	10.7
South West	5.5	12.0
West Midlands	5.1	15.0
East Midlands	4.5	12.4
Yorks and Humber	5.3	14.9
North West	6.7	15.7
North	7.9	18.3
Wales	7.4	16.6
Scotland	7.3	15.0
Northern Ireland	10.4	21.8
United Kingdom	5.4	13.2

TABLE 13.2 Regional unemployment 1979 and 1986, seasonally adjusted and excluding school leavers (Dept of Employment press release, 30 January, 1986, and *Employment Gazette*, 1979)

3 Male unemployment

Socio-economic group	1955–1977 %	1983 %
Professional, employers and managers	4	6
Intermediate and junior non-manual	8	10
All non-manual	6	8
Skilled manual	9	17
Semiskilled and unskilled manual	18	32
All manual	12	23
All males aged 18–64	10	18
Colour (males aged 18–59)		
White	9	17
Coloured	17	29
Males aged 18–24	21	35
25–39	9	16
40–59	9	12
60–64	7	17

TABLE 13.3 Male unemployment in the previous twelve months, 1975–7 and 1983, Great Britain. Percentages. (General Household Survey in *Social Trends 1980*, Tables 5.18 and 19, and *Social Trends 1985*, Table 4.26) (Data not published for females)

4 Ages of the long-term unemployed

People under		
	25	357,986
	25–34	316,026
	35–44	235,694
	45–54	240,924
	55–64	201,227

TABLE 13.4 Age distribution of long-term unemployed claimants in the UK at 10 October 1985. (Out of work and claiming benefit for more than twelve months.) (*Unemployment Unit Briefing*, Statistical Supplement, University of Edinburgh, January, 1986)

5 Figures in January, 1986 Sinfield and Fraser (1986) reported,

> On 9th January 1986 unemployment in the United Kingdom reached a new record total of 3,407,729. This gave a rate of 14.1%, the first time unemployment had reached 14% since the 1930s.

These data are according to the Department of the Environment definition.

3 Those vulnerable to unemployment

3.1 The vulnerable groups

Sinfield (1981) suggested that some groups are particularly vulnerable to become unemployed: these included:

1 *Those on low wages.* In a DHSS survey of 2,321 men registered as unemployed (Moylan and Davies, 1980), as many as 50 per cent had previously been receiving the lowest earnings in the national earnings distribution.
2 *Young people.* There is clear evidence of a much higher rate of unemployment among young people without any qualifications, and that they come particularly from families where the main wage-earner is a manual worker. See also Willis (1985).
3 *Older workers and those in poor health.* The employment hierarchy (Townsend, 1979), operates so that professional and administrative groups gain increasing rewards and privileges as they advance, so diminishing the power and opportunities of the older, weaker members of the community, and those in poorer health.
4 *Women.* Many women are still choosing not to register as unemployed. Moreover, many jobs formerly taken by women, e.g. low-paid, monotonous work in textile, clothing and footwear industries, are now not readily available.
5 *Those already unemployed.* There is evidence from Britain and other countries, that the experience of being unemployed makes it more likely that people remain unemployed.

3.2 A summary statement upon the research

Sinfield (1981) concluded:

> It is important to emphasise that those most likely to become unemployed are people in low-paying and insecure jobs, the very young and the oldest in the labour force, people from ethnic and racial minorities, people from among the disabled and handicapped, and generally those with the least skills and living in the most depressed areas.

4 Effects of becoming unemployed

4.1 The multiple impacts of unemployment

Several studies suggest the many functions of employment. Hayes and Nutman (1981), for example, suggested that work can be considered as:

1 A form of activity.
2 A source of income.
3 A means of structuring time.
4 Providing opportunities for mastery and creativity.
5 Providing an opportunity for social contacts.
6 Giving an opportunity for a sense of identity and purpose.

Each will be considered separately below.

1 **Work as a form of activity** Here the main issue is that there has been a disastrous drop in employment opportunities. In particular there has been an

unprecedented decline in job opportunities in the production sector, manufacturing, construction and the metal industry, and such growth as there has been has been in the service sector, e.g., clerical, communication and catering. (Department of Employment, 1985)

2 **Work as providing income: the impact of poverty**

1 The very great majority of people suffer a reduction of income when they are unemployed, and both government and industrial research shows the very high risk of poverty to the unemployed. Burghes (1981) has written,

> Together unemployment and poverty create a vicious trap of suffering. It is those with low incomes in work who are most likely to become unemployed; once out of work, unemployment pushes them further into poverty.

2 She pinpointed some ways in which this occurs:
(a) Entitlement to unemployment benefit depends on those out of work having paid enough national insurance contributions while in work. Many young people have never been in work.
(b) Entitlement to unemployment benefit is limited to 1 year.
(c) Supplementary benefits provide least adequately for the long term unemployed and for families with children. At the end of 1980, there were about three quarters of a million children dependent on an unemployed adult.

3 **Work as a means of structuring time** Many studies have examined the ways in which people who find themselves unemployed fill their time. Warr (1983) reported a study with 399 unemployed men which found that the more time-filling activities (sitting around at home, watching TV and looking around the shops) were reported as increased, the lower was psychological well-being – as measured by the General Health Questionnaire.

4 **Work as providing opportunities for mastery and creativity** Warr (1982), in an examination of psychological aspects of employment and unemployment, quoted the finding of e.g. Karasek (1979) that it is the lack of personal control of one's work activities which is most strongly predictive of low psychological well-being. By definition, unemployed people have absolutely no control over work activities.

5 **Work as providing an opportunity for social contacts** There is evidence that not only do people who become unemployed lose the social interactions implicit in the work setting, but the effect of this situation extends to the whole family. McLellan (1985), in a study of the effect of unemployment on the family, found the partners of unemployed men described,

> not joining in conversations with other mothers at the school gates in case subjects were brought up mentioning/requiring money, such as

Status in the labour market	Type of work experience	Work identity	Financial situation	Identity within the family
Full and part-time employees, male and female	Professional or white collar	Threatened	Secure	Not threatened
	Sheltered manual or skilled manual	Some threat	Short-term security	Threatened by long-term unemployment
	Work without shelters, usually semi-skilled and unskilled	No threat	Insecure	Threatened by short- and long-term unemployment
School-leavers seeking entry to labour market	None	Threat to realisation of work identity	Insecure	Access delayed to adult status and dependence on family enhanced
Females seeking part-time work	No recent experience or low-grade, white-collar and service work	No serious threat	Variable—threatens their position in family; threatens family if no other source of income	Role as household manager not threatened

FIGURE 13.1 Factors affecting the experience of unemployment (Ashton, 1986) Reprinted with permission.

outings, parties, clothing . . . most of these women had reduced their social interaction considerably and felt isolated.

6 **Work as giving opportunities for a sense of identity**

1 There is much evidence of the impact of unemployment in terms of loss of confidence and self-esteem. Many studies, e.g. Warr (1983), found that unemployed people experience significantly fewer positive feelings, and more strain, anxiety and depression. They concluded:

> making the transition into unemployment yields a marked reduction in psychological well-being, and regaining a job restores well-being very sharply.

2 In a confirming study, Warr, Banks and Ullah (1985) examined the experience of unemployment among black and white urban teenagers; they found distress levels significantly higher among both black and white seventeen-year-olds than among a comparable group of employed young people.

5 Effects of becoming unemployed

5.1 Loss of work as a bereavement experience

Hayes and Nutman (1981) quoted Parkes (1971) who viewed the loss of a job as comparable to a bereavement. (See Chapter 37, page 355) Parkes commented, 'Unemployment is a form of crippling which can be expected to have the same effects as other forms of loss. . . .'

5.2 Stages of adaptation to the loss of employment

1 Research studies suggest a broadly comparable sequence following loss of work among men who have been employed in full-time work for many years. Different researchers divide the sequence into more or fewer stages. Thus Harrison (1976) suggested the sequence shown in Figure 13.2.

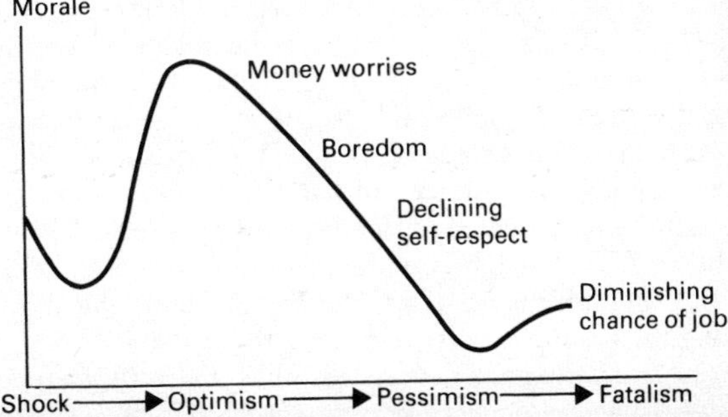

FIGURE 13.2 The phase model of unemployment. *Source:* Adapted from Harrison (1976) *Employment Gazette*, vol. 94.

2 Sinfield (1986) and others, however, have pointed out that such a sequence may not be accurate of people in part-time or short-time work; it will also be affected by factors such as availability of work, of personal support systems, and by many other variables such as individual cognitions and perceptions.

5.3 Individual responses to the loss of employment

Many researchers recognize that the response to unemployment is highly individual, and is likely to be mediated by the interactions of external and personal circumstances, for example:

(a) the industrial structure of the area
(b) the perceived future of the area in terms of work availability
(c) a sense of being the victim of circumstances and not personally responsible
(d) the response of relatives: wife, husband, parents, children
(e) the financial implications
(f) the frustration of personal aspirations
(g) the sense of 'loss of face'
(h) the extent of supportive networks and relationships

6 Further areas of research

6.1 Health and unemployment

1 There is controversy concerning the impact of unemployment upon health. Describing a major American study by Brenner (1976), Popay (1981) reported its finding that,

> Using data for unemployment over a 30-year period, a key finding of the study was that a one per cent increase in the unemployment rate in the USA, sustained over a period of six years, had been associated with approximately 36,887 extra deaths (including 920 extra suicides and 648 extra murders) and 4,227 extra state mental hospital admissions.

Popay reported that when Brenner repeated his work (Brenner 1980) with the British data, the effect on indicators of ill health seemed even stronger, although many have challenged his methodology.

2 Several studies in Britain and elsewhere have found an association between unemployment and poor health. In a small scale study, McLellan (1985) reported that sixteen of the twenty men, whose progress after job loss she investigated in depth, had consulted a GP with a new health problem since becoming unemployed. Warr (1983) in a larger study, using a measure of general health, found much higher distress among the unemployed than among the employed.

3 There is converging evidence, e.g. Sinfield (1980), of the damaging effects of unemployment upon the health, via poverty and stress, of the wives and children of men without work.

4 There are also indications (Sinfield, 1986) that many people who experience poor health are at risk of becoming unemployed.

6.2 Mental health and unemployment

McLellan (1985), reporting a small study by Fagin (1981), wrote,

> Following job loss, Fagin found that many male breadwinners experienced feelings of sadness, hopelessness, self-blame, lethargy, lack of energy, loss of self-esteem, insomnia, withdrawal and poor communication, suicidal thoughts, impulsive and sometimes violent outbursts, and increased use of tobacco and alcohol. Their wives too, often exhibited the same symptoms of anxiety, despair and apathy, and marital tension was found.

6.3 Suicide and unemployment

The evidence here is mixed. Although early studies found no association between unemployment and suicide, Kreitman and Dyer (1983) found unemployment was an important variable when identifying those at particular risk following parasuicide.

6.4 Use of the personal social services and unemployment

1 Westland (1986) has reported a survey undertaken with eight authorities in the light of the impact of unemployment. He reported:

> Eight authorities were surveyed: Sunderland, Harrow, Coventry, Manchester, Bradford, Tower Hamlets, Knowsley and Lambeth. Six social services activities were chosen: services for people with physical handicaps; for those with mental handicaps; those who have been or are mentally ill; children in care and leaving care; juvenile crime, and finally, referrals for financial advice and welfare rights.

2 In the sample of 796 cases referred in September 1984 to selected area offices, Westland noted:

> Only 7 per cent of the people referred were in paid employment. . . .
>
> Of the unemployed who were referred most were suffering long term unemployment. . . .
>
> Children in care and those leaving care were a strikingly underprivileged group. In one area 100 per cent of children of employable age in residential care were unemployed. . . . Young people from ethnic minorities were seen to be even more at risk than others.
>
> For physically and mentally handicapped people there was a similarly gloomy picture. . . .
>
> We found that the generalized effect of economic recession and unemployment is often not perceived by social services staff. . . .

References

Ashton, D. (1986), *Unemployment and Capitalism. The Sociology of British and American Labour Markets*, Brighton: Wheatsheaf Books, Ltd.

Brenner, H. (1976), *Estimating the Social Cost of National Economic Policy*, US Government Printing Offices, Washington, Paper no. 5.

Brenner, H. (1980), 'Mortality and the national economy', *The Lancet*, 15 September, pp. 568–73.

Burghes, L. (1981), 'Unemployment and poverty' in L. Burghes and R. Lister (eds), *Unemployment: Who Pays the Price?*, London: Child Poverty Action Group.

Burghes, L. and Lister, R. (eds), (1981), *Unemployment: Who Pays the Price?*, London: Child Poverty Action Group.

Department of Employment, (1985), Labour force survey: preliminary results for 1984, *Employment Gazette*, May, 1985, pp. 175–9.

Employment Gazette (1985), vol. 93, no. 7, Unemployment: Age and Duration, Department of Employment, London: HMSO.

Fagin, L. (1981), *Unemployment and health and families*, London, D.H.S.S.

Harrison, R. (1976), 'The demoralising experience of prolonged unemployment', *Department of Employment Gazette*, April 1976.

Hayes, J. and Nutman, P. (1981), *Understanding the Unemployed*, London: Tavistock Publications.

Hopson, B. and Adams, J. (1976), 'Towards an understanding of transition: defining some boundaries of transition dynamics' in J. Adams, J. Hayes and N. Hopson (eds), *Transition*, London: Martin Robertson.

Karasek, R. A. (1979), 'Job demands, job decision latitude, and mental strain: implications for job redesign', *Administrative Science Quarterly*, vol. 24, pp. 285–308.

Kreitman, N. and Dyer, J. (1983), 'Suicide and parasuicide' in R. E. Kendall and A. K. Zealley (eds), *Companion to Psychiatric Studies*, 3rd edn, Edinburgh: Churchill Livingstone.

McLellan, J. (1985), 'The effect of unemployment on the family', *Health Visitor*, vol. 58, pp. 157–61.

Moylan, S. and Davies, B. (1980), 'The disadvantages of the unemployed', *Employment Gazette*, August, pp. 830–1.

Parkes, C. M. (1971), 'Psycho-social transitions: a field for study', *Social Science and Medicine*, vol. 5, pp. 101–15.

Popay, J. (1981), 'Unemployment: a threat to public health' in L. Burghes and R. Lister (eds) (1981), *Unemployment: Who Pays the Price?*

Sinfield, A. (1980), 'The blunt facts of unemployment', *New Universities Quarterly*, vol. 34, Winter 1979–80, pp. 29–47.

Sinfield, A. (1981), *What Unemployment Means*, Oxford: Martin Robertson.

Sinfield, A. (1986), Personal communication.

Sinfield, A. and Fraser, N. (1986), 'Unemployment and poverty', *Modern Studies Association*, no. 36. In press.

Sorrentino, C. (1981), 'Unemployment in International Perspective' in B.

Showler and A. Sinfield (eds), *The Workless State*, Oxford: Martin Robertson.

Townsend, P. (1979), *Poverty in the United Kingdom*, London: Allen Lane.

Unemployment Unit Briefing, Statistical Supplement, University of Edinburgh 1986.

Warr, P. (1982), 'Psychological aspects of employment and unemployment', *Psychological Medicine*, vol. 12, pp. 7–11.

Warr, P. (1983), 'Job loss, unemployment and psychological well-being' in van de Vliert and V. Allen (eds), *Role Transitions*, New York: Plenum Press.

Warr, P., Banks, M. and Ullah, P. (1985), 'The experience of unemployment among black and white urban teenagers', *British Journal of Psychology*, vol. 76, pp. 75–87.

Westland, P. (1986), 'Power and the underprivileged', *Social Services Insight*, February 15–22, 1986.

Willis, P. (1985), *The Social Condition of Young People in Wolverhampton in 1984*. Wolverhampton Borough Council.

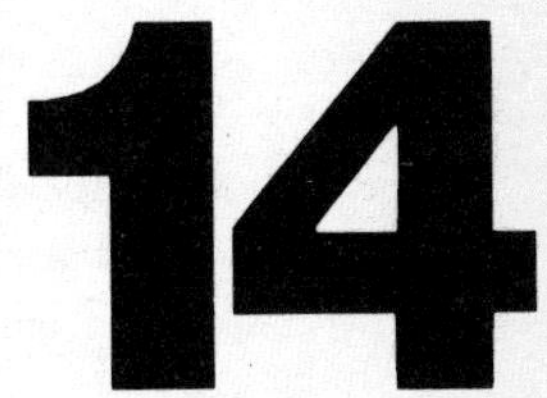

Research concerning people from ethnic minorities

Consultant: Usha Prashar, Director, National Council for Voluntary Organisations, London.

1 Some statistics

1.1 Communities within Britain

	Birthplace			
	United Kingdom	Outside United Kingdom	Not stated	Total
Ethnic origin				
White	48,728	1,792	254	50,774
West Indian or Guyanese	248	257	4	510
Indian	263	513	14	789
Pakistani	139	210	4	353

(contd overleaf)

	Birthplace			Total
	United Kingdom	Outside United Kingdom	Not stated	
Bangladeshi	26	55	1	83
Chinese	21	83	–	105
African	32	58	2	92
Arab	10	58	1	69
Mixed	149	47	1	198
Other	24	86	–	110
Not stated	656	34	261	952
All origins	50,297	3,196	541	54,035

Source: Labour Force Survey, 1983,
Office of Population Censuses and Surveys

TABLE 14.1 Population of Great Britain by ethnic origin and birthplace, 1983. Thousands. (*Social Trends*, 1985)

1.2 The predominance of the white population

The authors of *Social Trends* (1985) noted:

> About 94 per cent of the population in Great Britain in 1983 were of white ethnic origin. . . . About half the rest were known to be of West Indian, Guyanese, Indian or Pakistani ethnic origin. . . .

Belonging to groups which are numerically small, and of which many members experience discrimination and racism, contributes to the vulnerability felt by many ethnic minority communities.

2 Fields of research concerning the experience of people from ethnic minority groups

While there are a great many fields of such research, there will be a focus here upon the following fields:

1 Employment and unemployment
2 Housing
3 Education
4 Health and welfare
5 Racial attacks

3 Research concerning employment and unemployment

3.1 Employment and unemployment among peoples and sexes

This data is shown in Table 14.2 overleaf.

	Ethnic origin				All ethnic origins[2]
	White	West Indian or Guyanese	Indian/ Pakistani/ Bangladeshi	Other[1]	
Males					
In employment					
Employees[3]	75.4	64.3	61.8	66.6	74.7
– full-time	73.0	62.0	60.5	62.5	72.2
– part-time	2.3	2.1	1.3	3.7	2.3
Self-employed	11.3	2.5	14.6	12.6	11.3
All in employment[4]	88.4	72.4	78.5	83.6	87.9
Out of employment	11.6	27.6	21.5	16.4	12.1
Economically active (= 100%) (thousands)	14,484	149	329	156	15,356
Females					
In employment					
Employees[3]	82.7	75.4	65.1	73.2	82.0
– full-time	46.3	56.0	50.3	53.0	46.4
– part-time	34.9	18.8	13.3	20.0	34.0
Self-employed	5.2	1.0	10.6	7.3	5.2
All in employment[4]	89.9	82.0	78.4	85.4	89.6
Out of employment	10.1	18.0	21.6	14.6	10.4
Economically active (= 100%) (thousands)	9,920	135	145	113	10,484

[1] African, Arab, Chinese, other stated, and mixed.
[2] Includes ethnic origin not stated.
[3] Includes hours worked not stated.
[4] Includes employment status not stated.

Source: Labour Force Survey, 1983, *Office of Population Censuses and Surveys*

TABLE 14.2 Economic status of the economically active in Great Britain: by ethnic origin and sex. 1983. Percentages. (*Social Trends*, 1985)

3.2 A commentary on the above data

The authors of *Social Trends* commented that this table:

> shows that in 1983 88 per cent of economically active men of white ethnic origin were in employment, compared with 84 per cent of those of 'Other' minority ethnic origins, that is people of African, Arab, Chinese, other stated, or mixed origin, 79 per cent of those of Indian, Pakistani, or Bangladeshi ethnic origin, and only 72 per cent of those of West Indian ethnic origin.
>
> Among economically active women, 90 per cent of those of white ethnic origin were in employment in 1983, compared with 85 per cent of

'Other' minority ethnic origins, 82 per cent of those of West Indian ethnic origin, and 78 per cent of those of Indian, Pakistani, or Bangladeshi ethnic origin.

3.3 The experience of discrimination in the field of employment

1 **The rate of increased unemployment among black people** The authors of *Race and Immigration* (1983) reported that the *rate* at which unemployment has increased has . . . been significantly greater among black people than among white workers. They wrote,

> Thus, between 1974 and 1975, when unemployment generally rose by some 26.4%, among black people the rise was more than double at 57.4%. More recently, unemployment among black people increased by 11.5% in 1978–80, by 82.4% in 1980–81, and by 25% in 1981–82. This compared with rises in the same years of 2.5%, 66.2%, and 24.1% for unemployment as a whole.

2 **Why higher unemployment?** The same authors, noting the particularly high figures for unemployment among black women, and black young people, especially in urban areas, reported that several factors are suggested as contributing to this situation:

> the concentration of black workers in industries which are in decline, lack of qualifications, lack of knowledge of the English language, and discrimination.

They examined the empirical evidence for each factor in turn, and concluded,

> Discrimination, whether direct or indirect, would therefore appear to be the single most important factor in explaining disproportionately high black unemployment. Concentration in certain vulnerable industries may be a factor, but, as we have seen, this is itself originally attributable to racism in that black people came to Britain to do the work not wanted by white workers and have been largely confined to these sectors. Language problems may also be a factor, but, again as we have seen, language is frequently used to hide discrimination.

4 Research concerning housing

4.1 A major survey, including data on housing

1 Brown (1984) has reported a major national survey of the circumstances of black people by comparison with those of white. This survey, described in *Black and White Britain*, comprised 5,001 interviews with individual black (West Indian/Afro-Caribbean and Asian) people from 3,083 separate households and 2,305 interviews with individual white people, each from a separate household. Brown wrote that:

Both surveys are designed to be nationally representative of their respective populations of England and Wales.

4.2 Where people lived, and in what sort of housing

Information concerning tenure in major areas of black residence is shown in Table 14.3

Column percentages

	Inner London	Outer London	West Midlands Met. County	Leics, Notts and Derbys	West and South Yorks	Greater Manchester and Lancs	Berks, Bucks and Herts	Rest of England and Wales
White Households								
Owner-occupied	27	63	47	62	57	67	60	61
Rented from Council	43	24	41	30	35	22	35	29
Privately rented	21	9	11	7	5	9	5	9
Housing Association	8	3	2	1	2	2	1	1
West Indian Households								
Owner-occupied	27	48	34	(55)	(43)	46	(75)	50
Rented from Council	59	43	58	(25)	(25)	46	(22)	31
Privately rented	3	4	1	(16)	(18)	2	(4)	12
Housing Association	11	5	7	(5)	(14)	6	(–)	7
Asian Households								
Owner-occupied	34	75	76	84	91	80	83	78
Rented from Council	50	17	19	8	3	15	14	13
Privately rented	9	5	3	5	5	3	4	7
Housing Association	5	1	2	2	1	3	–	2

TABLE 14.3 Tenure in major areas of black residence by ethnic group (Brown, 1984)

4.3 Standard of amenities

Information concerning amenities in black and white households is shown in Table 14.1.

Column percentages

	White	West Indian	Asian	Indian	Paki-stani	Bangla-deshi	African Asian
Lack exclusive use of bath, hot water or inside WC	5	5	7	5	7	18	5
No garden	11	32	21	15	21	56	18
No central heating	43	38	44	37	66	56	27
No refrigerator	6	6	11	4	19	37	5
No washing machine	22	37	44	38	61	78	22
No telephone	24	24	24	18	34	44	14
Base: Households							
(weighted)	2694	1834	2851	1150	751	277	604
(unweighted)	2305	1189	1893	726	518	197	411

TABLE 14.4 Amenities by ethnic group (Brown, 1984)

4.4 Inner city residence and poor quality housing

Many additional studies, e.g. *Britain's Black Population* (1980), have reported the evidence that people of ethnic minority groups often find themselves in the poorest quality housing. This is often in the inner city, where housing is older, amenities fewer, and densities of occupation greater.

5 Research concerning education

5.1 The Report of the Swann Committee

1 Some conclusions and recommendations

1 The Report, *Education for All* (1985), concerned the education of children from ethnic minority groups. Among its Conclusions and Recommendations, it was reported:

> 2.1 West Indian children, on average, are under-achieving at school. . . . Asian children, by contrast, show on average, a pattern of achievement which resembles that of White children, although there is some evidence of variation between different sub-groups. . . . Bangladeshis in particular are seriously under-achieving. . . .
>
> 2.2 Low average IQ has often been suggested as a cause of under-achievement, particularly in the case of West Indians. This has long been disputed, and our own investigations leave us in no doubt that IQ is *not* a significant factor in under-achievement. . . .
>
> 2.3 School performance has long been known to show a close correlation with socio-economic status and social class, in the case of all children. The ethnic minorities, however, are particularly disadvantaged in social and economic terms, and there can no longer be any doubt that this extra deprivation is the result of racial prejudice and discrimination, especially in the areas of employment and housing. . . . A substantial part of ethnic minority underachievement, where it occurs, is thus the result of racial prejudice and discrimination on the part of society at large, bearing on ethnic minority homes and families, and hence, *indirectly* on children. . . .
>
> 2.4 . . . the rest, we believe, is due in large measure to prejudice and discrimination bearing *directly* on children, within the educational system, as well as outside it. . . .

2 Other issues noted from the Swann Report In its summary of the Swann Report, the Runnymede Trust, in its section on the concept of 'Education for All', reported that the essential steps in this argument were,

> . . . the fundamental change that is necessary is the recognition that the problem facing the education system is not how to educate children of ethnic minorities, but how to educate *all* children;

> . . . Britain is a multi-racial and multicultural society and all pupils must be enabled to understand what this means;
>
> . . . this challenge cannot be left to the separate and independent initiative of LEAs and schools: only those with experience of substantial numbers of ethnic minority pupils have attempted to tackle it, though the issue affects all schools and all pupils;
>
> . . . education has to be something more than the reinforcement of the beliefs, values and identity which each child brings to school;
>
> . . . it is necessary to combat racism, to attack inherited myths and stereotypes, and the ways in which they are embodied in institutional practices;
>
> . . . multicultural understanding has to permeate all aspects of a school's work; it is not a separate topic that can be welded onto existing practices;
>
> . . . only in this way can schools begin to offer anything approaching the equality of opportunity for all pupils which it must be the aspiration of the education system to provide.

5.2 Other important issues

1 **Research concerning teachers of ethnic minority pupils** Tomlinson (1984) has surveyed the field of teachers' views and experience of parents and children from ethnic minority groups. Among the studies she highlighted is that of Green (1982), which she summarized:

> Green studied the 70 white teachers of 940 white, 449 Asian and 425 West Indian pupils, and demonstrated that teachers' racial (or 'ethnocentric' as he described them) attitudes affect not only expectations about pupils but also actual classroom teaching. Teachers who were 'highly intolerant' spent more time with white boys, and then with Asian boys; Asian girls and West Indian boys got least teacher time. Highly tolerant teachers gave more time equally to boys and girls and more to West Indian boys. Green's study demonstrates powerfully that, on the whole, white and Asian children benefit substantially more from teacher attention in the classroom, whatever the tolerance level of the teacher, than children of West Indian origin.

2 **Lack of preparation for teaching children from minority ethnic groups** Tomlinson (1984), noting the difficulties that negative stereotyping of minority ethnic group children can lead to, pointed out that teachers

> have, by and large, received little help or preparation from their training to encourage more positive views. . . . There has never been a coordinated national policy to ensure that teachers received even minimal preparation for teaching in racially and culturally-mixed schools. . . .

3 **The need for more teachers and psychologists from ethnic minority cultures** Many researchers and reports have called for these: e.g. Coard (1971), The Rampton Report (1981) and Parekh (1983). They also called for active efforts by schools to take full account of the multi-racial nature of British society.

6 Research concerning health and welfare

6.1 Health care

1 The Policy Studies Institute survey did not find marked differences among Asian, Afro-Caribbean and white groups in terms of the extent of being registered with a General Practitioner; almost all were registered.
2 It was the view of more than 72 per cent of all groups and sexes sampled that people of Asian and West Indian origin were treated the same as white people by hospitals.

6.2 Welfare

1 **The Policy Studies Institute survey**

1 In terms of receipt of benefits, the survey found that twice as many black households as white receive unemployment benefit, reflecting the difficulties which black people have in finding work.
2 Brown (1984) commented that there is no evidence to suggest that Asian or West Indian households are receiving benefits beyond their entitlement; in fact, the proportion of Asian households receiving supplementary benefit and family income supplement is lower than might be expected.

2 **An examination of discrimination and social security** Gordon and Newnham (1985) drew upon material collected from a number of advice agencies and from previously published research in their study. Their investigation included consideration of the following issues,

(a) The connection between the entitlement to benefit and immigrant status.
(b) How immigration control is concerned with the control of the poor.
(c) Problems faced by black claimants as a result of the operation of immigration control, such as families divided by immigration rules, and the lack of information in different languages.
(d) The development in the UK of a system of internal immigration controls.

7 Some findings concerning racial attacks

7.1 A study in thirteen areas of Britain

1 A Home Office study, *Racial Attacks* (1981) examined the extent of racially motivated aggression towards people, both black and white, in thirteen police areas within Britain. A racial incident was defined as:

> an incident, or alleged offence by a person or persons of one racial group against a person or persons or property of another racial group, where there are indications of racial motive.

Notice of 2,630 incidents, involving 2,851 victims, was given.

2 The writers of the report stated:

> In absolute terms . . . racial attacks appear to constitute only a very small proportion of recorded crime (less than ¼%). However, the proportion does rise to about 3% if only offences of violence against the person and robbery are considered. . . . proportionately, the incidence of victimisation was much higher for the ethnic minority population, particularly the Asians, than for white people. Indeed the rate for Asians was 50 times that for white people and the rate for blacks was over 36 times that for white people.

3 The writers also noted:
   (a) Evidence of a fairly steady rise in the number of attacks reported since 1977, and a marked rise since 1980.
   (b) Indications that about 7,000 incidents with either 'strong' or 'some' evidence of a racial motive will be reported annually in England and Wales.
   (c) Closer agreement between victims, black, white and Asian, and the police, as to whether attacks were racially motivated, than had been anticipated.
   (d) Broad support for the views of other groups, e.g. that of the Joint Committee against Racialism, that many racial incidents are carried out by gangs of youths: e.g. 'white youths of the skinhead fraternity'.
   (e) The very real fears of ethnic minority and white victims and the urgent need for police intervention and protection.

7.2 The Policy Studies Institute survey

1 This survey (Brown, 1984) reviewed a larger sample than did the Home Office study (which was based only upon people who had contacted the police). Informants were asked about any incidents of assault, deliberate property damage and burglary of which they had been the victims in the previous sixteen to eighteen months.

2 Those asked about such incidents were,

White informants	2,265
West Indian informants	882
Asian informants	1,688

3 Results showed the following percentages (see Table 14.5 overleaf).

4 The survey monitored many other variables, including the beliefs and attitudes of participants towards protection by the police. Brown concluded that the results showed,

that there is among black people an alarmingly low level of confidence in the support from the police against racial attacks, and that this is particularly the case among West Indians.

<table>
<tr><th></th><th>White</th><th>West Indian</th><th>Asian</th></tr>
<tr><td>Per cent of informants that have been 'physically attacked, assaulted or molested in any way':</td><td></td><td></td><td></td></tr>
<tr><td>All</td><td>3</td><td>5</td><td>3</td></tr>
<tr><td>Men</td><td>4</td><td>6</td><td>3</td></tr>
<tr><td>Women</td><td>2</td><td>3</td><td>3</td></tr>
<tr><td>Inner London, Inner Birmingham, Inner Manchester</td><td>10</td><td colspan="2">5</td></tr>
<tr><td>Rest of London, W. Midlands M.C. and Greater Manchester M.C.</td><td>3</td><td colspan="2">4</td></tr>
<tr><td>Elsewhere</td><td>2</td><td colspan="2">3</td></tr>
<tr><td>Age group:</td><td></td><td></td><td></td></tr>
<tr><td>16–24</td><td>10</td><td colspan="2">7</td></tr>
<tr><td>25–34</td><td>3</td><td colspan="2">4</td></tr>
<tr><td>35–64</td><td>1</td><td colspan="2">2</td></tr>
<tr><td>65+</td><td>1</td><td colspan="2">2</td></tr>
</table>

TABLE 14.5 Victims of assault over past 16–18 months (Brown 1984) percentages.

References

Brown, C. (1984), *Black and White Britain. The Third PSI Survey*, London: Heinemann Educational Books.

Coard, B. (1971), *How the West Indian Child is Made Educationally Sub-normal in the British School System*, London: New Beacon Books, Ltd.

'Education for All'. A Summary of the Swann Report, (1985), London: The Runnymede Trust.

Education for All. The Report of the Committee of Inquiry into the Education of Children from Ethnic Minority Groups, (1985), (The Swann Report), London: HMSO.

Gordon, P. and Newnham, A. (1985), *Passport to Benefits?*, London: Child Poverty Action Group and the Runnymede Trust.

Green, P. A. (1982), 'Teachers' influence on the self-concept of pupils of different ethnic origins', (Unpublished Ph.D. thesis), University of Durham.

Home Office, (1981), *Racial Attacks*, London: Home Office.

Parekh, B. (1983), 'Educational opportunity in multi-ethnic Britain' in N. Glazer and K. Young (eds), *Ethnic Pluralism and Public Policy*, London: Heinemann Educational Books.

Race and Immigration, Runnymede Trust Bulletin, No. 159/September 1983, London: Runnymede Trust.

The Runnymede Trust and the Radical Statistics Group (1980), *Britain's Black Population*, London: Heinemann Educational Books.
Tomlinson, S. (1984), *Home and School in Multi-Cultural Britain*, London: Batsford Academic and Educational Ltd.
West Indian Children In Our Schools (1981), Interim Report of the Committee of Inquiry into the Education of Children from Ethnic Minority Groups (1981), (The Rampton Report), London: HMSO.

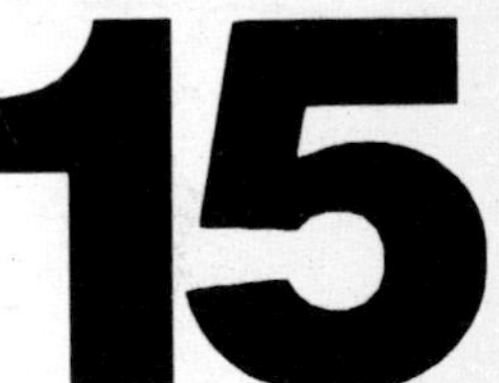

Research concerning people with physical handicaps

Full acknowledgment is made that this chapter draws extensively upon the book *Children with Disabilities and their Families: A Review of Research*, by Philp and Duckworth (1982).

1 Definitions

1.1 Early attempts at definitions

Philp and Duckworth (1982) report early distinctions between 'intrinsic' and 'extrinsic' handicap and between 'primary' and 'secondary' handicap: each formulation attempted to distinguish the primary medical situation from associated social and environmental factors.

1.2 A suggested terminology from the WHO trial scheme

1 The World Health Organisation, developing the work of Wood (1975) has published a classification based on three, interacting levels. Philp and Duckworth (1982) report these concepts (see Figure 15.1) and adopt the suggestion that 'disablement' should be the collective term.

2 The following definitions of terms are suggested:
   i. 'impairments' are abnormalities of bodily structure . . .
   ii. 'disabilities' are restrictions on the performance of . . . functions and activities . . .
   iii. 'handicaps' are disadvantages preventing the fulfilment of roles. . . .

Disease or Disorder	Disablement (experience summarized)		
→	Impairment →	Disability →	Handicap
intrinsic situation	experience exteriorized	experience objectified	experience socialized

FIGURE 15.1 The concepts in the World Health Organisation trial scheme.

2 Statistics

The table gives selected data for England:

	1980	1981	1982	1983	1984
General classes					
All ages: total	900.7	954.8	–	–	1102.6
Under 16	19.5	19.9	–	–	20.6
Very severely handicapped					
All ages: total	56.5	59.1	–	–	71.6
Under 16	–	5.8	–	–	5.8
Severely or appreciably handicapped					
All ages: total	353.4	374.9	–	–	454.4
Under 16	–	6.9	–	–	7.4
Other classified persons					
All ages: total	276.7	308.8	–	–	379.4
Under 16	–	3.3	–	–	4.1
Unclassified					
All ages: total	214.2	212.1	–	–	197.1
Under 16	–	4.0	–	–	3.4
Blind					
All ages: total	107.8	–	111.7	–	–
Under 16	2.0	–	2.0	–	–
Partially sighted					
All ages: total	51.4	–	58.0	–	–
Under 16	2.4	–	2.2	–	–
Deaf					
All ages: total	29.7	–	–	31.8	–
Under 16	3.1	–	–	3.3	–
Hard of hearing					
All ages: total	35.1	–	–	47.2	–
Under 16	1.1	–	–	1.6	–

TABLE 15.1 Persons registered as substantially and permanently handicapped. England. Thousands. (*Health and Personal Social Services Statistics for England*, 1985)

3 Research concerning the particular difficulties of people with disabilities and their families

3.1 Housing problems

1 The inadequacy of housing for families with disabled children

1. Summarizing several studies, Philp and Duckworth (1982) concluded that families with disabled children are more likely to have poor housing than families without disabled children, where the prevalence of disability has a social class bias: (e.g. that arising from spina bifida).
2. Several studies, e.g. Glendinning and Bradshaw (1977), have shown that between a third and a half of families with a disabled child live in council accommodation.
3. The Bristol studies by Butler and colleagues (1978) identify the main housing problem in terms of the mobility of the child; steps and stairs presented major difficulties, and 43 per cent of the children had to be carried upstairs.

2 The inadequacy of housing for adult disabled people

1. Shearer (1973) is among the many researchers who have shown that many disabled people seek accommodation in ordinary housing within the community – adapted to their particular needs.
2. She has advocated the Fokus model, developed in Sweden, as particularly constructive, and has written,

   > Since 1964, Fokus has built some 300 flats for disabled people, scattered through normal housing blocks all over the country. Staff are available at any time the residents want help . . .

3. She pointed out that 'the only people who know how the disabled want to live are the disabled people themselves', and she urged the inclusion of disabled people upon any groups and committees planning accommodation. Such practices, and the resultant accommodation are beginning to develop in Britain: for example, in Haringey, Sutton in Ashfield and Rochdale.

3.2 Problems of transport and mobility

1. Butler *et al.* (1978) found that 45 per cent of mothers with a disabled child never travelled on public transport. In terms of school transport, however, 88 per cent of parents of disabled children reported satisfactory arrangements.
2. Gormley and Walters (1981) conducted a postal survey of over 600 disabled individuals concerning their mobility needs. Some extracts of the summary of their conclusions are reported below:
   1. Disabled people go out infrequently, for short periods, and the types of trip they do make are largely restricted to essential shopping,

and visiting friends and relatives. Indoor mobility patterns are also severely limited in comparison with the general public. . . .

2 Information resources in the UK are poorly developed. Many disabled people . . . are not sure exactly what information they need, or where it can be reliably obtained. . . . There is an increasing need for a national, disinterested organisation to speak with one voice in detail to *all* disabled people about *all* types of mobility aids. . . .

3 Disabled people's incomes are still on average, low. Total weekly income from all sources to complete households containing disabled individuals are roughly equivalent to the weekly average pay of one member of the national workforce. Insufficient extra resources are available to meet added costs of mobility and other needs essential to normal life. For example, 45% of disabled people have spent money which did not come from government, charity or any other 'free' source on mobility aids. . . .

4 There is a favourable balance of opinion about the technical performance of modern devices to aid mobility, such as electric wheelchairs. . . .

5 . . . considerable evidence of improved relations between disabled people and the general public was uncovered by this study.

N.B. The Disabled Living Foundation and others are attempting to respond to the need for national organizations for disabled people, while some boroughs, e.g. Haringey, have established community transport facilities, such as Dial a Ride.

3.3 Social and emotional problems

1 The experience of stigma

1 Goffman (1968) has written a very well-known book on this subject: *Stigma*. He has explored the world of people who undergo stigmatizing experience, the responses of others to them, and the effects upon their families. He concluded:

> The central feature of the stigmatized individual's situation in life can now be stated. It is a question of what is often, if vaguely, called 'acceptance'. Those who have dealings with him fail to accord him . . . respect and regard. . . .

2 Many others, e.g. Finkelstein (1981), have reported the experience of discrimination suffered at the hands of society by the disabled, and the humiliation of being the objects of other people's specialist studies. . . .

3 Similarly, Philp and Duckworth (1982) reported the stress experienced by families with handicapped children because of the effects of social attitudes towards disability.

4 These writers quoted studies upon how parents respond to the role of being related to a stigmatized person – particularly that of Voysey (1975), who wrote empathically of the efforts of parents to offer ordinary, everyday parenting to their handicapped children, and of the 'negotiations' conducted with others over the visibility and severity of the disability. Voysey also noted the way in which various coping styles are responded to by others: e.g. 'coping splendidly', or 'not facing the facts'.

2 The experience of stress

1 Bradshaw and Lawton (1978), working with the families of handicapped children, noted stress effects of three kinds:
   (a) Physical strain
   (b) Financial strain
   (c) Emotional and psychosomatic symptoms.

2 Several studies, e.g. Cull (1974), indicated that many mothers of disabled children show signs of stress. From her study, Baldwin (1976) showed that only 22 per cent of mothers and 50 per cent of fathers in her sample felt that their physical or mental health had *not* been affected.

3 Philp and Duckworth (1982) from their examination of a wide range of studies, summarized the position thus:

> Taking all studies together, there is reasonably firm evidence that the parents of children with disablement are more likely than parents of children without disablement to suffer from stress, anxiety and depression.

3.4 Social isolation

Several studies have examined the general social isolation of disabled children, and Philp and Duckworth note the Report of Clarke and colleagues (1977) for the Warnock Committee on Special Education. This compared a group of disabled children with a group of controls, and the findings include evidence that children with disablement are,

(a) More likely to play alone.
(b) Slightly more likely to be alone with an adult.
(c) Likely to spend a similar time in a group with an adult and children.
(d) Less likely to engage in imaginative play.
(e) More likely to engage in non-specific activity, in listen-with others or watching others' activities.
(f) Equally likely to communicate with adults and children for a similar length of time.
(g) More likely to communicate less with other children.
(h) More likely to have one, rather than two-way, speech patterns.

3.5 Adjustment to disability

1 **Adjustment among disabled children** Philp and Duckworth (1982) have noted the review of research by Pless and Pinkerton (1975) upon the influence of chronic illness in childhood on the child's personality. The findings include the following:

1 Certain features of a disability, e.g. age of onset, severity, duration, affect the adjustment of the child.
2 Some characteristics of the child, personality, coping style and intelligence, influence adjustment to disability.
3 Coping is also influenced by the strength of, and other stresses upon, family relationships.
4 The attitudes of parents, especially the mother, are of crucial importance.

2 **Adjustment among disabled adolescents** The book by Anderson and Clarke (1982), *Disability in Adolescence*, has reported very fully upon the experience of disabled young people, and some of the stresses encountered. These include those associated with:

1 Aspects of their education: the frequent wish to attend ordinary schools.
2 Some aspects of their social life: friendship and the use of leisure time.
3 Relationships with the opposite sex: fears and aspirations.
4 The transition from school to adult life.
5 Fears and aspirations about employment or the lack of it.

3 **The meaning of disability to those affected by it** Thomas (1982) has described the sudden impact of the new identity thrust upon people following, e.g. an accident, while Oliver (1981) has questioned a number of studies based mainly upon psychological perspectives of disability: he suggested that the sociological perspective of symbolic interaction has been much neglected. Such a perspective emphasizes the *meaning* of an event such as a stroke or a physically disabling accident not only to the person primarily concerned, but also to those in that person's immediate circle.

4 Research concerning the particular needs of families with disabled members

4.1 Support when discussing the nature of a child's disability

1 **The need for sensitivity at the time of diagnosis** Mackeith (1973) has written of the great sensitivity called for by those who have to inform parents of their new-born child's disability, and of the mix of feelings which may be produced in parents:

1 Two biological reactions: protection of the helpless; rejection of the abnormal.
2 Two feelings of inadequacy: inadequacy at reproduction; inadequacy at rearing.

3 Three feelings of bereavement: at the loss of the normal child they expected . . . (a) anger, (b) grief; and (c) adjustment, which takes time.
4 Feeling of shock.
5 Feeling of guilt, which is probably less common than many writers state.
6 Feeling of embarrassment, which is a social reaction to what the parents think other people are feeling.

2 The need for on-going clarification and support

1 Philp and Duckworth (1982) reported that,

> There is a general feeling that parents should be told of the disorder or impairment as soon as it is known . . . (. . . National Association for Mental Health, 1971 . . .); however, since such information cannot be absorbed in one session, there is a common view among parents, and reported by for instance, Cull (1974) . . . that parents need to be able to come back and ask questions.

2 These authors also reported several studies, e.g. Hunt (1973) indicating that,

> Not only does information need to be individual and specific, it also needs to be clear, concise, non-technical and given consistently over an extended period of time.

4.2 Recognition of the difficulties of adjustment

1 Several researchers have noted the difficulties of the neo-natal period: for example, Kogan and Tyler (1973) suggested,

> that mothers of children with disablement often experience 'affect turn-off' because of the unrewarding nature of interaction with the child which stems, in turn, from the child's failure to develop independence.

2 Mattson (1972) has noted some difficulties of adjustment among disabled children:
   1 Over-dependency: marked by fearfulness and leading to a lack of friends; mothers may themselves be very protective.
   2 Over-independency: marked by daring and risk-taking.
   3 Isolation: marked by shyness and loneliness, among those children who see their condition as an injustice.

3 Several studies, e.g. Tinkelman (1976), have examined the personal responses of children to their own disabilities, and in some children have found anger, a sense of guilt or fear, as well as envy of the normality of others.

5 Research concerning the services provided for families with a disabled child

5.1 Involvement with professionals

1 **General practitioners** The average GP was found by Goddard and Rubissow (1977) to be likely to have only three disabled children in the practice at any one time; the few studies conducted suggest good relationships exist, with the GP seen as supportive.

2 **Hospital doctors** Philp and Duckworth (1982) noted the central importance of the consultant and his or her colleagues, and reported,

> From the evidence that exists on parents' experience with hospitals it would appear that the technical proficiency of the personnel is high, though parents sometimes feel that they rank low in humanity . . .

Further, parents disliked seeing a different doctor on each visit.

3 **Health visitors** Philp and Duckworth reported the study by Goddard and Rubissow (1977) to be the only one employing a control group; this found, 'children with disablement were visited, on average, 7.8 times per annum while controls were visited 4.7 times.'

Fox (1975) and Voysey (1975) reported that although mothers felt that health visitors lacked specialist knowledge and information, they did enjoy their visits and the support they offered.

4 **Social workers** Philp and Duckworth report from the studies by Butler and colleagues (1976, 1978) that only 23 per cent of families had received help from social workers in the year preceding interview in the earlier study and 51 per cent in the later. However, 56 per cent of the latter were dissatisfied with this service, complaining that the turnover was too high, that they were too young, inexperienced or over-worked with inadequate knowledge of benefits. Other studies have provided mixed evidence about the amount and helpfulness of contacts with social workers.

5 **Short-term care** Hewett's study (1970) with the families of children with cerebral palsy found that 41 per cent of parents had accepted short-term care for their child at some stage, and another 14 per cent said they would if offered. In Baldwin's (1976) study, however, 76 per cent of parents had never had their child cared for away from home, about 13 per cent had done so once, and 11 per cent had done so several times. Asked if they wanted more short-term care, 74 per cent said no.

6 **Long-term care** Pless (1969) found that parents were more likely to use this when the child had poor home circumstances or behaviour problems. Hewett (1976) found parents very reluctant to decide to seek long-term care or to send their child to a residential school.

7 **Financial provision** Bradshaw's (1978) report concerning the Family Fund, which gives financial help to the parents of disabled children, indicated

(a) The Fund was known to about half the families eligible, though only a third had applied.
(b) Applicants could be increased by half as much again if new efforts were made to tell eligible families about the Fund.

Concerning statutory benefits, e.g. the Attendance allowance and the Mobility allowance, it seemed in 1982 that some 10 per cent of families entitled to the former had not applied for it.

8 **Self-help groups and voluntary organizations** It has been found that in any sample of parents of physically impaired children about half will belong to a relevant voluntary organization (Hewett, 1970). Fewer parents of mentally handicapped children seem to join such organizations.

References

Anderson, E. M. and Clarke, L. (1982), *Disability in Adolescence*, London: Methuen.

Baldwin, S. (1976), *Some Practical Consequences of Caring for Handicapped Children at Home*, University of York: Social Policy Research Unit.

Bradshaw, J. (1978), 'The Family Fund: An Initiative in Social Policy', PhD Thesis, University of York.

Bradshaw, J. and Lawton, D. (1978), *Tracing the causes of stress in families with handicapped children*, University of York, Social Policy Research Unit.

Brechin, A., Liddiard, P. and Swain, J. (eds) (1981), *Handicap in a Social World*, London: Hodder & Stoughton and The Open University.

Butler, N., Gill, R. and Pomeroy, D. (1976), *Housing problems of handicapped people in Bristol*, University of Bristol: Child Health Research Unit.

Butler, N., Gill, R., Pomeroy, D. and Fewtrell, J. (1978), *Handicapped children – their homes and life styles*, University of Bristol: Department of Child Health.

Clarke, M. M., Riach, J. and Cheyne, W. M., (1977), 'Handicapped children and pre-school education', University of Strathclyde: Report to Warnock Committee on Special Education.

Cull, A. M. (1974), 'A study of the psychological concomitants of a chronic illness in childhood', PhD Thesis, University of Edinburgh.

Department of Health and Social Security (1986) *Health and Personal Social Services Statistics for England, 1985 edition*, London: HMSO.

Finkelstein, V. (1981), 'To deny or not to deny disability' in A. Brechin, P. Liddiard and J. Swain (eds), *Handicap in a Social World*, London: Hodder & Stoughton and The Open University.

Fox, A. M. (1975), 'Families with handicapped children – a challenge to the caring professions', *Community Health*, vol. 6, pp. 217–23.

Glendinning, C. and Bradshaw, J. (1977), 'Housing handicapped children and their families', University of York: Social Policy Research Unit.

Goddard, J. and Rubissow, J. (1977), 'Meeting the needs of handicapped children and their families: the evolution of Honeylands, a family support unit, Exeter', *Child: Care, Health and Development*, vol. 3, pp. 261–73.

Goffman, E. (1968), *Stigma: Notes on the Management of a Spoiled Identity*, New York: Prentice-Hall.

Gormley, R. and Walters, L. (1981), 'Mobility needs of disabled people in the U.K.' in A. Brechin, P. Liddiard and J. Swain (eds), *Handicap in a Social World*.

Hewett, S. (1976), 'Research on families with handicapped children: an aid or an impediment to understanding', *Birth Defects*, vol. 12, no. 4, pp. 35–46.

Hewett, S. (with Newson, J. and Newson, E.) (1970), *The Family and the Handicapped Child*, London: Allen & Unwin.

Hunt, G. M. (1973), 'Implications of the treatment of myelo-meningocele for the child and his family', *Lancet*, vol. 2, pp. 1308–10.

Kogan, K. L. and Tyler, H. B. (1973), 'Mother–child interaction in young physically handicapped children', *American Journal of Mental Deficiency*, vol. 77, pp. 492–7.

Mackeith, R. (1973), 'The feelings and behaviour of parents of handicapped children' in D. Boswell and J. Wingrove (eds), *The Handicapped Person in the Community*, London: Tavistock Publications and The Open University.

Mattson, A. (1972), 'The chronically ill child: a challenge to family adaptation', *Medical College of Virginia Quarterly*, vol. 8, pp. 171–5.

National Association for Mental Health (1972), 'The birth of the abnormal child: telling the parents', *Lancet*, vol. 2, pp. 1075–7.

Oliver, M. (1981), 'Disability, adjustment and family life – some theoretical considerations' in A. Brechin, P. Liddiard and J. Swain (eds), *Handicap in a Social World*.

Philp, M. and Duckworth, D. (1982), *Children with Disabilities and their Families: A Review of Research*, Windsor: National Foundation for Educational Research and Nelson.

Pless, I. B. (1969), 'Why special education for physically handicapped pupils?', *Social and Economic Administration*, vol. 3, pp. 253–63.

Pless, I. B. and Pinkerton, P. (1975), *Chronic Childhood Disorder – Promoting Patterns of Adjustment*, London: Henry Kimpton.

Shearer, A. (1973), 'Housing to fit the handicapped', *The Guardian*, 26 June, p. 16.

Sheridan, M. D. (1965), *The Handicapped Child and his Home*, London: National Children's Home.

Thomas, D. (1982), *The Experience of Handicap*, London: Methuen.

Tinkelman, D. G., Brice, J., Yoshida, G. N. and Sadler, J. E. (1976), 'The impact of chronic asthma on the developing child: observations made in a group setting', *Annals of Allergy*, vol. 37, pp. 174–9.

Voysey, M. (1975), *A Constant Burden: the Reconstitutions of Family Life*, London: Routledge & Kegan Paul.

Warnock Committee (1978), *Special Education Needs: Report of the Committee of Enquiry into the Education of Handicapped Children and Young People*, Cmnd 7212, London: HMSO.

Wood, P. (1975), *Classification of Impairments and Handicaps*, Document WHO/ICDO/REV CONF/75.15, Geneva: WHO.

World Health Organization (1980), *International Classification of Impairments, Disabilities and Handicaps*, Geneva: World Health Organization.

PART 3

Research concerning youth work and the youth service

16 Research concerning youth work and the youth service

Consultant:* *Ray Fabes, Senior Lecturer, Youth and Community Development Course, Leicester Polytechnic.

1 Some features of the youth service

1.1 Origins

The phrase 'Youth Service' is used to denote a wide range of voluntary and local authority provision for the leisure-time education and recreation of young people between 14 and 21 years of age, excluding students' organisations and youth sections of political parties. Responsibility for securing the provision of youth facilities was vested in local education authorities under the 1944 Education Act. (Report of the County Working Party on the Youth Service, Warwickshire County Council, 1985).

1.2 A description

The written evidence of the National Youth Bureau to the Department of Education Review of the Youth Service (1981) stated:

> The administrative title 'Youth Service, is used to denote a wide range of provision for, and responses to, the social education, recreation and leisure time activities of young people aged between 14 and 20 through a partnership between voluntary organizations and the statutory sector. (*Young People, the Youth Service and Youth Provision*)

1.3 Aspects of the development of the Youth Service

In a research project on the organization and purpose of the Youth Service in England and Wales, Eggleston (1976) pinpointed five phases of development:

1 The establishment phase: 1939–1944
2 The reconstruction and development phase: 1944–1960
3 The expansionist era: 1960–1965
4 The experimental phase: 1965–1972
5 The community phase: 1972 to the present.

1.4 Some distinguishing features

1 The statutory sector is now usually, but not always, administered by education departments; it employs full-time and part-time qualified and unqualified youth leaders, who join with volunteers in a wide variety of activities with or led by, the young people themselves.

2 *Experience and Participation. The Report of the Review Group on the Youth Service in England* (1982) highlighted as specific methods and resources of the Service:
   1 *The experiential curriculum. . . .*
   2 *Participation in decision making. . . .*
   3 *Voluntaryism* both in membership and in the adult worker role. . . .
   4 *A non-directive relationship between workers and young people. . . .*

3 The same Report suggests five 'offerings' which the Service should make available:
Association: . . . a place to go, a place to meet, a place to be with friends. . . .
Activities: . . . things to do . . . opportunities of fresh experience. . . .
Advice: . . . the whole process of providing information, advice and personal counselling.
Action in the Community: . . . community action . . . in many shapes and forms.
Access to Life and Vocational Skills.

2 Some statistics and other data concerning the youth service

2.1 The extent of involvement in the Youth Service

The Editorial of *Youth and Policy*, Autumn, (1984) considered evidence of the involvement of young people in the Youth Service, and reported a number of surveys included in, for example:

1 **The Albemarle Report (1960)** The Editorial noted that this report had found that the 'most optimistic' rate of attachment to the service was one in three in the age-range fifteen to twenty.

2 **The Crowther Report (1960)** The Editorial noted that the Crowther surveys showed that middle-class young people attend youth clubs and similar groups at a much higher rate than their working-class counterparts. (These surveys referred to broad-based youth provision, while other reports referred more specifically to education-based provision.)

3 **The Milson-Fairbairn Report (1969)** The Editorial concluded that this report, *Youth and Community Work in the 70's*, considered the Albemarle estimate of a 33 per cent involvement by the fourteen to twenty age group was 'optimistic' by 1968. Booton (1984) noted the findings that higher proportions of boys than girls belonged to youth groups; that in the fourteen to twenty age group the ratio of voluntary to statutory sector membership

was almost three to one; and that the main involvement was between those aged thirteen and sixteen.

4 **The Bone and Ross Report** (**1972**) The Editor noted that this report, *The Youth Service and Similar Provision for Young People*, endorsed earlier findings concerning specific youth club attachment. He observed:

> Early leavers were less likely to be attached. This was important because it raised the question whether school leaving age (eg: class, fundamentally) is the real key to understanding participation, or sex, as had been previously thought.

Fabes (1985) has noted:

> One can also consider Bone and Ross in a wider context in that they report that 65% of young people (14–20) went to a club, participated in a team, society or similar group and nearly all, 95%, had passed through such groups before the age of 21.

5 **The Thompson Report** (**1982**) This Review, *Experience and Participation*, drew heavily on data from *Young People in the 80s*, a survey of the leisure choices of a sample of 1,270 young people, from the North, Midlands and South of England. The sample contained:

Caucasians	70%
West Indians	15%
Asians	15%

The Editorial summarized:

> Only 3 in 10 (29%) of the 14 to 19 age group were found to be attached to a youth club. . . . Usage of youth clubs was found to be age, sex and class determined. . . . Of the 14–16 age group, nearly 2 in 5 (38%) were currently involved, compared with less than 1 in 5 (19%) of the 16+. Around one-third (32%) of boys attended, and just over one quarter girls (26%). The unemployed were more likely still to use youth clubs than those in work (29% to 19%). . . .

2.2 Estimated number of 'Youth workers' in England and Wales

1 Estimates from the Thompson Report (1982)
This Report offered the following approximate figures overleaf:
2 Some additional estimates
Fabes and Ritchie (1984), using figures drawn from the Thompson Report (1982), estimated that of full-time paid youth workers, whom they number at 8,600:
(a) 3,500 are based in Local Education Authority Youth and Community Centres (40% located on school campuses).

Employed by	Full-time officers	Full-time workers	Part-time workers	Unpaid volunteers
Local authorities	900	2,400	15,000	100,000
Voluntary bodies	600	1,100	16,500	400,000 workers 23,000 officers

TABLE 16.1 Estimated staffing of the Youth Service. Re-printed from *Experience and Participation* (1982)

(b) 1,500 are national and regional voluntary youth organisation staff.
(c) 1,100 are staff who are grant-aided and seconded to projects and voluntary associations.
(d) 1,000 are staff in the field of play and recreation.
(e) 1,000 are staff on short term special projects: Community Relations Councils, etc.
(f) 300 work as 'detached' youth workers.
(g) 200 work in Young Volunteer Organisations.

N.B. Staff in areas (d) to (g) inclusive are rarely staffed by workers having a two-year qualifying course of training.

3 Fabes (1985) has commented:

> Thus the response by adults to working with young people is to a great extent undertaken voluntarily and at best on a part-time paid basis. The training offered to part-time and volunteer workers has been studied by Newell and Butters (1978) in *Realities of Training*.

4 A major study of the careers of ex-students of community and youth work courses in England and Wales has been made by Holmes (1981) in *Professionalisation. A misleading myth?*

2.3 Expenditure on the Youth Service 1978–83

Smith (1985) summarized his findings:

> The report shows quite clearly that financial support to the local education authority youth services is varied and inconsistent. There appears to be no rational basis for the allocation of resources. Adjacent local authorities, having similar populations of young people in comparable circumstances, fund the youth service at very different levels. The highest spending authority spends 17 times as much per young person as the lowest spending authority.
>
> In many ways the expenditure data cast doubt on whether it is really possible to refer to a national youth service properly funded and supported across the country.

3 Research studies concerning youth work and young people

3.1 Further findings from Young People in the 1980s

This survey included extensive information about the sample of young people interviewed:

(i) **Those aged fourteen to sixteen** Aspirations included:

Enjoyment of social interaction with the peer group and with the opposite sex.
Having access to stimulating and exciting activities.
Being accorded significance and being listened to.

Problems included:

Uncertainty about self-image.
Lack of financial independence.
Lack of perceived significance in relation to adults and peers.
Anxiety about coping with challenges of development, including sex, alcohol and fighting.

(ii) **Those aged seventeen to nineteen** Satisfactions included:

Greater independence from parental constraints.
Increasing confidence and a stronger sense of identity.
Greater financial independence (if employed).

Problems included:

Lack of financial independence if unemployed.
Lack of status.
Racial conflict (for ethnic minorities).
Potential involvement with police (males only).

3.2 A study of participation in youth clubs by young women

Smith (1984) conducted a national survey on this issue, which revealed,

Of those in official membership of mixed clubs:

33% noted an equal distribution of young women and men,
63% noted a higher proportion of male club members,
4% noted a higher proportion of female club members.

On club activities nights:

4% said they had equal numbers of young women and men attending,
79% said they had a higher proportion of young men attending,
7% said they had a higher proportion of young women attending.

On club disco nights:

23% equal numbers attending,
58% higher proportion of young men,
18% higher proportion of young women.

3.3 Involvement of ethnic minority young people in the youth service

Cheetham and colleagues (1980) drawing upon publications such as *Youth in Multi-Racial Society* (1980), reported:

> The studies of the former C.R.C. ten years after the Hunt Report found that only about 33% of black adolescents had used youth clubs in the past and only about 11% were still attending some kind of club. Asians were less likely to have used a club than West Indians or Cypriots, irrespective of whether they were born in Britain or abroad.

3.4 An example from the voluntary sector

Fabes (1985) has noted:

> The shortage of research concerning the voluntary sector of the youth service needs to be noted in any overview, for the analysis offered by Springhall, Fraser and Hoare (1983) in their history of the Boys' Brigade, suggests that the reasons quoted for joining that uniformed organisation were explicitly because it met some of the aspirations noted in *Young People in the 80s*.
>
> *Social Trends* 1987 gives an analysis of the members of organisations for young people which suggests that over the period 1971–1985 there were significant increases in the Army Cadet Force (39–44,000), in the National Association of Youth Clubs affiliated clubs (319–567,000) and in the YMCA (48–80,000, males and females). It does not offer a comparable analysis for the statutory sector. It should also be noted that the falling birth rate after 1964 has led to a decline in club membership since 1981.

4 The shortage of research upon youth work and young people

4.1 The shortage and limitations of existing research

Baldock (1982), in a survey of the research literature in this field, noted the skewed nature of such research as exists and highlighted:

1 **The 'youth as a problem' focus of much research** He suggested that such a focus reinforces public preoccupation with unruly and troublesome young people.

2 **The neglect of the wider scene and the family** He quoted McRobbie's (1980) critique of this research literature and reported her comment:

> If we look at the structured absences in this youth literature it is the sphere of the family and domestic life that is missing. . . . Only what happened out there on the streets mattered. . . . I don't know of a study that considers, never mind prioritises, youth and the family.

4.2 The present and future of research

Fabes (1985) has commented:

> What little research has been completed has mainly focused upon white, male, working class young people in the major connurbations in Britain. The findings seem far too general to influence decisions about youth work in this country. Arguments being used to influence policy decisions seem to be based mainly on deficit, deprivation and pathology models, and proposals for resource allocation seem to be dominated by a range of political considerations which bear little or no relation to any empirical base. (See Smith, 1984; Davies, 1979, 1981)

He added:

> The consultation, in November, 1985, which reviewed the responses to the N.Y.B. survey on *Research Priorities in Youth Work* (1984) suggested the following areas to the National Advisory Committee on Youth Work: responses to, and action with, young people (i.e. action research); policy change affecting the youth service; and staff development, training and re-training. In the light of this the research scene may look very different in a few years' time.

References

Baldock (1982), 'Research literature on youth and youthwork', *Youth and Policy*, vol. 1, pp. 1–5.

Bone, M. and Ross, E. (1972), *The Youth Service and Similar Provision for Young People*, London: HMSO.

Booton, F. (1984), 'Data', *Youth and Policy*, vol. 10, pp. 25–6.

British Information Services (1974), *The Youth Service in Britain*, London: Central Office of Information.

Commission for Racial Equality (1980), *Youth in Multi-Racial Society: The Urgent Need for New Policies*, London: CRE.

Central Advisory Council on Education (1960), *15 to 18*, (The Crowther Report), London: HMSO.

Cheetham, J., James, W., Loney, M., Major, B. and Prescott, W. (1980), *Social and Community Work in a Multi-Racial Society*, London: Harper & Row.

Davies, B. (1979), *From Social Education to Life and Social Skills – In Whose Interests?*, Leicester: National Youth Bureau.

Davies, B. (1981), *Restructuring Youth Policies in Britain – The State We're In*, Leicester: National Youth Bureau.

Department of Education and Science (1982), *Experience and Participation.* (The Thompson Report), London: HMSO.
Department of Education and Science (1982), *Young People in the 80s*, London: HMSO.
Editorial analysis, *Youth and Policy*, (1984), vol. 10, pp. 25–6.
Eggleston, J. (1976), *Adolescence and Community*, London: Edward Arnold.
Fabes, R. (1985), Personal communication.
Fabes, R. and Ritchie, N. (1984), 'A snapshot of "Youth Workers" in England and Wales', Unpublished (Leicester: National Youth Bureau).
Holmes, J. (1981), *Professionalisation – a misleading myth?* Leicester Polytechnic and Youth Work Unit: National Youth Bureau.
McRobbie, A. (1980), 'Settling accounts with subcultures: a feminist critique', *Screen Education*, no. 34, p. 41.
Ministry of Education (1960), *The Youth Service in England and Wales*, (Albemarle Report), London: HMSO.
National Youth Bureau (1981), *Young People, the Youth Service, and Youth Provision*, Leicester: National Youth Bureau.
National Youth Bureau (1984), *Research Priorities in Youth Work. A Discussion Document*, Leicester: National Youth Bureau.
Newell, S. and Butters, S. (1978), *Realities of Training*, Leicester: National Youth Bureau.
Smith, D. I. (1985), *Expenditure on the Youth Service 1979–1983. A Consultative Document*, Leicester: National Youth Bureau.
Smith, D. I. (1985), Personal communication.
Smith, D. R. (1984), *GREA Today: Gone Tomorrow?* Leicester: National Council of Voluntary Youth Services.
Smith, N. (1984), *Youth Service Provision for Girls and Young Women*, Leicester: National Association of Youth Clubs.
Springhall, J., Fraser, B. and Hoare, M. (1983), *Sure and Steadfast – a History of the Boys' Brigade 1883–1983*, London: Collins.
Warwickshire County Council (1985), *The Way Ahead.* County Education Department, Warwickshire County Council.
Yeung, K. (1985), *Working with Girls*, Leicester: National Youth Bureau.
Youth Service Development Council (1968), *Immigrants and the Youth Service*, (The Hunt Report), London: HMSO.
Youth Service Development Council (1969), *Youth and Community Work in the 70s*, (The Milson-Fairbairn Report), London: HMSO.

PART 4

Research concerning women's issues

17 Research concerning women's experience of violence, including rape

N.B. There is clear overlap between these research fields. For clarity, definitions and information on prevalence are given on the fields together, while other research is reported separately.

1 Definitions of terms

1.1 Legal definitions

The law considers 'violence' in terms of 'assault' and 'battery'; definitions are offered by Smith and Hogan (1983):

> *Assault*: An assault is any act by which one person intentionally or recklessly, causes another person to apprehend immediate and unlawful personal violence.
>
> *Battery*: A battery is any act by which one person, intentionally or recklessly inflicts personal violence upon another person.

1.2 A general definition

Gayford (1975) has written of battered women:

> A battered wife may be defined as any woman who has received deliberate, severe and repeated demonstrable physical injury from her marital partner. . . . The term 'marital partner' means either the spouse or the cohabitee.

1.3 A legal definition of rape

Cross and Jones (1984) have written:

> the definition of rape . . . is now provided by s 1 of the Sexual Offences (Amendment) Act 1976. . . . The section provides that a man commits the actus reus of rape if he has unlawful sexual intercourse with a woman who at the time of the intercourse does not consent to it . . .
>
> Moreover, an apparent consent is not a real consent, and rape is committed in the following cases:
>
> (a) Where submission is procured by personal violence or threats of personal violence.
> (b) Where the consent is obtained by fraud as to the nature of the act.
> (c) Where consent is obtained by impersonating the woman's husband.

(d) Where the female is so mentally deficient or young or drunk that her knowledge and understanding are such that she is not in a position to decide whether to consent or not.

2 Prevalence of violence to women, including rape

2.1 Official statistics of violence to women – and men, for comparison

England & Wales Percentages and thousands

	Percentages		Estimated[1] numbers (thousands)	
	Males	Females	Males	Females
Age				
0–9	*3*	*4*	3.0	2.8
10–15	*14*	*13*	15.8	9.6
16–24	*37*	*32*	39.9	23.2
25–44	*27*	*26*	29.2	18.8
45–59	*15*	*15*	16.4	10.9
60 or over	*4*	*11*	4.8	8.1
All ages	*100*	*100*	109.1	73.4

1 Attempted murder, wounding endangering life, other wounding, assault, rape, buggery, indecent assault, robbery, and theft from the person, recorded by the police.

TABLE 17.1 Victims of selected notifiable offences: by sex and age, 1984 (*Social Trends*, 1987)

2.2 The Report from the Select Committee on Violence in Marriage

This contains a section on *The scale of the problem*,

> Little indeed is known about how much violence in marriage there is, and whether or not it is increasing. What is clear is that the number of battered wives is large. . . . Several estimates, all on small samples . . . and using different definitions, have been made . . . the Parliamentary Under-Secretary of State, Welsh Office . . . thought that there might be perhaps 5,000 battered wives in Wales each year, out of a figure of 680,000 married women. . . . Most witnesses agreed (and this is almost certainly correct) that all strata of society are involved . . .

2.3 Official statistics of rape and indecent assault on a female

	1981	1982	1983	1984	1985
Rape	326	412	330	359	450
Indecent assault on a female	3,258	3,391	3,235	3,147	3,315

TABLE 17.2 Offenders found guilty at all courts or cautioned for indictable sexual offences, by offence. England and Wales. (*Criminal Statistics*, 1985)

2.4 Inadequacy of the official statistics

There is a marked shortage of research in this field. All concerned seem to agree that the official figures seriously underestimate true prevalences.

3 Research concerning violence against women

3.1 A British study of battered wives

Gayford (1975) recorded the physical injuries of 100 women who attended a hospital casualty clinic:

1	Bruising	100 women
2	Bruising and laceration	44
3	Laceration, with razor, knife or bottle	17
4	Hit with a clenched fist	100
5	Repeated kicking	59
6	Strangulation	9
7	Burns and scalds	11
8	Fractures of nose, teeth or ribs	24
9	Found unconscious	9
10	Retinal damage	2

Gayford wrote:

> with 23 of the women and 51 of their husbands being exposed to models of family violence in their childhood, there is support for Steinmetz and Straus (1974), in claiming that violence passes on through the generations. . . . Fear must be expressed for the 315 children of the 100 women reported, as many males are developing the prodromal signs of violence . . .

3.2 Wife battering as part of family violence

McClintock (1978) reported that in a large-scale study of urban violence in England, which examined crime in districts broadly representative of a quarter of the total population, some 15 per cent of all indictable crimes against the person were committed within the family. Of salient features emerging from 1,527 cases of family violence recorded by the police in 1970, he wrote:

> Almost three-quarters of the victims were females (1128 or 74%), the remaining male victims numbering 399 (26%). Thus while the prevalence of the battered female, or more particularly the battered wife, is confirmed, it should not be overlooked that there is a substantial proportion of battered husbands in the group as well as fathers battered by sons. . . .

3.3 An American study of family violence

1 Gelles (1974) in a study of eighty families in which he interviewed sixty-six wives and fourteen husbands, investigated

(a) The severity and frequency of violence.
(b) Experience of and exposure to violence as children.
(c) Education and occupation of wife and details of children.
(d) External constraints on the action of the wife.

2 Gelles then examined variables affecting the wife's decision to stay with or leave a violent husband, and concluded:
(a) The less severe, and the less frequent the violence, the greater the probability of staying and not seeking help.
(b) The more the wife was hit by her parents as a child, the more inclined she was to stay.
(c) Wives who did not seek help were less likely to have completed high school, and more likely to be unemployed.

3 Gelles summarized:

> We conclude that the fewer resources a woman has, the less power she has, and the more entrapped she is in her marriage, the more she suffers at the hands of her husband without calling for help outside the family.

3.4 Some Scottish data

1 Dobash and Dobash (1978) conducted studies in selected areas of Scotland. Their findings included the following information upon 3,020 instances of violent behaviour reported to the police:

	% of cases
Men attacking men	38.7
Wife beating	26.2
Men beating women not their wives	9.8
2 Of 1.044 cases of violence within families	
Wife beaten	75.8
Child beaten	10.7
Husband beaten	1.1
3 Causes of wife beating in 106 typical cases	
Sexual jealousy	45.0
Money troubles	17.0
Rows over housework/husband's meals, etc.	16.0
Husband's drinking	6.0

TABLE 17.3 Summary of data concerning assault and wife-beating (Dobash and Dobash, 1978, *Sunday Times*, 9 March, 1980)

4 The increasing acceptance of a multi-variate model of violence against women

4.1 Rejection of single factor models

Increasingly, researchers are rejecting single factor models, in which wife (and child) abuse are seen as stemming from e.g. the pathology of abusers, from stress or from social class factors. Of this last Gelles (1979) has written:

> It is difficult to conceive of violent acts between family members as arising out of a single causal factor, such as a psychopathic or genetic condition, because of the various social and social psychological elements that are associated with occurrences and patterns of family violence.

4.2 Proposed multi-variate model

Gelles (1974) proposed an interactive model (See Figure 17.1) wherein a large number of variables, sociological, psychological and situational, interact to contribute to the probability of family violence. They include,

1 Norms which tolerate and mandate violence.
2 Structural sources of violence. Lower socio-economic groups bear the brunt of stress from unemployment and low income. While family violence is found among all classes of society, it may be a more frequent response among those bearing the greatest frustrations and stresses.
3 Sexual inequality: Of this, Gelles has written:

> Our research on family violence illustrates that violence between husband and wife is common when men cannot hold down the dominant position that they see society mandating for them.

4 Socio-psychological factors: Of these, Gelles wrote:

> Our research indicates that there are two main social–psychological forces which are associated with family violence. The first is the fact that the family serves as a training ground for violence. Research on murderers . . . child abusers . . . and wife abusers all confirm the hypothesis that the more violence he experiences in growing up, the more likely an individual is to use violence as an adult. In fact, the more violence a woman experiences as a child in her family of orientation, the more likely she is to be a *victim* of violence in her family of procreation. . . .
>
> A second factor which increases the extent of violence in the family is privacy.

5 Research concerning responses to violence to women

5.1 The shortage of research

1 *The Report from the Select Committee on Violence in Marriage* (1975) noted the serious lack of information and research in this field.

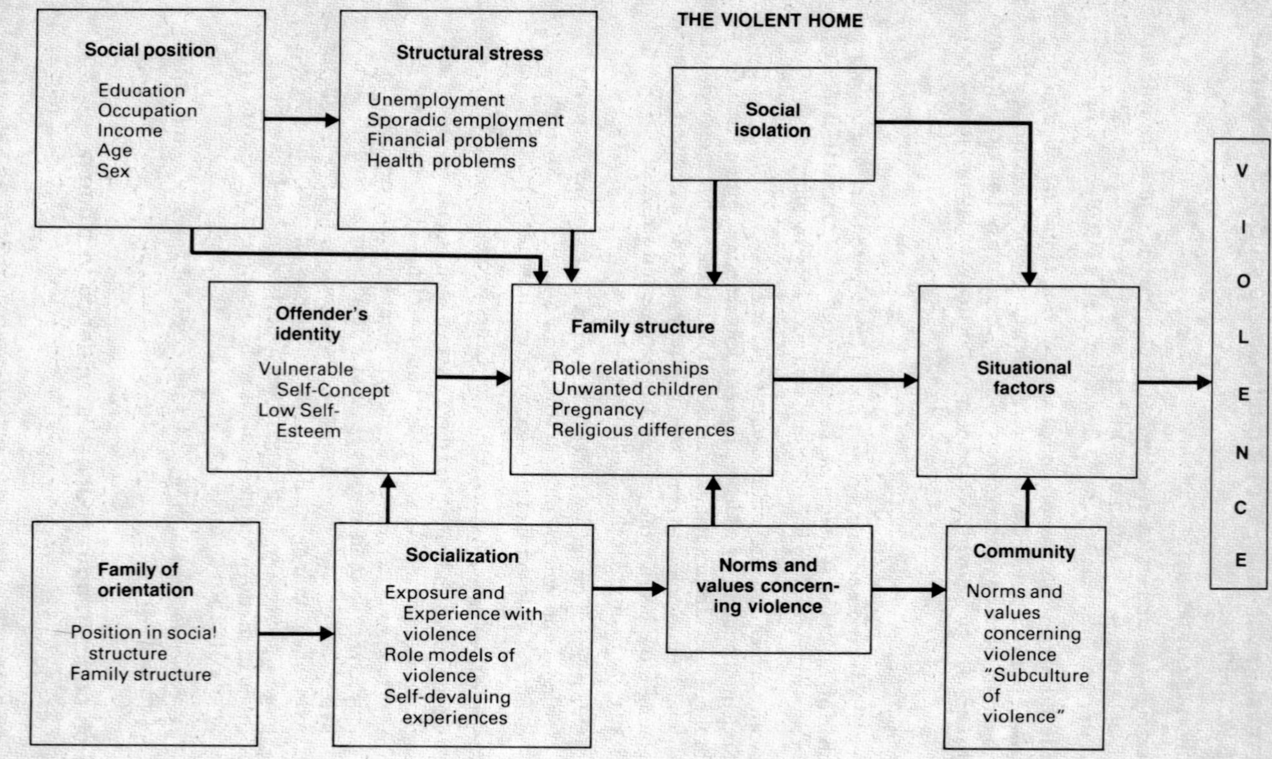

FIGURE 17.1 A model of intrafamily violence. From R. Gelles (1974). *The Violent Home*. Beverly Hills, CA: Sage Publications. Used by permission of the author.

2 There are very few studies upon intervention with those who practise violence, but see Howells (See Chapter 41, page 382).

5.2 Studies of provision for women subjected to violence

1 **A study of a Women's Centre** The study by Pahl (1978) of the Women's Centre in Canterbury showed that within one year, November 1975 to November 1976, no less than 130 women sought refuge there, with 200 children.

2 **A study by the Women's Aid Federation** This study, *Leaving Violent Men*, (1981) gathered data on refuges in England and Wales, and on their residents.

(a) Information about numbers The authors reported:

> 1 The 150 refuges traced in England and Wales had accommodated an estimated 11,400 women and 20,850 children between September 1977 and September 1978 and had turned away many more. The women using refuges ranged in age from 17 to 70, and at any one time there were approximately 900 women and 1700 children living in them.
>
> 2 The vast majority of women had left home to escape physical violence to themselves and sometimes also to their children (27%) . . .

(b) Information upon the duration of battering The authors wrote:

> As the violence had usually started when women were in their early 20s it was generally the case that the older a woman was, the longer she had suffered. . . . Other research has shown that the severity of the violence tends to increase over the course of the relationship . . .

6 Some research findings concerning rape and sexual assault

1 **An early American study** A study by Amir (1971) examined police files for the years 1958 to 1960 and gathered data relating to 646 victims of rape. His conclusions are paraphrased in the following:

1 70 per cent of rapes were planned.
11 per cent of rapes were partially planned.
16 per cent of rapes were an 'explosive event'.

2 277 of the 646 victims (43 per cent) were subjected to rape by more than one man.

3 Sexual humiliation, including fellatio and repeated rape, were features of 27 per cent of rapes: this was more common in white intraracial rapes than black.

4 43 per cent of rapists were total strangers to their victims.
10 per cent of rapists had a general knowledge of their victims.

47 per cent of rapists knew, were friendly with or related to their victims.

5 56 per cent of rapes occurred at the home of rapist or victim
15 per cent of rapes occurred in cars
18 per cent of rapes occurred outdoors
11 per cent of rapes occurred elsewhere

2 **A London inquiry of rape and sexual assault** A major investigation conducted by Women Against Rape and reported by Hall (1985) distributed 2,000 questionnaires in thirty-two London boroughs, mainly in inner London and obtained a cross section of 1,236 respondents. Table 17.4 shows some of the results obtained.

	Number of women	% of 1,236 respondents
Raped	214	17
Sexually assaulted	379	31
Raped or sexually assaulted	448	36
Raped or sexually assaulted once only	281	23
Raped or sexually assaulted more than once	167	14
Attempted rape	243	20
Raped or sexually assaulted by a gang or pair of men	11	1
Raped in marriage or common law marriage	110	9
Raped or sexually assaulted because of race or nationality	17	1
Raped or sexually assaulted in own home	128	10
Raped or sexually assaulted before age 16	200	16

TABLE 17.4 Rape and sexual assault experienced by respondents to the Women's Safety Survey (Hall, 1985)

7 Research concerning responses to rape offences

7.1 A study concerning imprisonment and conviction

Toner (1977) studied the responses to the offence of rape in selected periods in the UK and commented:

> Only a very small percentage of men who commit rape get punished for it by imprisonment. Half the men who are tried for rape do not eventually go to prison for the crime. It is hard to believe that half the men who have been tried have been wrongly prosecuted.

7.2 Studies concerning the re-conviction rate of rapists

1 Toner (1977) further reported:

> Of men convicted in 1951, 49% were subsequently reconvicted, 27 per cent for crimes of violence or sexual offences. Of men convicted of rape in 1961, 50 per cent were reconvicted, 30% for crimes of violence or sexual offences.

2 Soothill, Jack and Gibbens (1976) conducted a twenty-two-year follow-up of men convicted of rape in 1951, and found that 15 per cent were convicted of further sexual offences.

3 These researchers suggest three broad divisions among these rapists:
- (a) Those in whom rape is part of a general aggressive personality, whose behaviour is likely to be intensified by heavy drinking.
- (b) Those who were convicted of paedophiliac offences, and who may subsequently commit lesser such offences.
- (c) Those for whom 'rape stands out in relative isolation' – the act of an inhibited and frustrated man who acted impulsively.

References

Amir, M. (1971), *Patterns in Forcible Rape*, University of Chicago Press.

Cross, R., Jones, P. (1984), *Introduction to Criminal Law*, 10th edition by J. Card, London: Butterworth.

Curzon, L. B. (1979), *A Dictionary of Law*, London: Macdonald and Evans.

Dobash, R. E. and Dobash, R. (1978), *Violence Against Wives*, London: Open Books, and New York: Free Press, Macmillan Publishing Co., Inc.

Gayford, J. J. (1975), 'Wife battering: a preliminary survey of 100 cases', *British Medical Journal*, 25 January 1975, pp. 194–7.

Gelles, R. J. (1974), *The Violent Home*, Beverly Hills: Sage Publications.

Gelles, R. J. (1976), 'Abused wives: why do they stay?', *Journal of Marriage and the Family*, vol. 38, pp. 659–68.

Gelles, R. J. (1979), *Family Violence*, Beverly Hills: Sage Publications.

Hall, R. (1985), *Ask Any Woman*, Bristol: Falling Wall Press.

Home Office (1984), *Criminal Statistics* 1984, London: HMSO.

McClintock, F. H. (1978), 'Criminological aspects of family violence' in J. P. Martin (ed.), *Violence and the Family*, Chichester: Wiley.

Martin, J. P. (1978), *Violence and the Family*, Chichester: Wiley.

Pahl, J. (1978), *A Refuge for Battered Women*, London: HMSO.

Select Committee on Violence in Marriage (1975), London: HMSO.

Smith, J. C. and Hogan, B. (1983), *Criminal Law*, London: Butterworth.

Soothill, K., Jack, A. and Gibbens, T. C. (1976), 'Rape: a twenty two year cohort study', *Medicine, Science and the Law*, vol. 16, pp. 62–9.

Steinmetz, S. K. and Straus, M. (1974), *Violence in the Family*, New York: Harper & Row. (Originally published by Dodd, Mead & Co.)

Toner, B. (1977), *The Facts of Rape*, London: Hutchinson.

Women's Aid Federation (1981), *Leaving Violent Men*, London: WAF.

PART 5

Research concerning the family and family life

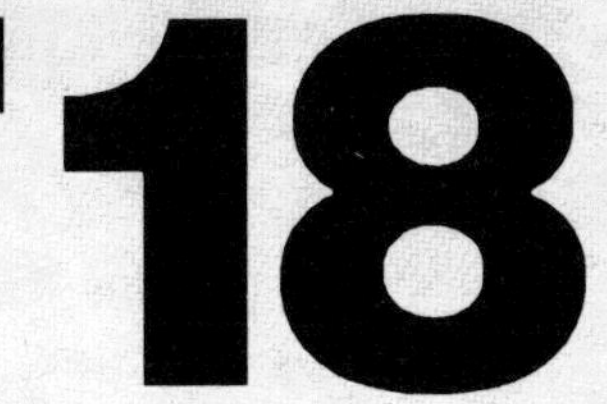

Research concerning aspects of family life, marriage and divorce

Consultant: Dr Jack Dominian, Consultant Psychiatrist, Central Middlesex Hospital, London.

1 A possible definition of a family

(A) set of parents and children, or of relations, living together or not. (*Concise Oxford Dictionary*)

2 Some relevant statistics

Below are some tables illustrating aspects of family life, marriage and divorce.

2.1 Households in Great Britain: by type. Selected years.

	Percentages		
	1961	1971	1981
No family			
One person			
Under retirement age	4	6	8
Over retirement	7	12	14
Two or more people			
One or more over retirement age	3	2	2
All under retirement age	2	2	3
One family			
Married couple only	26	27	26
Married couple with dependent children	38	35	31
Married couple with independent children only	10	8	8
Lone parent with at least one dependent child	2	3	5
Lone parent with independent child(ren) only	4	4	4
Two or more families	3	1	1
Total households (thousands)	16,189	18,317	19,493

TABLE 18.1 Households by type in Great Britain. (*Social Trends*, 1985. OPCS.)

2.2 Implications of Table 18.1

Commenting on the above table, the authors of *Happy Families?* (1980) a discussion paper on the family noted of the data up to that time:

1 Nearly a quarter of all households are 'no family' households.
2 Of these, the largest group is single elderly people living alone.
3 44% are married couples with dependent children – the 'typical family'.
4 Most British families are therefore not 'typical'.
5 There is great diversity in family patterns.

2.3 Marriage

1 Selected data

United Kingdom	1961	1971	1981
Marriages (thousands)			
First marriage for both partners	340	369	263
First marriage for one partner			
Bachelor/divorced woman	11	21	32
Bachelor/widow	5	4	3
Spinster/divorced man	12	24	36
Spinster/widower	8	5	3
Second or later marriage for both partners			
Both divorced	5	17	44
Both widowed	10	10	7
Divorced man/widow	3	4	5
Divorced woman/widower	3	5	5

TABLE 18.2 Marriage in Great Britain. (*Social Trends*, 1987, OPCS.)

2.4 Divorce

1 Selected data

	1961	1971	1981
England and Wales			
Petitions filed (thousands)			
By husband	14	44	47
By wife	18	67	123
Persons divorcing per thousand married people	2.1	6.0	11.9
Percentage of divorces where one or both partners had been divorced previously			
England and Wales	9.3	8.8	17.1

TABLE 18.3 Divorce in England and Wales. (*Social Trends*, 1985, OPCS.)

2 **Numbers of children of divorcing couples** The authors of *Social Trends* (1984) reported:

> Six out of every ten couples divorcing in 1981 had children under 16. Altogether there were 169 thousand children under 16 in families in Great Britain where the parents divorced in 1981. . . . Two thirds of these children were aged under 11, and a quarter were under 5.

3 Research concerning relationships within marriage

3.1 The changing expectations of marriage

Dominian (1968) pointed out the expectation in many communities that marriage nowadays shall be egalitarian, and wrote:

> It is a reciprocal relationship based on understanding, in which authority, power, and decision-making are shared. It reflects the pronounced changes in women's position achieved in this century and the tendency for modern marriage to seek solutions in its day to day survival on the basis of mutual interaction . . .

3.2 Studies concerning the happiness of marriage

1 Argyle (1985) has summarized several features of social interaction between husband and wife who claim to be happily married:
   (a) Pleasing verbal acts, e.g. compliments; few negative ones, especially criticism.
   (b) Pleasing non-verbal acts: a kiss, helpful behaviour.
   (c) Enjoyable sex life.
   (d) A lot of time spent together, e.g. in leisure activities.
   (e) Agreement over finances.
   (f) A problem solving approach to decisions and difficulties.

2 Argyle and Henderson (1985) have also summarized what their research suggests as important 'rules' for both spouses:
   1 Show emotional support
   2 Share news of success
   3 Be faithful
   4 Create a harmonious home atmosphere
   5 Respect the other partner's privacy
   6 Address the partner by first name
   7 Keep confidences
   8 Engage in sexual activity with the other partner
   9 Give birthday cards and presents
   10 Stand up for the other person in his/her absence
   11 Talk to the partner about sex and death
   12 Disclose personal feelings and problems to the partner
   13 Inform the partner about one's personal schedule
   14 Be tolerant of each other's friends

15 Don't criticise the partner publicly
16 Ask for personal advice
17 Talk to the partner about religion and politics
18 Look the partner in the eye during conversation
19 Discuss personal financial matters with the partner
20 Touch the other person intentionally
21 Engage in joking or teasing with the partner
22 Show affection for one another in public
23 Ask the partner for material help
24 Show distress or anxiety in front of the partner
25 Repay debts and favours, and compliments.

Additional rules for the husband
1 Look after the family when the wife is unwell
2 Show an interest in the wife's daily activities
3 Be responsible for household repair and maintenance
4 Offer to pay for the partner when going out together

Additional rules for the wife
1 Show anger in front of the partner
2 Don't nag

4 Research concerning marital breakdown

4.1 Antecedents of marital breakdown

Newcomb and Bentler (1981) reported that from American studies, several variables seem important:

1 Demographic variables: age at marriage and parental divorce

(a) *Age at marriage* Newcomb and Bentler confirmed British data that marrying at a young age is associated with marriage breakdown.

(b) *Separation or divorce of parents* The evidence here is mixed. Some studies, e.g. Mott and Moore (1979) found an increased probability of divorce among the second generation, but others, e.g. Thorne and Collard (1979) in Britain, found no increased probability.

2 Personality Newcomb and Bentler (1981) summarized findings in this area and suggested that high levels of competition, individualism and ambition in a person were all associated with high levels of marital unhappiness and instability: e.g. Bentler and Newcomb (1978). These features may lower the priority and commitment an individual gives to a marriage.

3 Premarital sexual experience There is some evidence that premarital sexual behaviour has a detrimental influence on a subsequent marriage; e.g. Shope and Broderick (1967). Newcomb and Bentler (1983) suggested that one possible explanation is that the amount and likelihood of pre-marital sexual experience may predict the occurrence of extra-marital sexual behaviour – known to be a factor in marital disruption.

4 Relationship factors contributing to marriage happiness

(a) Equal matching between marriage partners, e.g. in terms of age, race and/or religion and expectations of marriage.
(b) Ways of dealing with disagreement and conflict. Readiness to disclose feelings seems positively linked to successful marriage.
(c) Egalitarian marital roles for partners.

5 Other variables

(a) Short acquaintance or courtship period. e.g. Thorne and Collard (1979) found this linked with low marriage happiness.
(b) Premarital cohabitation. Newcomb and Bentler (1978) found no differences between marriages preceded or not preceded by cohabitation in terms of divorce rates or happiness.
(c) Communal marriage. Jaffe and Kanter (1979) found this a severe stress, contributing to marital breakdown.

4.2 Processes of divorce and separation

1 Precipitating events: British findings In a major study of the multiple variables associated with divorce, Thorne and Collard (1979) pinpointed:

(a) The higher-than-average divorce rate of socio-economic class 5 seemed to be linked with acute environmental disadvantage, particularly disadvantaged housing.
(b) A lower-than-average divorce rate where both partners were associated with a particular religion, and especially where both were church-goers.
(c) Short courtships, especially where the marriage was opposed by parents, were associated with divorce.
(d) Teenage marriage and pre-marital pregnancy, especially in association with socio-economic class 5, were high risk factors for divorce.
(e) Early parenthood, especially when arising from pre-marital pregnancy, was linked with major marital difficulties in the first year of marriage.

N.B. Marital difficulties which subsequently ended in divorce, frequently began in the first year of marriage. A protective factor, in all the above, was parental support for the young couple.

2 Precipitating events: American findings Newcomb and Bentler (1981) reported that researchers had found problems such as adultery, alcohol abuse and financial difficulties were stated by divorced people as major causes of their marital disruption.

3 **Components of divorce or separation** Bohannon (1970) suggested that these are:

(a) The emotional divorce, often accompanied by the well-documented stages of grief, and personal trauma.
(b) The legal divorce.
(c) The parental divorce, and planning the children's future.
(d) The economic divorce, concerning finances and property.
(e) The community divorce, affecting social networks.
(f) The psychic divorce, involving establishing oneself as an individual.

5 Research concerning conciliation and/or reconciliation

5.1 Studies concerning family and marital therapy

For research in this field, see Chapter 38 page 361.

5.2 Studies focusing primarily upon conciliation

Popay, Rimmer and Rossiter (1983) reported:

> Conciliation, as opposed to reconciliation, focuses on assisting parties to reach *agreed* decisions on specific issues arising from the *established* breakdown of their relationship. . . .
>
> Research does suggest that conciliation services can successfully reduce conflict. In a study of a year's cases of one service, full agreement was reached on all disputed matters – the divorce itself, children, money and property – in 81% of cases. . . . One in six of the cases in fact resulted in reconciliation. (Davis, 1982)

6 Research concerning adjustment and relationships after divorce or separation

6.1 Stepfamilies: data from the National Child Development Study

1 Ferri (1984) reported an extensive longitudinal study of children growing up in 'reconstituted' or stepfamilies, by comparison with those growing up with both natural parents, or a natural mother or father alone. The data were gathered when the young people concerned were aged sixteen:

Children living with a natural mother and stepfather:	455
Children living with a natural father and stepmother:	136
Children living with both natural parents:	9,767
Children living with natural mother alone:	830
Children living with natural father alone:	152

2 In her summary Ferri (1984) concluded,

> the development of children with stepmothers did not differ very

> markedly from that of their peers in unbroken families or of those living with lone fathers. . . . The findings relating to children with *stepfathers*, however, were rather less reassuring. These children, and particularly the boys, frequently compared unfavourably with those in unbroken families. . . . This suggests that the arrival of a stepfather may not be a solution to all of the difficulties of fatherless families. . . .

6.2 Studies recognizing the strength of the extended family

Burgoyne and Clark (1982), in their study of forty Sheffield families, highlighted the fact that there are still many communities where the nuclear family is far from being the norm, and where children can potentially enjoy greater security in a variety of extended and 'reconstituted' or blended families.

6.3 Studies concerning the effects of divorce upon children: a longitudinal American study

Wallerstein and Kelly (1980), in *Surviving the Breakup*, described a longitudinal, but uncontrolled, study with sixty families who sought counselling and who had 136 children aged from one to twenty-two years between them. Information was gathered at the time of divorce and at five-year follow-up. From the wealth of data, the following is selected:

(a) **Immediate circumstances and distress**

(i) 36 per cent of the children faced the divorce constructively and coped successfully. The authors reported that these youngsters confirmed their view that unsatisfactory marriages can still provide a setting for successful parenting and loving relationships between parent and child.

(ii) 48 per cent came to the divorce as 'adequate or average children' who coped as best they could.

(iii) 13 per cent entered the divorce period already coping with clear psychological problems.

(b) **Responses at different ages** The authors reported that children under eight characteristically responded with grief, bewilderment, sadness, fear and behaviour typical of younger children. Older children often displayed a 'fully conscious, intense anger', as well as by active attempts to master and cope with the situation.

(c) **Responses and circumstances at five-year follow-up** The authors reported that even after five years 29 per cent of the children were 'party to intense bitterness between parents; an even larger group continued to be aware of limited friction or anger.'

Wallerstein and Kelly wrote of their general findings that those components which seemed particularly important in affecting outcome included:

(1) the extent to which the parents had been able to resolve and put aside their conflicts and angers;
(2) the course of the custodial parent's handling of the child and the resumption or improvement of parenting within the home;
(3) the extent to which the child did not feel rejected in relationship to the non-custodial or visiting parent;
(4) the range of personality assets or deficits which the child brought to the divorce;
(5) the availability to the child of a supportive human network;
(6) the absence of continuing anger and depression in the child; and
(7) the sex and age of the child.

The authors added that it was not uncommon for two children in the same family to respond in different ways: for one child to improve and the other to deteriorate.

6.5 Broken homes and anti-social behaviour

1 **The distinction between family breakup and family discord** Rutter (1975) reported the findings, from several separate studies, that the risk of anti-social behaviour was much increased if parents divorced or separated, but that the risk is only slightly raised if the parent died. He wrote:

> this suggests that it may be family discord and disharmony rather than the break-up of the family as such, which leads to anti-social behaviour. . . . In fact it appears that delinquency may actually be commoner in unhappy, unbroken homes than it is in harmonious but broken ones. In short it may be concluded that it is the ongoing disturbance in family relationships which does the damage rather than the family break-up.

2 **Types of family discord which may lead to problems** Rutter (1975) pinpointed:

(a) Children may be harmed by open hostility or lack of affection, but particularly by the former.
(b) The effect is worse if the child is involved in disputes.
(c) The effect is worse if the disputes go on over years.
(d) The ill effects are not irreversible; improvement in relationships can be very restorative.
(e) The child is particularly at risk if one or both parents has a severe personality disorder.
(f) A good relationship with one parent can be compensatory.

References

Argyle, M. and Henderson, M. (1985), *The Anatomy of Relationships*, London: Heinemann.

Bentler, P. M. and Newcomb, M. D. (1978), 'Longitudinal study of marital success and failure', *Journal of Consulting and Clinical Psychology*, vol. 46, pp. 1053–70.

Bohannon, P. (1970), *Divorce and After*, Garden City, New York: Doubleday and Co.

Bumpass, L. and Sweet, J. (1972), 'Differentials in marital stability', *American Sociological Review*, vol. 9, pp. 225–54.

Burgoyne, J. and Clark, D. (1982), 'Reconstituted families' in R. N. Rapoport, M. P. Fogarty and R. Rapoport (eds), *Families in Britain*, London: Routledge & Kegan Paul.

Carter, H. and Glick, P. C. (1976), *Marriage and Divorce: A Social and Economic Study*, Cambridge, Mass.: Harvard University Press.

Central Statistical Office (1984), *Social Trends 14*, London: OPCS.

Concise Oxford Dictionary (1977), London: Book Club Associates and Oxford University Press.

Davis, G. (1982), 'Conciliation or litigation?', *Legal Aid Group Bulletin*, April 1982, pp. 11–13.

Dominian, J. (1968), *Marital Breakdown*, Harmondsworth: Penguin.

Dominian, J. (1982), 'Families in divorce' in R. N. Rapoport, M. P. Fogarty and R. Rapoport (eds), *Families in Britain*.

Duck, S. and Gilmour, R. (1981), *Personal Relationships. 3: Personal Relationships in Disorder*, London: Academic Press.

Ferri, E. (1984), *Step Children*, Windsor: N.F.E.R.-Nelson Publishing Company.

Goode, W. J. (1956), *After Divorce*, New York: Free Press.

Jaffe, D. T. and Kanter, R. M. (1 979), 'Couple strains in communal households: A four factor model of the separation process' in G. Levinger and O. C. Moles (eds), *Divorce and Separation*, New York: Basic Books, Inc.

Levinger, G. and Senn, D. J. (1967), 'Disclosure of feelings in marriage', *Merrill-Palmer Quarterly*, vol. 13, pp. 237–49.

Mott, F. L. and Moore, S. F. (1979), 'The causes of marital disruption among young American women: An inter-disciplinary perspective', *Journal of Marriage and the Family*, vol. 42, pp. 335–65.

Newcomb, M. D. and Bentler, P. M. (1981), 'Marital breakdown' in S. Duck and R. Gilmour (eds), *Personal Relationships 3: Personal Relationships in Disorder*.

Popay, J., Rimmer, L. and Rossiter, C. (1983), *One Parent Families. Parents, Children and Public Policy*, London: Study Commission on the Family.

Rutter, M. (1975), *Helping Troubled Children*, Harmondsworth: Penguin.

Shope, D. F. and Broderick, C. B. (1967), 'Level of sexual experience and predicted adjustment in marriage', *Journal of Marriage and the Family*, vol. 29, pp. 424–7.

Study Commission on the Family (1980), *Who divorces?*, London: Routledge & Kegan Paul.

Wallerstein, J. S. and Kelly, J. B. (1980), *Surviving the Breakup*, London: Grant McIntyre.

19 Research concerning one-parent families

Consultant: Dr Carol Smart, Lecturer in Sociology, University of Warwick.

1 Definition

A one-parent family is a group of one or more children dependent upon a lone parent, mother or father.

2.1 Official statistics: composition of one-parent families

See Table 19.1 on page 173.

2.2 Broad statistics

1 According to the 1981 Census figures, there are just under one million one-parent families.
2 One in seven families with children is a one-parent family. Between 1971 and 1981 the number of lone parents has increased by 68 per cent and the number of children in one-parent families by 53 per cent from 1 million to 1.53 million.

2.3 Additional statistics: type of one-parent family

In 1983, 89.3 per cent of one-parent families were headed by women, and 10.7 by men. Their circumstances were as follows:

	Lone mothers	Lone fathers
Unmarried	19.1%	)
Divorced	39.8%	) 10.7%
Separated	18.3%	)
Widowed	12%	)

TABLE 19.2 Circumstances of lone mothers and lone fathers (*General Household Survey*, 1984)

Great Britain — Percentages and numbers

	Marital status of lone mothers													
	Single		Widowed		Divorced		Separated		All lone mothers		All lone fathers		All one parent families	
	1973 –75	1980 –82	1973 –75	1980 –82	1973 –75	1980 –82	1973 –75	1980 –82	1973 –75	1980 –82	1973 –75	1980 –82	1973 –75	1980 –82
Household composition														
Living alone	36	54	88	90	74	83	78	80	72	77	70	85	72	78
Living with parents	49	33	7	2	15	5	13	9	18	11	11	6	17	11
Living with relatives	7	5	4	6	4	3	3	4	4	4	8	3	5	4
Living with non-relatives														
Male	7	6	2	2	7	8	5	6	5	6	1	0	5	5
Female	1	2	0	–	–	2	1	1	–	1	10	6	2	2
Sample size (= 100%) (numbers)	182	285	256	211	350	553	302	290	1,090	1,339	183	174	1,273	1,513

TABLE 19.1 One-parent families: by household composition (*Social Trends 15*, (1985)

2.4 Additional statistics: family size

The figures for family size in 1980–1 were as follows:

	Lone mothers	Lone fathers
1 child	57%	55%
2 children	32%	33%
3 or more children	12%	12%

TABLE 19.3 Family size in one-parent families (*Information sheet no. 5, National Council for One-Parent Families* November, 1983)

3 Research concerning the circumstances of one-parent families

3.1 Income and spending

1 In 1983, the average disposable income of a one-parent family was £92.48 per week, compared with £187.65 for a comparable two-parent family. One-parent families thus had about half the financial resources of two-parent families although many of their costs were as high.

2 In 1983, there were 475,000 lone parents with 794,000 children aged under sixteen receiving Supplementary Benefit.

Unmarried mothers dependent on Supplementary Benefit:	80.8%
Separated wives dependent on Supplementary Benefit:	82.0%
Divorced mothers dependent on Supplementary Benefit:	42.5%
Widows dependent on Supplementary Benefit:	5.8%

N.B. Figures are approximations.

3.2 Supplementary benefit: one-and two-parent families

Table 19.4 shows the comparative figures in July, 1985

Income relative to supplementary benefit level	One Parent Families		Two Parent Families	
	Families	Children in Families	Families	Children in Families
(i) below level	60,000	110,000	200,000	450,000
(ii) at level	370,000	620,000	250,000	540,000
(iii) above but within 110 per cent	<10,000	<10,000	130,000	290,000

TABLE 19.4 Comparative incomes relative to Supplementary Benefit levels of one-parent and two-parent families. (*Hansard*, 26 July, 1985)

3.3 Employment

In 1981, 25 per cent of lone mothers worked full-time and 22 per cent worked part-time.

3.4 Housing

1 In 1981, 126,000 one-parent families shared their accommodation with other people. 86.8 per cent had a home of their own.
2 Figures for council/own home are as follows:

	Council homes	Own homes
Lone mothers	56%	33%
Lone fathers	40%	47%
Two-parent families	24%	68%

TABLE 19.5 Housing: one- and two-parent families (*One parent families 1984. Annual Report and Accounts 1983–1984*)

3.5 Interaction of these variables and social disadvantage

1 There have been a number of studies stemming from the data gathered in the National Child Development Study, which has followed the progress of over 11,000 children born in one week in March, 1958. Ferri (1976) has reported much of this data in a well-known book, *Growing Up in a One Parent Family*, which drew attention to some of the circumstances reported in section 3, above.
2 Using data from the same study, Wedge and Prosser (1973) selected three variables as fundamental when describing 'social disadvantage':
   1 Family composition: one parent or large family.
   2 Low income.
   3 Poor housing.

   In their book, *Born to Fail?*, Wedge and Prosser described as 'socially disadvantaged' those children who experienced all three of these conditions.
3 Smart (1985) has noted, however, that it is likely that these three variables are actually linked, rather than independent of each other. She commented,

> a one-parent family or large family is socially disadvantaged because it is poor (i.e. on an income insufficient to meet its needs). The problem with separating them out as if they were independent variables is that it appears that there is something 'essentially' amiss with one-parent families just as there is with low income or poor housing. . . . Whilst it is true that many children in one-parent families are socially disadvantaged this is because lone parenthood is linked so often to poverty.

4 The interactions of these variables are illustrated in Figure 19.1. Wedge and Prosser (1973) reported:

> One child in 16 was the proportion of disadvantaged among all children in Britain, but in individual regions the prevalence varied. In Southern England there was only one in 47 children. In Wales and in Northern England, on the other hand, there was one in every 12.
>
> But the most disturbing proportion was found in Scotland, where one in every 10 children was disadvantaged.
>
> 11% of the eleven-year-old British children lived in Scotland, but 19% of disadvantaged children were found there.

5 In the light of the increasing number of one-parent families and of increasing hardship, these figures are now likely to be even more serious.

4 Research concerning other aspects of the circumstances of one-parent families

Popay, Rimmer and Rossiter (1983), considering the particular circumstances of one-parent families, examined some aspects of their circumstances.

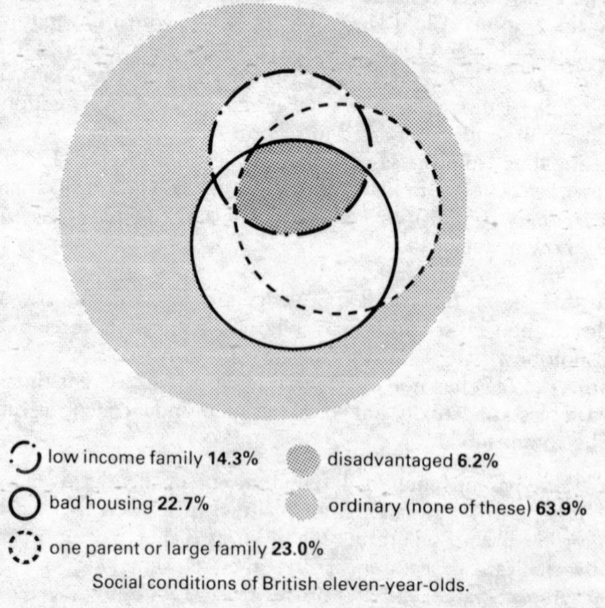

FIGURE 19.1 Social conditions of British eleven-year-olds (Wedge and Prosser, 1973)

4.1 Perceptions of one-parent families

1 These authors quoted the *Report of the Committee on One Parent Families* (the Finer Report, 1974), which although several years old now, still notes some relevant issues:

> To fail in marriage nowadays is to go bankrupt in a business of life in which everyone engages and in which the large majority at least appear to be successful. So it is likely that a family in which a mother or father has to bring up children single-handed will think of itself and be treated by others, as a little cluster of deviants from the marital norm.

They commented,

> one parent families are not a homogeneous group and to varying extents public attitudes still reflect a hierarchy of acceptability or legitimacy, according to the 'cause' of lone parenthood, which goes back many years.
>
> The Finer Committee noted that this hierarchy – with sympathy and pity for widows and widowers turning into varying degrees of moral disapprobation for the separated and divorced parent and unmarried mother – was 'becoming irrelevant in the face of the imperative recognition that what chiefly matters in such situations is to assist and protect dependent children, all of whom ought to be treated alike, irrespective of their mother's circumstances'.

2 Popay, Rimmer and Rossiter (1983) suggested several factors contribute towards biased perceptions of one parent families:

(a) **Media images** They suggested that some groups have received disproportionate media coverage, so distorting public perceptions – in particular,

(i) The plight of the lone *father* – as distinct from that of the mother.
(ii) Welfare 'scroungers'.

(b) **Social surveys** They reported a number of surveys, e.g. that conducted by MORI (1982), indicating considerable and continuing ambivalence upon whether the mothers of young children should work.

(c) **Professional attitudes** Popay, Rimmer and Rossiter suggested that the implication of some literature written for professional groups, including doctors and, in America, teachers, is that the one-parent family is 'deviant', and they wrote,

> In the professional literature, such families are often referred to as 'broken homes', or atypical, disintegrated, incomplete or disorganized families . . . this 'pathological' imagery may colour the response of many professionals.

(d) **How one-parent families see themselves** These authors reported, 'Research on the experience of lone parenthood in the early 1970s described situations of social rejection, acute loneliness, uncertainty and material deprivation.' They went on to report several studies, e.g. Hart (1976), indicating the position of divorced and separated wives still to be a stigmatized one in society; they noted the wide range of attitudes towards unmarried motherhood within different cultural groups in Britain.

4.2 Experience in one-parent families

While questioning some of the indicators of well-being often used to assess development in 'ordinary' families, and noting that some studies, e.g. Thomas (1968), found few differences between children from one- and two-parent families. Popay, Rimmer and Rossiter (1983) examined a number of research studies of children's experience in one-parent families under a number of headings.

1 **The absence of a parent** They noted a number of conclusions of the Finer Committee, based upon evidence submitted to it: from the then Association of Educational Psychologists, 'the lack of a father appears to have detrimental effects on the social and psychological development of the child, but it is too early to say just what these effects are', and from the British Medical Association, 'it would seem that there are compensatory mechanisms which allow children to be as emotionally healthy in one parent families as in two parent families.'

They drew attention to the conclusion of Rutter (1972) that it was not the separation of itself which might be damaging to children in one-parent families, but the circumstances leading up to and accompanying the parting. Thus, marked conflict before the separation, followed by recriminations against an absent partner which might produce a conflict of loyalty in the children, could all be unhelpful to them and productive of insecurity and stress. They noted, however, that such stress could also stem from other factors such as parental violence, mental illness or drink-related problems.

2 **Further studies** Popay, Rimmer and Rossiter (1983) quoted the work of Murchison (1974), who drew upon data from the National Survey of Health and Development, a longitudinal study undertaken in 1946, 1958 and 1970. Findings included the following:

(a) Children in families in which one parent had died before the child was 6, but where the remaining parent had not remarried tended to do better than those where the parent had remarried or had cohabited.
(b) Children whose parent had remarried were associated with greater disadvantage than those who had not.
(c) The most disadvantaged children were those living with fathers alone, with foster parents or relatives or in institutions.
(d) A higher proportion of illegitimate children, particularly those living

> alone with one parent, were below average for their age in general knowledge and creativity.

There are also indications of rather poorer health among children from one- rather than two-parent families. (The Black Report, 1981)

3 **The impact of financial disadvantage** Popay, Rimmer and Rossiter (1983) noted the associations between a number of variables and financial disadvantage. For example, they quoted the findings of Murchison (1974), which found an association between delinquency and marital separation but,

> when matched for income and for parental criminality or for family size there was no clearly significant difference between delinquents and non-delinquents in the incidence of such separations.

These authors also emphasized the clear evidence, e.g. from the Black Report (1981), indicating that health is closely linked to socio-economic circumstances – which are themselves grounded upon income, property, conditions of work and education.

4 **These authors' conclusions** Popay, Rimmer and Rossiter summarized their overview of the research in this field by indicating the complexity of the field and the far-from-consistent findings which emerge. They concluded,

> The development process would appear to be adversely affected by unstable family backgrounds but once established a one parent family situation need not inevitably be unstable any more than two-parent families will inevitably provide security.

References

Central Statistical Office (1984), *Social Trends 14*, London: HMSO.

Ferri, E. (1976), *Growing Up in a One Parent Family*, Windsor: National Foundation for Educational Research.

Finer, R. M. (1974), *Report of the Committee on One Parent Families*, Cmnd 5629, London: HMSO.

Hart, N. (1976), *When Marriage Ends*, London: Tavistock.

Inequalities in Health (1981), (The Black Report), London: Department of Health and Social Security.

MORI (1982), 'A woman's place', *The Sunday Times*, poll conducted in association with MORI, 2 May 1982.

Murchison, N. (1974), 'Illustration of the difficulties of some children in one parent families' in R. M. Finer, *Report of the Committee on One Parent Families*.

National Council for One Parent Families (1984), *One Parent Families 1984: Annual Report and Accounts, 1983–1984*, London.

Popay, J., Rimmer, L. and Rossiter, C. (1983), *One Parent Families: Parents, Children and Public Policies*, London: Study Commission on the Family.

Rutter, M. (1972), *Maternal Deprivation Reassessed*, Harmondsworth: Penguin.

Smart, C. (1985), Personal communication.

Thomas, M. M. (1968), 'Children with absent fathers', *Journal of Marriage and the Family*, vol. 30, p. 89.

Wedge, P. and Prosser, H. (1973), *Born to Fail?*, London: Arrow Books, in association with the National Children's Bureau.

PART 6

Research concerning young people in difficulties

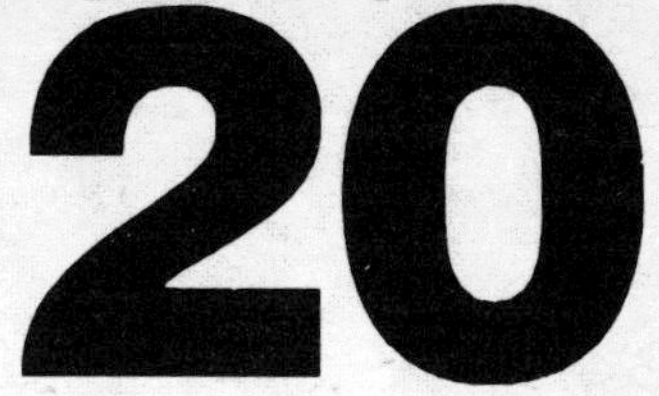

Research concerning young people and emotional disorders

Consultant: Professor Michael Rutter, Professor of Child Psychiatry, Institute of Psychiatry, University of London, London.

1 A general classification

1 The International Classification of Diseases published by the World Health Organization (ICD 9) contains an extensive classification of psychiatric disorders experienced by children and adolescents. Rutter (1975) has devised a simplified table of some of the diagnostic categories.

2 This classification, shown in Table 20.1, is based upon the empirical evidence for certain diagnostic groups, and shows some of the circumstances associated with them. Emotional disorders, the focus of this chapter, is one diagnostic group.

3 Some of these disorders are dealt with in more detail in other chapters:

Conduct disorders	Chapter 21
Hyperkinesis/hyperactivity	Chapter 21
Schizophrenia (adult forms)	Chapter 35

While this chapter will focus upon emotional disorders, there will be inevitable and necessary overlap with other chapters.

2 The prevalence of psychiatric disorders among children and young people

2.1 Studies of children in the Isle of Wight and Inner London

1 **The focus of the studies** This large-scale series of studies (Rutter and colleagues, 1975a, 1975b) compared characteristics and circumstances of 1,689 ten-year-old children growing up in an Inner London Borough with those of 1,279 ten-year-old children growing up on the Isle of Wight. Extensive data using a range of measures were gathered from both home and school settings.

	Variables						
Diagnostic Groups	Age of onset	Sex	Reading difficulties	Organic brain dysfunction	Family discord	Response to treatment	Adult state (if impaired)
Emotional	any	=	–	±	–	++++	neurosis/depression
Conduct	any	male	++	±	++	+	delinquency/personality disorder
Hyperkinetic	<5 years	male	+++	+	+	+	personality disorder/ psychosis
Autism	<2½ years	male	+++	++	–	+	language and social impairment
Schizophrenia	>7 years	=	+	±	±	+	relapsing or chronic psychosis
Development	infancy	male	+++	+	–	++	educational difficulties

TABLE 20.1 Variables differentiating diagnostic categories (Rutter, 1975). (Reproduced by permission of Penguin Books Ltd.)

2 Some findings

Setting where 10-year-olds were studied.	Total population	Estimated number with disorder in the total population	Estimated prevalence (%)
Isle of Wight	1,279	153	12.0
Inner London Borough	1,689	428	25.4

TABLE 20.2 Prevalence of psychiatric disorder among ten-year-olds in two areas (Rutter and colleagues, 1975)

3 The Family Adversity Index

1 From the sociological, psychological and psychiatric data gathered it was possible to devise tables of stress factors associated with child psychiatric disorder and behavioural deviance. See Table 20.3.

1. Father: unskilled/semiskilled job
2. Overcrowding or large family size
3. Marital discord and/or broken home
4. Mother: depression/neurosis
5. Child ever 'in care'
6. Father: any offence against law

TABLE 20.3 Family Adversity Index (Rutter, 1978)

2 Rutter (1978) reported that if a stress appeared alone, there was no significantly associated risk of problems for the child, but if two or more stresses occurred together, there was an interaction effect which markedly inflated the risk of problems for the child – far beyond what a simple summation of risk would suggest.

4 A summary comment upon these findings Rutter (1978) offered the following summary:

> The results were much the same however psychiatric disorder or behavioural deviance were assessed: the rate was twice as high in Inner London as on the Isle of Wight. This was so for both boys and girls and for both emotional and conduct disorders . . .
>
> The difference in the prevalence . . . is almost entirely explicable in terms of the much greater frequency of family adversity in the two areas.

2.2 Studies of young people

1 Prevalence studies

1 Rutter (1979) reported several studies investigating the prevalence of emotional and conduct disorders among young people. He noted, for example, Lavik's (1977) survey of the psychiatric state of adolescents in Oslo compared with a rural area. In Oslo, one in five adolescents showed psychiatric problems but in the rural area only 8 per cent did so.

2 Rutter (1979) also noted from studies of over 2,000 fourteen-year-olds in the Isle of Wight that the prevalence of psychiatric disorder was 10 to 15 per cent: a further group of teenagers reported marked distress which had not been recognized by either parents or teachers. This raised the prevalence rate to 21 per cent.

2 Types of disorder The disorders experienced by these 21 per cent of young people were:

Emotional disorder: anxiety, depression, etc.	40%
Conduct disorder: aggressive and destructive behaviour	40%
Mixed emotional and conduct disorders	20%

3 Variables protecting some young people from difficulties

3.1 Studies of resilience

1 Findings from the Isle of Wight/Inner London studies These studies (see 2.1) gave pointers to variables likely to protect a child or young person from serious difficulties:

(a) A low stress level within the home.
(b) Compensating good circumstances, e.g. at school.
(c) Temperamental features: easy adaptable children are less vulnerable than awkward, negativistic ones.
(d) Heredity: some children may be genetically less likely to succumb to environmental stress than others.
(e) Good relationships with at least one parent.

2 Findings among acutely disadvantaged children Research reviewed by Garmezy (1983) of black children living in urban ghettoes examined which children remained able to function well despite poverty and prejudice; the evidence suggested important factors were:

(a) Features of the child's disposition; the children were seen as stable, competent and with a positive sense of self.
(b) Family cohesion and warmth; even where fathers were absent, mothers offered a well-structured environment, and generous personal praise.

(c) Support figures, e.g. in school, who served as positive models for the children.

3 **Longitudinal studies** Werner *et al.* (1982) followed a cohort of children born on one of the Hawaiian islands from birth to early adulthood, and reported that resilient children were characterized by three factors:

(a) Personality dispositions in infancy and early childhood described as 'active' and 'socially responsive'.
(b) Family cohesion, marked by close personal relationships and parents who are supportive but set firm guidelines for children.
(c) The presence of external support from peers, older friends, teachers and others.

3.2 Convergence of evidence concerning resilience in children

It is rare for studies from such diverse settings to produce such similar evidence; moreover, it is rare for three variables to emerge so consistently as being of such importance – namely:

(a) Features of the child's temperament or disposition.
(b) Family cohesion and warmth.
(c) Supportive figures in the school or local environment.

3.3 A summary comment

It thus appears that while psychosocial stress, such as growing up in a family where there is marital discord, unemployment, poverty or overcrowding, *particularly where these stresses are cumulative*, can place a child at risk of psychiatric disorder, nevertheless, protective factors of the kind shown in 3.2 above, can reduce this risk.

4 Specific emotional disorders among young people: anxiety, phobias, obsessive-compulsive conditions and depression

4.1 Definition of emotional disorders

Rutter (1975) has written:

> Emotional disorders, as the name suggests, are those in which the main problem involves an abnormality of the emotions such as anxiety, fear, depression, obsessions, hypochondriasis and the like.

4.2 Temperamental differences and children's vulnerability

1 Studies in different communities, e.g. Thomas, Chess and Birch (1968) in New York and Graham, Rutter and George (1973) in London have found evidence of distinctive patterns of characteristics among babies and young children. Rutter (1977) has noted that 'emotionally intense'

children, who 'tend to be irritable and negative in mood' are more at risk of psychiatric disorder than 'the easy, adaptable, regular child of positive mood'.

2 Rutter (1977) noted the tensions and anxiety which can arise between children and parents of differing temperaments as they pass through the developmental stages of language acquisition, and gaining control of bladder and bowel. These anxieties can sometimes undermine confident parenting.

4.3 Anxiety-related disorders

1 **Anxiety-related disorders at different ages** Both anxiety and fear are natural among infants, children and adolescents and adults, but may take particular forms at different ages. Hersov (1977, 1985) has written that while fear during infancy in early childhood is often related to actual events, such as separation from major attachment figures or having to meet strangers, as the child grows older, fantasy and imagination come to play a greater role. Thus fears may become linked to possible future dangers or impulses to action.

He noted that fears concerning school (such as worries about position in class, teachers or speaking in public) increase from age nine to twelve years. There is also an increase in fears about social relationships, worries about money, and vague fears about identity.

2 **Precipitated or reinforced anxiety** Hersov has reported the evidence that some anxiety states are precipitated by a specific frightening experience, such as a hospital operation (Langford, 1937), the death of a friend or relative or an accident. In other cases, there is contagion of anxiety from chronically anxious parents. (Eisenberg, 1958).

4.4 Other anxiety-related disorders: phobias

1 **A definition of phobic states** Hersov (1985) quoted the definition of Marks (1969)

> Phobic states are emotional disorders in which there is an abnormally intense dread of certain objects, or of specific situations that normally do not have that effect.

2 **Prevalence of phobias** Hersov (1977) reported the finding of Rutter and colleagues (1970) that specific situational phobias were the most common among ten-year-old children, equally frequently among boys and girls. Such phobias were rarely the only symptom in children with emotional disorders; this emphasized the need for detailed clinical assessment.

3 **School phobia/school refusal (as one form of non-attendance at school)** Rutter

(1975) has conceptualized school phobia as an anxiety-related disorder, precipitated by a number of possible factors.

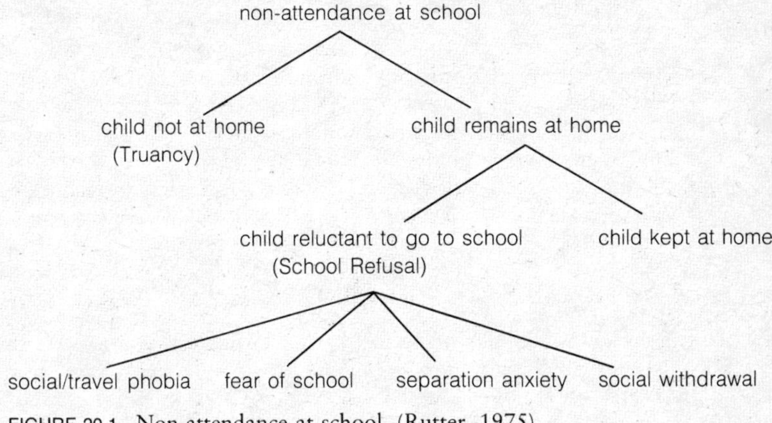

FIGURE 20.1 Non-attendance at school. (Rutter, 1975).

The distinctions to be made between forms of non-attendance at school are shown in Figure 20.1; this highlights the need for very careful assessment and treatment/management.

4.5 Further anxiety-related disorders: obsessive-compulsive conditions

1 Hersov (1977, 1985) reported these as relatively common in the form of simple rituals in pre-school and school age children, especially among the particularly shy or conscientious. So long as they are not reinforced by a great deal of adult attention, they often fade away. He also noted the evidence that many children with obsessive-compulsive features in his sample came from homes particularly concerned with cleanliness, etiquette and morality.

2 Concerning adolescents with these disorders, Hersov noted that they were often lacking in social skills. This can lead to increasing isolation from normal peer group activities, leading to misery which can exacerbate the obsessive symptoms. Obsessional thought and behaviour may also develop as secondary features in a depressive disorder.

4.6 Depression

1 Depression in young children: the shortage of research

1 Rutter (1986) advocated a developmental approach to the study of depression. He noted the shortage of research upon depression in early childhood, and the uncertainties as to whether normal grief reactions

and the protest-despair-detachment sequence noted by Bowlby (1969) as characteristic of very young children admitted alone to e.g. hospital, should be included within the depressive syndrome.

2 Of older children he wrote:

> In the Isle of Wight general population study of 10-to-11-year-old children (Rutter, Tizard and Whitmore 1970/1981), 13% showed a depressed mood at interview, 9% appeared preoccupied with depressive topics, 17% failed to smile, and 15% showed poor emotional responsiveness. . . . The same children were reassessed at 14–15 years with very different findings . . . depressive feelings being considerably more prevalent. Over 40% of the adolescents reported substantial feelings of misery and depression during a psychiatric interview, 20% reported feelings of self-depreciation, 7–8% reported that they had suicidal feelings, and 25% described ideas of reference.

Rutter noted the much higher prevalence of depression among post-pubertal than among pre-pubertal children, and he quoted the study by Pearce (1978), who studied a sample of 547 children referred to the Maudsley Hospital. This showed that among the pre-pubertal children, depressive symptoms were twice as common in boys, while after puberty they were twice as common in girls.

2 **Vulnerability to depression** Hersov (1977) has suggested that as a result of genetic factors and/or early experience some children seem more likely than others to respond to stressful events with more lasting moods of sadness. These may continue even though the child's life experience takes a turn for the better.

3 **Possible explanations for these changes** Rutter (1986) has suggested that one or more of the following may be implicated in the increase of depression at puberty:

(a) Hormonal changes associated with puberty.
(b) Genetic factors, since there is evidence of their involvement in emotional disorders.
(c) An increase in the number of environmental stressors at puberty.
(d) Variations in vulnerability or protective factors – e.g. family factors may be supportive or may constitute a stress.
(e) Differential opportunities to express or discharge emotions.

5 Treatment of specific emotional disorders in young people: anxiety, phobias, obsessive-compulsive conditions and depression

5.1 Principles which should underlie a therapeutic approach

Hersov (1985) has written that Reisman (1973) has devised a useful summary of these:

1 Therapy should be based on a careful assessment of the actual psychological mechanisms which underlie each child's problems, rather than on the basis of theoretical considerations;
2 the psychotherapy situation should be structured to facilitate communication and the therapist should allow the child ample opportunity to express his feelings and beliefs;
3 the therapist should communicate his understanding of the child and his wish to be of help;
4 the therapist and child should define the purpose or goal of their meeting;
5 the therapist must make clear what is ineffective or inappropriate in the child's behaviour;
6 when dealing with behaviour that is dependent on social interaction, the therapist may modify it by focusing directly on the interactions where they take place (this may mean conjoint family interviews, group therapy or contact with school teachers according to where the problem lies); and
7 treatment should end when the advantages of ending outweigh the advantages of continuing: (this may mean finishing before the child is fully better).

5.2 The treatment of anxiety

Hersov (1977) suggested that treatment would be likely to include a variety of approaches, often in combination. Some children will need individual psychotherapy aimed at the origins of the anxiety, and it will often be brief and focused. (Rosenthal and Levine, 1971).

Hersov also suggested that behavioural methods to teach children how to relax and how to deal with situation-specific anxiety may be useful. (Montenegro, 1968). (See also Chapter 32, page 305) Hersove indicated that in certain circumstances medication can contribute to a reduction in anxiety.

5.3 The treatment of phobias

1 Hersov (1985) has written,

> Many techniques have been used in the treatment of phobias; these include psychotropic drugs, abreaction, psychotherapy and various forms of behaviour therapy. Behavioural methods constitute the treatment of choice in the case of monosymptomatic phobias. However, more complex phobic disorders often require a combination of approaches which include behavioural methods, environmental manipulation and psychotherapy.

2 He went on to report the conclusion of Miller, Barrett and Hampe (1974) that the treatment of phobias in children can be reduced to four essentials:

(a) Establishing a helping relationship, through interviews with child and parents, and showing a conviction that one can help.
(b) Stimulus clarification: pinpointing cues and triggers to the phobic reaction.
(c) Desensitization to the stimulus: e.g. teaching parents gently to encourage children to face feared situations.
(d) Confrontation of the stimulus; this may be via progressive steps up a hierarchy from least feared to most feared setting.

5.4 The treatment of obsessive-compulsive conditions

Hersov (1985) reported that until the advent of behaviour therapy, psychotherapy with the child together with parental counselling was the main treatment, and that this is still seen as helpful when there is marked general anxiety. Recently, however, there has been good evidence, from Bolton, Collins and Steinberg (1983), of the helpfulness of behavioural approaches (response prevention) in relieving obsessional-compulsive conditions, but used in the context of work with the family.

5.5 The treatment of depression

Hersov (1977) summarized these, indicating that depression in school-age children is often associated with a range of acute and chronic stresses within and without the home. Individual and family therapy is often helpful, to help child and family develop more successful ways of coping with stress. Where there is a clear-cut depression preventing a child from functioning at home or at school, then medical advice upon medication is necessary.

5.6 Absence of relationship between childhood emotional disorder and adult neurosis

Reviewing this field, Rutter (1985) has reported that many children with emotional disorders go on to become well-functioning adults, and that it is unusual for children with an emotional disturbance to go on to develop, for example, an anti-social personality disorder.

References

Bolton, D., Collins, S. and Steinberg, D. (1983), 'The treatment of obsessive-compulsive disorder in adolescence', *British Journal of Psychiatry*, vol. 142, pp. 456–64.

Bowlby, J. (1969), *Attachment and Loss, 1. Attachment*, London: Hogarth Press.

Eisenberg, L. (1958), 'School phobia: a study in the communication of anxiety', *American Journal of Psychiatry*, vol. 114, pp. 712–18.

Garmezy, N. (1983), 'Stressors of childhood' in N. Garmezy and M. Rutter (eds), *Stress, Coping and Development in Children*, Stanford,

California, Center for Advanced Study in the Behavioral Sciences, McGraw Hill Book Company.

Graham, P., Rutter, M. and George, S. (1973), 'Temperamental characteristics as predictors of child behaviour disorders in children', *American Journal of Orthopsychiatry*, vol. 43, pp. 328–39.

Hersov, L. (1977), 'Emotional disorders' in M. Rutter and L. Hersov (eds), *Child Psychiatry: Modern Approaches*, Oxford: Blackwell Scientific Publications.

Hersov, L. (1986), 'Emotional disorders' in M. Rutter and L. Hersov (eds), *Child and Adolescent Psychiatry: Modern Approaches* (2nd edition), Oxford: Blackwell Scientific Publications.

Langford, W. (1937), 'Anxiety attacks in children', *American Journal of Orthopsychiatry*, vol. 7, pp. 210–18.

Lavik, N. J. (1977), 'Urban-rural differences in rates of disorder. A comparative population study of Norwegian adolescents' in P. J. Graham (ed.), *Epidemiological Approaches in Child Psychiatry*, London: Academic Press.

Marks, I. (1969), *Fears and Phobias*, London: Heinemann.

Miller, L. C., Barrett, C. L. and Hampe, E. (1974), 'Phobias of childhood in a prescientific era' in A. Davids (ed.), *Child Personality and Psychopathology: Current Topics*, New York: Wiley.

Montenegro, H. (1968), 'Severe separation anxiety in two pre-school children: successfully treated by reciprocal inhibition', *Journal of Child Psychology and Psychiatry*, vol. 9, pp. 93–103.

Pearce, J. (1978), 'The recognition of depressive disorder in children', *Journal of the Royal Society of Medicine*, vol. 71, pp. 494–500.

Reisman, J. (1973), *Principles of Psychotherapy with Children*, London: Wiley.

Rosenthal, A. and Levine, S. (1971), 'Brief psychotherapy with children: process of therapy', *American Journal of Psychiatry*, vol. 128, pp. 141–6.

Rutter, M. (1970), 'Sex differences in children's responses to family stress' in R. J. Anthony and C. Koupernik (eds), *The Child in his Family*, New York: Wiley.

Rutter, M. (1975), *Helping Troubled Children*, Harmondsworth: Penguin.

Rutter, M. (1977), 'Individual differences' in M. Rutter and L. Hersov (eds), *Child Psychiatry: Modern Approaches*, Oxford: Blackwell Scientific.

Rutter, M. (1978), 'Family, area and school influences in the genesis of conduct disorders' in L. A. Hersov, M. Berger and D. Shaffer (eds), *Aggression and Anti-social Behaviour in Childhood and Adolescence*, Oxford: Pergamon Press.

Rutter, M. (1979), *Changing youth in a changing society, Patterns of adolescent development and disorder*, London: The Nuffield Provincial Hospitals Trust.

Rutter, M. (1980), *Scientific foundations of developmental psychiatry*, London: Heinemann Medical Books.

Rutter, M. (1985), 'Psychopathology and development: Links between childhood and adult life' in M. Rutter and L. Hersov (eds), *Child and Adolescent Psychiatry* (2nd edition), Oxford: Blackwell Scientific Publications.

Rutter, M. (1986), 'The developmental, psychopathology of depression: Issues and perspectives' in M. Rutter, C. Izard and P. Read (eds), *Depression in Young People: Developmental and Clinical Perspectives*, New York: Guilford Press.

Rutter, M. and Hersov, L. (1976), *Child Psychiatry: Modern Approaches*, Oxford: Blackwell Scientific Publications.

Rutter, M. and Hersov, L. (1985), *Child and Adolescent Psychiatry: Modern Approaches* (2nd edition), Oxford: Blackwell Scientific Publications.

Rutter, M., Cox, A., Tupling, C., Berger, M. and Yule, W. (1975a), 'Attainment and adjustment in two geographical areas: I. The prevalence of psychiatric disorder', *British Journal of Psychiatry*, vol. 126, pp. 493–509.

Rutter, M., Tizard, J. and Whitmore, K. (eds) (1970), *Education, Health and Behaviour*, London: Longman. (Reprinted 1981, New York: Kreiger, Huntington.)

Rutter, M., Graham, P., Chadwick, O. and Yule, W. (1976), 'Adolescent turmoil: fact or fiction?', *Journal of Child Psychology and Psychiatry and Allied Disciplines*, vol. 17, pp. 35–56.

Rutter, M., Yule, B., Quinton, D., Rowlands, O., Yule, W. and Berger, M. (1975b), 'Attainment and adjustment in two geographical areas: III. Some factors accounting for area differences', *British Journal of Psychiatry*, vol. 126, pp. 520–33.

Thomas, A., Chess, S. and Birch, H. G. (1968), *Temperament and Behaviour Disorders in Children*, New York: Universities Press.

Werner, E. E. and Smith, R. S. (1982), *Vulnerable but Invincible: A Study of Resilient Children*, New York: McGraw-Hill.

21 Research concerning young people and conduct disorders

Consultant: Professor Martin Herbert, Department of Psychology, University of Leicester.

1 A grouping within a general classification

Conduct disorders constitute one of the categories in the classification of children's disorders devised by Rutter (1975), and which is based upon empirical evidence. (See page 184). Several disorders will be considered, although non-attendance at school is clearly a broader category than the others. Thus, the disorders under consideration are:

1 Aggressiveness/destructiveness
2 Hyperkinetic behaviour/hyperactivity
3 Non-attendance at school

N.B. Although there is clearly some overlap, it is not intended to consider here behaviour which offends against the law. For this field, see Chapter 28, page 269.

2 Research concerning the prevalence and persistence of conduct disorders

The evidence from the various studies is mixed:

2.1 Data from the National Child Development Study

1 This British longitudinal study examined the progress of all traceable children born in the week 3–9 March, 1958. The original figure was about 17,000 births in England, Scotland and Wales, although this figure decreased as it became difficult to trace all the children. Data was gathered upon many aspects of the children's development, including separate ratings of the child's behaviour at home and at school, at ages seven, eleven and sixteen.
2 Fogelman (1983) has summarized findings upon many aspects of the children's progress. In respect of behaviour, rated at home and at school, the 13 per cent of children with the highest ratings were considered as showing 'deviant' behaviour. Fogelman noted that the figure of 13 per cent was necessarily arbitrary.
3 Some of the researchers' conclusions are paraphrased below. They noted:

(a) Moderate (0.31–0.48) correlations between ratings at different ages.
(b) Only very small groups of children (about 2.2 per cent) remained in the 'deviant' group at all three ages, seven, eleven and sixteen.
(c) School ratings indicated more girls in groups which were normal and more boys in the groups which were 'deviant' at all three ages.
(d) More children from bigger families (more than three children in the family at or below the age of seven) joined the deviant group (on the home rating) and more stayed in the deviant group (on the school rating).

4 Reflecting on the above, the researchers commented:

> What can be said with assurance from these results is that, in interpreting research studies, they give considerable warning against assuming a static and pathological stage for children identified as deviant.

2.2 Data from the Isle of Wight/Inner London Borough studies

1 Ten-year-olds

1 These studies, (see Chapter 20, page 183), compared the characteristics and circumstances of 1,279 ten-year-olds, growing up on the Isle of Wight, with those of 1,689 ten-year-olds growing up in an Inner London borough.
2 Children were screened for a range of disorders and, of the samples, 14.2 per cent of the boys, and 5.1 per cent of the girls in the Inner London borough, compared with 9.0 per cent of the boys and 3.0 per cent of the girls in the Isle of Wight, were considered as having a conduct disorder.

2 Fourteen-to-fifteen-year-olds Rutter (1979) reported that about 21 per cent of the sample of 2,000 young people screened in the Isle of Wight experienced marked distress or disorder. Of these, 40 per cent displayed conduct disorders, and a further 20 per cent mixed emotional and conduct disorders.

2.3 Data from other studies

An American longitudinal study.
A study by Robins (1966, 1972) involved 542 children seen at St. Louis Child Guidance Clinic, who were followed up when they were on average forty-three years old. Herbert (1978) summarized:

> Frequent anti-social behaviour in childhood (such as stealing, truancy and lying) was a very powerful predictor of poor adult outcomes. . . . This extremely poor prognosis was most likely when the antisocial

behaviour in childhood was most frequent and varied, and when it was shown outside the family and the child's own circle of friends.

3 Research into the origins of conduct disorders

3.1 Aggressive and destructive conduct disorders

1 **A description** Herbert (1978) has written:

> Conduct disorders . . . include . . . disruptiveness, boisterousness, fighting, attention seeking, restlessness, negativism, impertinence, destructiveness, irritability, temper-tantrums, hyperactivity, profanity, jealousy and uncooperativeness.

2 **Difficulties of delineating conduct disorders** Herbert (1978) continued,

> Most children manifest these 'problems' to some extent. The diagnostic problem lies in the fact that there is no clear-cut distinction between the characteristics of 'abnormal' children and other children; the differences are relative – a matter of degree.

3.2 A multi-variate/systems, model of contributory factors

The evidence suggests that a multi-variate/systems model encompassing many interacting contributory factors, is the most appropriate. Some of the research conducted from these interacting perspectives is reported below.

1 **Socio-economic and sociological factors**

(a) Many studies have indicated the association between children's behaviour problems and parental poverty, poor quality housing in inner city areas, unemployment and general disadvantage; e.g. Wilson (1974); Rutter (1978).

(b) Other studies, e.g. Dunning, Maguire, Murphy and Williams (1982) have suggested that some boys from deprived areas, excluded from the opportunities and employment available to the more privileged, find status and release from boredom by fighting with supporters of opposing football teams.

2 **Variables linked with socialization experiences**

(a) A major longitudinal study West and Farrington (1973, 1977) conducted a longitudinal study of 411 London boys. Factors contributing to the developing of aggression and delinquency were examined, but the latter will not be considered here. Data was gathered about annually from parents during the six years when the boys were aged eight to fourteen; teachers completed questionnaires on the boys at ages eight, ten, twelve and fourteen; and 95 per cent of the sample were themselves interviewed at ages fourteen,

sixteen and eighteen. Concerning aggressiveness, Farrington (1978) reported: '36.4% of the 44 boys rated aggressive by their teachers at age 8 were among the 76 boys highest on self-reported aggression at age 18.'

In the course of a detailed summary of the findings, Farrington suggested that some of his evidence suggests that: 'harsh parental attitude and discipline, criminal parents, separations, low family income, daring and low I.Q. were all significantly related to aggressiveness at 8–10.'

Farrington acknowledged, however, the many weaknesses of the study and the great need for further, more detailed research into the factors contributing to the development of aggressiveness.

(b) *The stresses encountered by parents* Herbert (1978), writing from the standpoint of social learning theory (see Chapter 9, page 71), has noted the difficulties encountered by parents, often isolated and stressed, in providing firm and consistent management for active and challenging children. In a study comparing Indian and English children, all aged between nine and twelve, Kallarackal and Herbert (1976) found the Indian children more stable and less unruly than the English, and attributed this in part to the way the parents managed their children. They wrote,

> We do think that the quality of Indian family life may positively help to reduce the risk of developing deviant behaviour in Indian children. . . . Indian parents were found to be insistent on close supervision of children and firm discipline at home.

3 **Variables pinpointed by a social learning theory analysis** Bandura and Walters (1959) compared twenty-six aggressive youths aged fourteen to seventeen with twenty-six non-aggressive youths matched for age, I.Q., socio-economic status and social background, focusing particularly upon the parenting practices of each group. They noted that the parents of the aggressive young people were more likely:

to use physical punishment
to disagree with each other
to be cold and rejecting to their sons

Bandura further reported:

> Parents of non-aggressive adolescents rarely reinforced their sons for resorting to physical aggression in response to provocation. Parents of aggressive delinquents, on the other hand, tolerated no aggressive displays whatsoever in the home, but condoned, actively encouraged and reinforced provocative and aggressive actions toward others in the community.

4 **Studies of the impact of television violence** The evidence in this field is inconclusive but Rutter and Cox (1985) have concluded from their overview of the evidence that:

> It seems reasonable to infer that films and television may have *some*

impact on attitudes and behaviour and hence that they may play a small part in the predisposition to violent behaviour. However, the effect seems likely to be greatest in young children, in those already showing psychosocial problems, and in situations where the influence of the media is consonant with other influences in the home.

5 **Cognitive and situational variables** Howells (1981) has reported studies highlighting the contribution of cognitive and situational variables in precipitating an aggressive encounter. (See Chapter 41, page 382). The same variables almost certainly apply to children and young people.

3.3 Hyperkinetic/hyperactive behaviour

1 **Difficulties of exact diagnosis** Herbert (1978) has written:

> There are no necessary and sufficient criteria for the diagnosis of hyperactivity . . . the majority of factor-analytic investigations . . . have failed to isolate a specific *hyperactive* syndrome in the medical sense of a disease entity. Rather the 'symptoms' of hyperactivity emerge as part of a conduct disorder.

He continued,

> The behaviour problem has the following elements: serious disobedience and failure to heed; defiance; 'excesses' of behaviour and predominance of negative mood (whiny petulance, excessive crying, screaming, tantrums); . . . extreme attention seeking; commanding behaviour (pestering, nagging, demanding, clinging, etc.). . . . From the parents' point of view the child seems out of control.

2 **Discrepancies of diagnosis between Britain and America** Herbert reported the very high number of children diagnosed as 'hyperactive' in the USA, about five to ten per cent of school-aged children according to O'Malley and Eisenberg (1973). In the Isle of Wight study only three among 2,199 children were so diagnosed.

3.4 Research with particular relevance to hyperactivity

Here, too, a multi-factorial model seems clearly necessary.

1 **Studies concerning possible genetic contributions** Herbert (1981) highlighted the studies by Thomas, Chess and Birch (1968) which, in a longitudinal investigation of 136 babies as they grew into children, noted marked individual differences of temperament among them. On the basis of actually observed behaviours, they found clusters of children with different temperaments; the clusters fell out broadly as follows:

- Difficult children: characterized by irregular patterns of sleeping and feeding, withdrawal and intense reactions.

- Easy children: characterized by regularity of patterns, adaptable behaviour, and mild reactions to e.g. novelty.
- Slow to warm up children: characterized by mixed patterns with negative response of mild intensity and slow adaptability to e.g. novelty.
- Children not fitting into any of the above groupings.

2 **Studies of possible organic factors** Research continues into the possibility that some substances such as lead from petrol fumes and food additives may contribute to hyperactivity.

3 **Variables from social learning theory**

1 Factors such as the unwitting rewarding of demanding and restless behaviours in children and inconsistent management of them by isolated and exhausted parents probably make a major contribution to the persistence of very active behaviour: (Patterson, 1976; Barkley, 1981; Herbert, 1981).

2 Herbert has suggested the following factors as key features of such children:

- The child's high level of arousal and excess activity.
- His poor performance (socialization) at home and his low attainment at school.
- His distractibility and low attention span.
- Behaviour problems: disobedience, attention-seeking and imperious behaviour.
- A history of few rewards and many punishments; he is likely to have had many experiences of failure.
- His great need for attention and success; he will often seek attention, even if it is in the form of punishment.
- His social isolation, since he is often rejected because of aggressiveness to his peers.
- His parents are likely to be demoralized and lacking in confidence through exhaustion: they may reject the child.
- The lack of mutually rewarding behaviour between parent and child.

3.5 Truancy and attempts to understand it

1 **Prevalence** Pugh (1976) has described this as absence from school without parental knowledge or consent, and has reported that there is evidence from the National Child Development Study that the rate at age eleven is 1.2 per cent, while at age sixteen it is 20 per cent.

2 **The need for a multi-variate, systems, model** Brown (1983) has criticized attempts to examine truancy from a single perspective: e.g. the maladjusted truant, the truant-producing family, the truant-producing community, the truant-producing school. From a systems perspective it seems clear that no

single variable is responsible for truancy: rather an attempt to understand this form of non-school attendance in terms of multiply interacting variables seems far more appropriate. Cognitive and perceptual factors, such as 'What is the point of going to school? It won't get me a job!' seem of particular relevance.

4 Research into intervention in conduct disorders

4.1 The very serious shortage of research

1 There is a *very* great shortage of sound research concerning effective ways of intervening in conduct disorders. Rather there are a few small-scale studies, with isolated and specific groups of young people which have not been fully replicated. The sociological analyses which have been conducted and which stress the contribution of disadvantage and lack of employment, are obviously of profound importance.
2 Just as a multi-variate, systems, model seems to offer the best way of understanding conduct disorders, so it may well be that a multi-dimensional strategy of intervention is called for to respond to them. Such a strategy clearly needs careful evaluation.
3 In default of research upon such a multi-dimensional model, a few primarily psychological studies are reported below.

4.2 Intervention in aggressive/destructive behaviour

1 **Studies drawing on principles of social learning theory** The best designed and reported studies appear to yield to an analysis in terms of principles of social learning theory. Thus Bandura (1973) reported: 'Following the general rule that problems are best treated in the environment in which they occur, hyperaggressive behaviour has been successfully eliminated in children by their parents.' (Allison and Allison, 1971) Other studies, e.g. by Patterson and colleagues (1975) have shown that parents can successfully reduce aggressive behaviour among their children, and that these improvements persist.

2 **The need for careful assessment of conduct disorders** Herbert (1981) has stressed the importance of assessment taking account of many variables, and has suggested the guidelines shown in Fig. 21.1. See also Chapter 9, page 71.

3 **Teaching young people to manage their own aggressiveness** While there is an encouraging body of research relating to those adults who actively seek to control their own anger and violence, (see page 382), only occasional studies have so far demonstrated that the same cognitively-based approaches can be taught to children and young people. This remains an under-explored area.

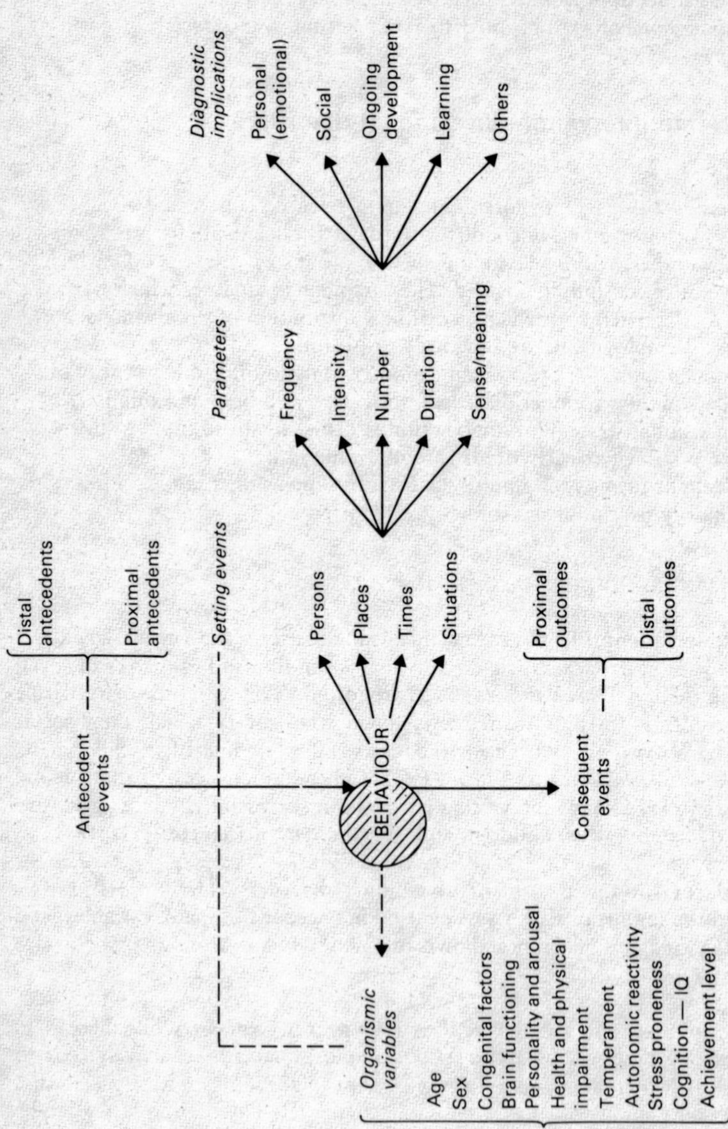

FIGURE 21.1 General assessment guidelines in the field of children's conduct disorders (Herbert, 1981)

4.3 Intervention in hyperkinetic/hyperactive behaviour

1 **The use of medication** In the United States, extensive use is made of medication with, according to the inquiry by Barkley (1981), extremely calming effects upon the children concerned. He and other researchers, however, seriously question the desirability and ethics of such a practice. Medication seems to be used rarely in the UK for such problems: Herbert (1981).

2 **The use of particular diets** Claims are made (e.g. Feingold, 1974) for the efficacy of diets excluding certain foods/additives. These claims are still being explored.

3 **Studies drawing on principles of social learning theory** There is some evidence, Rinn and Markle (1977) and Herbert (1981) of the usefulness of teaching parents how to manage the behaviour of their hyperactive children using principles of reinforcement, time out and contingency management. Further research is however needed into the detail of this approach – a task embarked upon by Horton (1982) – and into how to maintain parental practice of newly learned skills.

References

Allison, T. S. and Allison, S. L. (1971), 'Time out from reinforcement: Effect on sibling aggression', *Psychological Record*, vol. 21, pp. 81–6.

Bandura, A. (1973), *Aggression: a Social Learning Analysis*, New York: Prentice-Hall.

Bandura, A. and Walters, R. H. (1959), *Adolescent Aggression*, New York: Ronald Press.

Barkley, R. A. (1981), *Hyperactive Children*, New York: The Guildford Press.

Brown, D. (1983), 'Truants, families and schools: a critique of the literature on truancy', *Educational Review*, vol. 35, pp. 225–35.

Dunning, E., Maguire, J., Murphy, P. and Williams, J. M. (1982), 'The social roots of football hooligan violence', *Leisure Studies*, vol. 1, pp. 139–56.

Farrington, D. P. (1978), 'The family background of aggressive youths' in L. A. Hersov, M. Berger and D. Shaffer (eds), *Aggression and Anti-Social Behaviour in Childhood and Adolescence*, Oxford: Pergamon Press.

Feingold, B. (1974), *Why Your Child Is Hyperactive*, New York: Random House.

Fogelman, K. (1983), *Growing up in Great Britain: Papers from the National Child Development Study*, London: National Children's Bureau, Macmillan.

Herbert, M. (1978), *Conduct Disorders in Childhood and Adolescence: A Behavioural Approach to Treatment*, Chichester: John Wiley.

Herbert, M. (1981), *Behavioural Treatment of Problem Children. A Practice Manual*, London: Academic Press.

Horton, L. E. (1982), 'Comparison of instructional components in behavioural parent training. A review', *Behavioral Counseling Quarterly*, vol. 2, pp. 131–47.

Howells, K. (1981), 'Social relationships in violent offenders' in S. Duck and R. Gilmour (eds), *Personal Relationships. 3 Personal Relationships in Disorder*, London: Academic Press.

Kallarackal, A. M. and Herbert, M. (1976), 'The adjustment of Indian immigrant children' in *Growing Up: A New Society Social Studies Reader*, London: IPC.

O'Dell, S. (1974), 'Training parents in behaviour modification. A review', *Psychological Bulletin*, vol. 81, pp. 418–33.

O'Malley, J. E. and Eisenberg, L. (1973), 'The hyperkinetic syndrome', *Seminars Psychiatrica*, vol. 5, p. 95.

Patterson, G. R. (1976), *Living with Children*, Champaign, Illinois: Research Press.

Patterson, G. R., Reid, J. B., Jones, R. R. and Conger, R. E. (1975), *A Social Learning Approach to Family Intervention. Vol. 1. Families with Aggressive Children*, Eugene, Oregon: Castalia Publishing Company.

Pugh, G. (1976), *Truancy*, Highlight No. 23, London: National Children's Bureau.

Rinn, R. and Markle, A. (1977), 'Parent effectiveness training: a review', *Psychological Reports*, vol. 41, pp. 95–109.

Robins, L. N. (1966), *Deviant Children Grown Up*, Baltimore: Williams and Wilkins.

Robins, L. N. (1972), 'Follow up studies of behaviour disorders in children' in H. C. Quay and J. S. Werry (eds), *Psychopathological Disorders of Childhood*, New York: Wiley.

Rutter, M. (1975), *Helping Troubled Children*, Harmondsworth: Penguin.

Rutter, M. (1978), 'Family, area and school influences in the genesis of conduct disorders' in L. A. Hersov, M. Berger and D. Shaffer (eds), *Aggression and Anti-Social Behaviour in Childhood and Adolescence*, Oxford: Pergamon Press.

Rutter, M. (1979), *Changing Youth in a Changing Society: Patterns of Adolescent Development and Disorder*, London: The Nuffield Provincial Hospitals Trust.

Rutter, M. and Cox, A. (1985), 'Other family influences' in M. Rutter and L. Hersov (eds), *Child and Adolescent Psychiatry: Modern Approaches* (2nd edition), Oxford: Blackwell Scientific Publications.

Thomas, A., Chess, S. and Birch, H. G. (1968), *Temperament and Behaviour Disorders in Children*, London: University of London.

West, D. J. and Farrington, D. P. (1973), *Who Becomes Delinquent?* London: Heinemann.

West, D. J. and Farrington, D. P. (1977), *The Delinquent Way of Life*, London: Heinemann.

Wilson, H. (1974), 'Parenting in poverty', *British Journal of Social Work*, vol. 4, pp. 241–54.

Research concerning bed-wetting (enuresis)

22

Consultant:* *Professor Martin Herbert, Professor of Clinical Psychology, Department of Psychology, University of Leicester.

1 Definitions

There is no single accepted definition of enuresis. Diagnosis and definition tend to reflect the definer's own views. Thus the following may be regarded merely as provisional.

> *Enuresis*: Bed-wetting of a stated frequency, such as once a week, by a child over a stated age – often 4 or 5 years – in whom no obvious organic (physical) abnormality has been found. Wetting can also occur by day.

2 Prevalence

2.1 The broad picture

Differences in definition have led to discrepancies in statistics. Morgan (1981) has devised the graph shown in Figure 22.1 which accords with data from international studies.

3 Research concerning the origins of bed-wetting

3.1 Sociological factors

Miller (1960) studying 750 children in Newcastle for a period of several years, noted that children who wet the bed were more likely to:

1 come from large families
2 be second children
3 come from socio-economic classes 4 and 5
4 be subject to over-crowding in the home.

3.2 The contribution of psychological factors: the association with stress

Douglas (1973) reported on the National Children's Bureau longitudinal study of over 4,300 children born in one week in 1946, and examined the number of stressful events in the first four years of life, and any associated pattern of bed-wetting. There were correlations/associations between bed-wetting and:

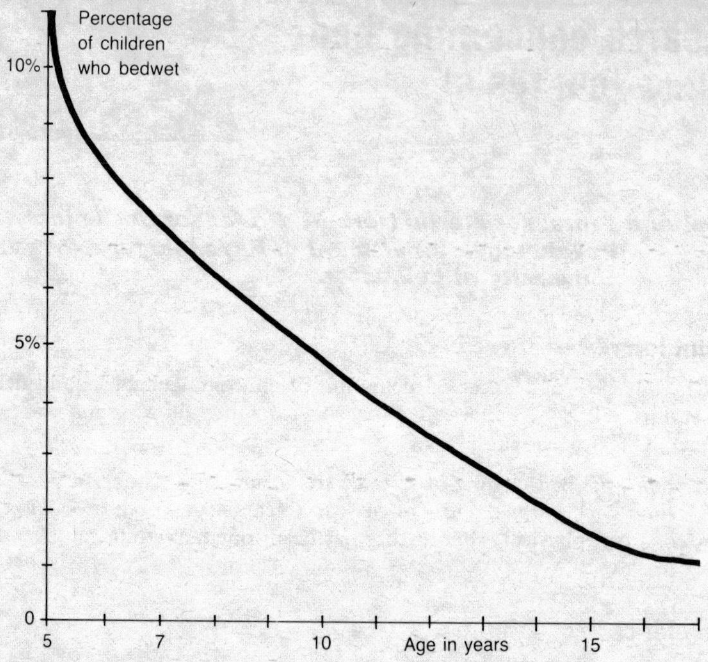

FIGURE 22.1 The frequency of bedwetting. From *Childhood Incontinence*, by R. Morgan, published by the Disabled Living Foundation, 1981.

1 Break-up of the family through death, divorce or separation.
2 Temporary separation from the mother.
3 The birth of a younger brother or sister.
4 Moving house or home.
5 Admission to hospital.
6 Accidents.

The implication of this is that stressful situations affect some, but by no means all, children. Those most likely to be affected by stress may be those who already have a genetic vulnerability.

3.3 The contribution of genetic factors

Bakwin (1973) reported the study by Hallgren (1960) of identical twins and their patterns of bed-wetting. This suggested a genetic contribution, and Bakwin examined 338 pairs of same-sex twins in an effort to confirm or refute Hallgren's findings. He found:

1 Bed-wetting was equally common in identical and non-identical twins.
2 The male–female ratio was 1.7:1.0.
3 Identical twins were found *both* to be bed-wetters more often than were non-identical twins.

3.4 The contribution of other factors

1 **Small bladder capacity** Zaleski, Gerrard and Shokeir (1973) examined previous studies of bed-wetters and in addition conducted their own study with 223 ordinary children and 75 who wet the bed, all aged four to fourteen years. All these studies confirmed that children who wet the bed:

1 Have smaller bladder capacities than non-wetters.
2 Pass urine more frequently than non-wetters.
3 Have bladders that are functionally, but not structurally small.

2 **Possible urinary tract infection** Stansfeld (1973) in his review of studies reported: 'About 16% of children with a urinary tract infection will present with enuresis, and a successful treatment of the infection will stop the enuresis in about 30%.'

3.5 Summary of the research findings

In their review of the evidence of how children become dry, MacKeith, Meadow and Turner (1973) summarized the position thus:

> We conclude that children become dry at night in the following way. At birth some partial mechanisms are already present. In the next four years, maturation takes place in the central nervous system, making the behaviour of nocturnal bladder control possible. This behaviour is not dependent on training or learning. It is destined to emerge during the first four years, providing nothing acts at the time of maturation to inhibit its emergence. Such negative factors may be transient or continuing stresses, amongst which unsuitable toilet training is probably important. The emergence of nocturnal bladder cannot be accelerated, but it can be retarded. A few children become dry at night by the age of one year, a large proportion in the second and third years. . . .
>
> In children under the age of five, but not in older children, delayed maturation is one of the factors leading to the delayed appearance of nocturnal dryness. . . . Genetic factors probably play a part by affecting either the age of maturation of necessary mechanisms or the development of nocturnal bladder capacity.

4 Research concerning the management of bed-wetting

4.1 The use of medication

McGonaghy (1969) compared five forms of treatment, in terms of their short- and long-term effectiveness:

1 Prescription of imipramine.
2 Prescription of amphetamine.

3 Prescription of placebo.
4 Random waking (to control for the giving of attention).
5 Behavioural/conditioning, using the bell and pad.

Behavioural conditioning was found to be the most effective, followed by the prescription of imipramine. Behavioural/conditioning was also found to be superior at one year follow-up.

4.2 Comparison of behavioural treatment with psychotherapy

Two studies, De Leon and Mandell (1966) and Werry and Cohrssen (1965) compared the relative effectiveness of two treatments: psychotherapy and behavioural treatment with the bell and pad. In both studies the latter group reached the criterion set for success significantly more frequently.

4.3 Further research into behavioural treatment

Turner (1973) reviewed seventeen studies of behavioural treatment, involving 1,067 children, and where the criterion for success was seven consecutive dry nights. He found success rates of 64.8 per cent to 100 per cent. All children were followed up for periods ranging from one month to sixty-three months, and while there was an average relapse rate of 27 per cent across the studies, many of these relapsed children, some of whom had wet only once in seven months, responded to a second intervention with bell and pad.

Turner (1981) regards behavioural/conditioning treatment with the bell and pad as the 'treatment of choice' i.e. the most effective treatment, for bed-wetting.

4.4 The use of the 'Dry-Bed' method

Azrin and Foxx (1974) developed a form of intensive behavioural training for children unresponsive to other methods; this requires a specially trained therapist, and a very structured pattern of intervention. Initial results with twenty-four chronically enuretic children were very successful. Other studies have tended to confirm the usefulness of this approach, and have involved enabling parents to work with their children using training manuals. This very encouraging field of work is currently being developed.

References

Azrin, N. H. and Foxx, R. M. (1974), *Toilet Training in Less Than a Day*, London: Macmillan.

Bakwin, H. (1973), 'The genetics of enuresis' in I. Kolvin, R. C. MacKeith, and S. R. Meadow (eds), *Bladder Control and Enuresis*, London: Heinemann Medical Books.

De Leon, J. and Mandell, W. (1966), 'A comparison of conditioning and psychotherapy in the treatment of functional enuresis', *Journal of Clinical Psychology*, vol. 22, pp. 326–8.

Douglas, J. W. B. (1973), 'Early disturbing events and later enuresis' in I. Kolvin, R. C. MacKeith and S. R. Meadow (eds), *Bladder Control and Enuresis*, London: Heinemann.

Hallgren, B. (1960), 'Nocturnal enuresis in twins', *Acta Psychiatrica et Neurologica Scandinavica*, vol. 35, p. 73.

McGonaghy, N. (1969), 'A controlled trial of imipramine, amphetamine, pad and bell conditioning and random awakening in the treatment of nocturnal enuresis', *Medical Journal of Australia*, vol. 2, pp. 237–9.

MacKeith, R., Meadow, R. and Turner, R. K. (1973), 'How children become dry' in I. Kolvin, R. C. MacKeith and S. R. Meadow (eds), *Bladder Control and Enuresis*, Spastics International Medical Publications, London: Heinemann Medical Books.

Miller, F. J. W., Court, S. D. M., Walton, W. S. and Knox, E. G. (1960), *Growing up in Newcastle upon Tyne*, London: Oxford University Press.

Morgan, R. (1981), *Childhood incontinence*, London: Disabled Living Foundation/Heinemann Medical Books.

Stansfeld, J. M. (1973), 'Enuresis and urinary tract infection', in I. Kolvin, R. C. MacKeith and S. R. Meadow (eds), op. cit., pp. 102–3.

Turner, R. K. (1973), 'Conditioning treatment of nocturnal enuresis' in I. Kolvin, R. C. MacKeith and S. R. Meadow (eds), op. cit., pp. 195–210.

Werry, J. S. and Cohrssen, J. (1965), 'Enuresis: an etiologic and therapeutic study', *Journal of Pediatrics*, vol. 67, pp. 423–39.

Zaleski, A., Gerrard, J. W. and Shokeir, M. H. K. (1973), 'Nocturnal enuresis: the importance of a small bladder capacity' in I. Kolvin, R. C. MacKeith and S. R. Meadow (eds), pp. 95–101.

PART 7

Research concerning services and settings with statutory implications

23

Research concerning aspects of statutory child care, including residential care

Consultant:* *Chris Payne, Lecturer/Consultant in Social Services Development, National Institute for Social Work, London.

1 A description of 'care'

1 Comprehensive provisions have been enacted for the care and welfare of children by local authorities where the child's welfare requires it. It is the local authority's duty, under certain circumstances, to receive a child into its care. Further, resolutions may be passed in certain circumstances concerning children in care that parental rights and duties shall vest in the local authority. Where it is believed that a child or young person is being ill-treated, or neglected, or has fulfilled one of a list of other conditions, and is in need of care and control, a local authority may institute court proceedings for a care order to be made.

2 *Care* in the above context can mean that a child is placed in a children's home or community home, is boarded out with foster parents, or is allowed to be under the charge or control of a parent, guardian, relative or friend.

3 In general, in the above, local authority means a County Council, a Metropolitan district council, or a London borough council. Children are those under eighteen, although some of the above duties (e.g. reception into care) only apply to those under seventeen.

2 Numbers of those in care

2.1 Official statistics

England				Thousands
	1980	1981	1982	1983
Total of all children in care	95.3	92.3	88.7	82.2
By age groups				
Under 5	10.1	9.6	9.6	8.7
5–15	62.1	59.9	56.5	51.8
16 and over	23.0	22.7	22.6	21.7
Manner of accommodation				
Boarded out (fostered)	35.2	35.7	36.9	36.5
In lodgings or residential employment	1.8	1.8	1.9	2.1
In community homes provided, controlled or assisted by local authorities:				
with observation and assessment facilities	5.0	4.7	4.4	3.6
with education on the premises	5.2	4.6	3.9	3.2
residential nurseries providing accommodation for children under the age of 7	0.7	0.4	0.3	0.2
other homes	18.0	16.7	15.1	13.0
Voluntary homes	3.1	2.8	2.2	1.7
Accommodation for handicapped children	2.9	3.0	2.8	2.5
Hostels	0.5	0.5	0.4	0.3
Under charge of parent, guardian, relative or friend	17.3	17.1	16.1	14.9
Other accommodation	5.5	4.9	4.6	4.1

TABLE 23.1 Children in care of local authorities: by age groups, and manner of accommodation. (*Health and Personal Social Services Statistics for England*, 1985). Figures are rounded.

2.2 Noteworthy points from the above data

1 The decrease in the number of children taken into care, especially among the under fives and children of five to fifteen years.
2 The decrease in the number of community homes.
3 The decrease in the number of voluntary homes (i.e. run by voluntary organizations).
4 The increase in boarding out (fostering).

2.3 Areas of research to be considered

1 Research concerning children in foster care is examined in Chapter 25, page 238, while research concerning children who are adopted is reported in Chapter 26, page 247.

2 This chapter will examine aspects of research within the general child care field, particularly the residential care field.

3 Group provision for children, whether in statutory care or not

3.1 The group care of children

1 Ainsworth and Fulcher (1981) have delineated the group care field, thus:

> It incorporates those areas of service – institutional care, residential group living (including but not necessarily requiring twenty-four hour, seven days per week care) and other community-based day services (covering lesser time periods) – that supply a range of developmentally enhancing services for groups of customers.

The above description referred to the care of children, but can of course be applied to the care of other groups of people.

2 The same authors describe group care as being, at one and the same time:
1 an occupational focus
2 a field of study
3 a domain of practice.

These writers adopt a systems approach, and have devised a framework showing areas of day services and of group care across the systems of health care, education, social welfare and justice. (See Table 23.2 and Figure 23.1).

Health care	*Education*	*Social welfare*	*Justice*
Day hospitals Day clinics Health centres Day nurseries	Youth and community centres Recreation and leisure centres Day nurseries Day schools Intermediate treatment units Alternative schools	Day care/ playgroups Activity programmes Intermediate treatment units Day nurseries	Community service centres Day and project centres Intermediate treatment units

TABLE 23.2 Types of day services across systems. (Ainsworth and Fulcher, 1981)

3.2 Difficulties in evaluating residential care

1 There are major difficulties in researching complex situations involving changing populations of residents and care staff. Durkin and Durkin (1975) have identified four models:
1 Descriptive studies
2 Outcome and follow-up studies

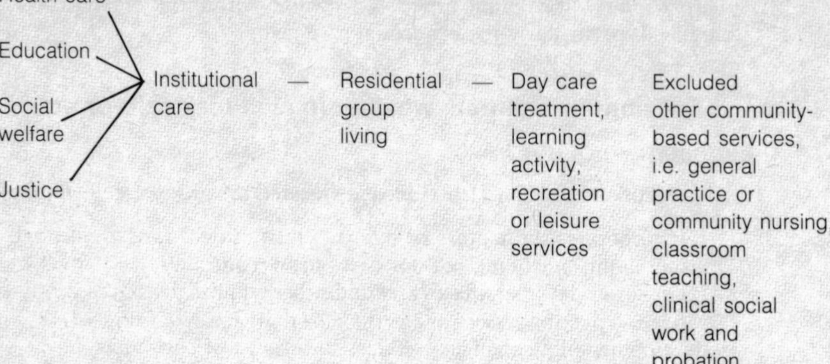

FIGURE 23.1 The group care field across systems. (Ainsworth and Fulcher, 1981)

3. Process evaluations
4. Systems analyses

2 Whittaker (1979) has proposed three models of evaluation:
1. Single subject designs
2. Goal attainment procedures: goals set *with* those concerned.
3. Consumer evaluation: e.g. *Who Cares* (Page and Clark, 1977). See page 219.

3 Payne (1981) has suggested the following models:
1. The 'classical' experimental design, with experimental and control groups, which often emphasize outcome.
2. The 'critical appraisal' model, involving enabling participants to understand the social situation, to take part in the evaluation and to help bring about change. Within this framework, Payne (1981) distinguished:
   (a) Self evaluation, where projects develop their own criteria for evaluation.
   (b) Individual case model, characterized by involving people in agreeing objectives, how to meet them and what will constitute the evidence of attainment. (This is comparable to the goal-attainment model, found useful in a number of forms of evaluation.)
   (c) Evaluation by 'informed observers' who visit a programme and feed back their findings.

4 Research on the residential care of children

4.1 Introductory studies

Payne (1981) noted the shortage of studies, but reported the work of Dinnage and Pringle (1967), who reviewed much previous research upon substitute care for children.

1 **Some early conclusions** Summarizing their conclusions, Dinnage and Pringle (1967) wrote,

> To sum up: there is considerable agreement that the child in care typically – but not of course always – has suffered from both emotional and intellectual handicaps, and functioned in most ways more poorly than his counterpart who is not in care. The unsuitability of residential care for small children is also confirmed, both by intensive current studies and by data on older children with a history of early entry into care.

2 **Later studies** Studies of children's progress in a variety of forms of care have increasd in a number of countries, e.g. Wolins (1974). In Britain, Prosser (1976) reviewed both the American and the sparse British research on the care of children in residential settings, and while noting the further conclusion by Dinnage and Pringle in 1967 that, 'prolonged institutionalization during the early years of life leaves a child very vulnerable to later stress', she added, 'today there appears to be no new evidence which contradicts this.'

Prosser noted, however, the mixed nature of the evidence from such studies as had been conducted, and the shortage of research upon the effects of residential care, associated with, for example, different ages of admission, length of stay and patterns of treatment.

4.2 Later studies of the group care of children

Berridge (1985) has suggested that such studies as have been conducted fall into three groups:

1 Empirical studies of social work practice – including consumer surveys
2 Theories of residential care
3 Evaluations of outcome

These will be considered below.

1 **Empirical studies: social work practice**

1 Berridge has highlighted several studies; these include that of Berry (1975) who, Berridge reported,

> included a group of 11 children's homes in her larger study of 44 residential establishments. Unfortunately the homes were not randomly selected and the fieldwork was undertaken by students on residential placements. Nevertheless, Berry found that two of the 11 children's homes were providing 'positive' daily care; in five, child care was felt to be 'good enough'; but in the remaining four, the homes' care was felt to be 'more negative'.

2 Berridge also noted the DHSS Social Work Service Survey (1982) of thirty children's homes in the London Region. He summarized,

> The report concludes that, although there is variation in provision,

the majority of homes were felt by social work advisers to be adequately meeting children's needs even though some homes continued to be aloof from their neighbourhoods.

3 Berridge (1985) himself made a comparative study of twenty children's homes and identified four broad categories of residents:
(a) short-term reception cases
(b) children awaiting long-term places, usually fostering
(c) those having experienced disrupted care for most of their lives
(d) adolescents in care maintaining close family contact
Among the many issues raised by his study, Berridge highlighted three relating to child care practice:
(a) the changing residential task
(b) problems of maintaining children's family links
(c) difficulties associated with leaving care
He also noted two broader professional issues:
(a) problems of achieving continuity, e.g. in education
(b) the relationship between residential care and fostering

2 **Empirical studies: consumer surveys** Berridge noted the importance of 'consumer surveys', i.e. studies of those who grew up in care, and in particular those of Kahan (1979) and Page and Clark (1977). The latter publication, *Who Cares?* is compiled from the discussions of fourteen young people and four adults who grew up in care; they devised a Charter of rights for young people in care, and a statement of 'Things we want to change'. The latter included:

1 Give us a chance to find a voice and to speak and mix with ordinary people so that public attitudes about care can be changed for the better.
2 Give all young people in care a chance to attend their own six-monthly review. Give us a say in who attends, beside the social worker, his boss and the people we live with. . . . Give all children in care a voice in their life.
3 Do away with the order book and special voucher system for buying our clothing.
4 Help residential workers and field social workers to find ways of working more closely together.
5 Bring pocket money and clothing allowance into line nationally.
6 Help us to have a realistic approach to sex education and personal relationships.
7 Help us to sort out our education while we're young.
8 Make sure every young person in care really understands his situation and why he cannot live with his family.
9 Ask local authorities to decide whether or not corporal punishment is allowed in their children's homes.
10 Find ways of letting us help children younger than ourselves. Give us something to work for while we're in care.

The difficulties of young people leaving care have been reported by e.g. Brearley *et al.* (1982) and Stein and Carey (1986).

3 Theories of residential care

1 Firth (1985) has reported the classification made by Davis (1982) of models of residential care. This classification can be applied to residential care for a range of people in need, including children:
   (a) Family – substitute care: this seeks to model itself on ordinary family life and to provide care 'as good as' family care.
   (b) Family – alternative care: this does not seek to emulate the family, but deliberately provides a different framework: e.g. therapeutic communities.
   (c) Family – supplement care: this, suggested Firth, 'is an attempt to use residential provision in a more flexible way than has been done previously.' It seeks to offer shared care with the family, for example, by offering short periods of 'respite care', so that, basically, the person may remain within the community.

2 Firth has summarized the strengths and weaknesses of each model, noting, for example, the limited power of residential staff in the selection of residents even though such decisions can have major implications for their work. She also noted the tensions which can arise between residential workers and the families of residents, and the many demands made upon the skills and resources of both residential and field workers in their work.

4 Evaluations of outcome

(a) *Outcome studies focusing upon the young people*

1 Reinach and Roberts (1979) conducted a follow-up of sixty-five children admitted to an Observation and Assessment Centre in Hampshire during its first year, 1973–4. Investigating the question of whether professional intervention in the lives of these children actually led to happy outcomes, they concluded that, while acknowledging the shortcomings of their research, it seemed that:
   (a) fifteen (23 per cent) of young people had had positive and happy outcomes.
   (b) thirty-six (55 per cent) experienced some positive periods interspersed with more problematic times in and out of care.
   (c) fourteen (22 per cent) had had negative outcomes, with repeated short-stay breakdowns with foster parents, relatives, lodgings, hostels and Detention Centres. Many were drifting at the time of the study.

2 Berridge (1985) reported the study by Lasson (1980) who investigated a sample of long-stay children in children's homes concentrating on their family links. She found that,

> the natural parents remain highly important for children who live in

residential settings. Children who were visited by their parents were more settled in their placements than those of their peers who retained no such contact.

(b) Outcome studies focusing upon inter-generational effects

1 Rutter, Quinton and Liddle (1983) conducted two studies, one 'retrospective' and one 'prospective' concerning the outcomes of a child's being admitted to care. The latter study followed up 150 children who, in 1964, lived in one of two Children's Homes run on group cottage lines, by comparison with that of 106 children from the same area of inner London, who lived throughout with their families and were never in care.
2 The follow-up groups were defined as those aged between twenty-one and twenty-seven in January 1978; data was obtained from 91 per cent of the 'ex-care' group and from 80 per cent of the contrast group.
3 These researchers' summary, in respect of the women only, included the following:

> First, there can be no doubt that adverse experiences in childhood do indeed predispose to poor parenting in early adult life. Furthermore, this association is quite a strong one – poor parenting was five times as common in the institution-reared group as in the . . . comparison group . . . and overt parenting breakdown was *confined* to the 'ex care' group. . . .
>
> But, although strong, the association was far from inevitable. About a quarter of the institution sample showed good parenting in spite of all their adverse experiences in early life. . . .

4 Rutter, Quinton and Liddle examined a wide range of related issues, and the subtleties of the impacts of multiple variables. They noted:

(i) Poor parenting as part of a broader pattern of poor psycho-social functioning.
(ii) The poor outcome, in terms both of parenting and of psycho-social functioning, for young people from institutional backgrounds who were showing disturbed behaviour in childhood and adolescence.
(iii) The beneficial outcome of a stable and harmonious relationship with a marital partner.

5 A study of social work decisions in child care

5.1 Studies summarized in the report

This report, published by the DHSS (1985), examined social work decisions in child care in general. It drew upon nine inter-related studies:

1 A study by Packman, Randall and Jacques (1986) of 361 cases of children admitted to care in two contrasting local authorities.
2 A study by Millham, Bullock, Hosie and Haak (1985) of 450 children, and their experiences in care. Among its conclusions relating to these authorities were:

> If a child remains in local authority care for longer than five weeks, it has a very strong chance (two out of three cases) of still being in care two years later;
>
> The maintenance of close contact with their families is the best indicator that a child will leave local authority care rapidly;
>
> Children and adolescents, even if their chances of returning home are slight, function better psychologically, socially and educationally if they remain in regular contact with their families.

3 A study by Vernon and Fruin (1985) concerning 185 children – some in care already and some coming into care, and how crucial decisions were made at key points in their experience. The authors reported that the study, 'found that social workers did not actively plan what should happen to children once they came into care.'
4 A study by Fisher, Marsh, Phillips and Sainsbury (1986) of the perceptions and experiences of care of seventy-nine children, their parents and social workers. Readers are referred to the study for an account of their important conclusions.
5 A study by Rowe, Cain, Hundleby and Keane (1984) concerning 200 children in long-term foster care, compared with those whose foster parents adopt them. (See Chapter 24, page 241)
6 A study by Sinclair (1984), concerning statutory reviews of children in care.
7 A study by Hilgendorf (1981), concerning the process of decision-making in care order cases, and focusing on 150 social workers and fifty lawyers.
8 A study by Adcock, White and Rowlands (1983), concerning 267 children affected by S.3 of the Children Act·1975.
9 An unpublished research report by Stevenson and Smith, concerning the implementation of S. 56 of the Children Act 1975 as it related to 339 cases from eleven authorities.

5.2 A summary of the main findings of the research

The compilers of the report highlighted 'six main messages':

'1 The depth, complexity and long-standing nature of child care problems makes them fiendishly difficult to deal with. . . . Yet the main responsibility lies with those on the lowest rung of the hierarchy who usually lack the seniority and power to gain access to key resources.
2 At present the system tends to constrain rather than support and 'caring

for the carers' receives little attention in social services departments . . . there is also a lack of well-thought out relevant policies which would provide a general framework of support.

3 Our huge bureaucratic structures make it difficult to provide good enough parenting for the individual child in care.
4 It seems very apparent that the deep emotional problems generated by the separation/care experience receive insufficient attention (parents feel ignored and direct work with children is minimal).
5 There is no adequate, comprehensive research, practice or value base which would help practitioners to decide when admission to care would be appropriate and for which groups of children. . . . There has been virtually no monitoring of outcomes and child care lacks even the level of research attention given to delinquency.
6 There is an overwhelming impression of social workers' passivity and their feelings of helplessness and being at the mercy of events and actions of other people and other agencies. . . . But the combined messages from these nine research studies do seem to be that social workers and their seniors are not offered the opportunity to acquire the sophisticated skills, knowledge and qualitative experience to equip them to deal confidently with the complex and extremely emotive issues raised by work with children and families.'

6 Research upon care-givers

6.1 A study of students training for residential work

1 Millham, Bullock and Hosie (1980) followed the progress of 201 people training for residential work with young people upon six full-time courses. They gathered both pre- and post-course data from 138 respondents, and gathered follow-up data from forty.
2 They found,
   (a) Of the forty people who returned the follow-up questionnaire after one year, '27 (68 per cent) of our respondents had ceased working directly and constantly in therapeutic or caring roles.'
   (b) Thirty-eight experienced difficulties on returning to their work situations, including the feeling that colleagues were not interested in what they had to offer.
   (c) Most valued their training and said that it gave them more confidence in working with children, but they were more aware of e.g., bureaucratic frustrations.
   (d) Training which was family-oriented seemed very beneficial in extending the students' understanding of the network of interactions of which the child was part.

7 Resources for staff development

A comprehensive survey of references and additional material as they relate to the residential care of children and other groups may be found in Douglas and Payne (1985).

References

Adcock, M., White, R. and Rowlands, O. (1983), *The Administrative Parent: A study of the assumption of parental rights and duties*, London: British Agencies for Adoption and Fostering.

Ainsworth, F. and Fulcher, L. C. (eds) (1981), *Group Care for Children: Concepts and Issues*. London: Tavistock Publications.

Oxford Berridge, D. (1985), *Children's Homes*, Oxford: Basil Blackwell.

Berry, J. (1975), *Daily Experiences in Residential Life: A Study of Children and their Care-givers*, London: Routledge & Kegan Paul.

Brearley, P., Black, J., Entridge, P., Roberts, G. and Tarran, E. (1982) *Leaving Residential Care*, London: Tavistock Publications.

Davis, A. (1982), *Residential Care: A Community Resource*, London: Heinemann.

Department of Health and Social Security, *Health and Personal Social Services Statistics for England*, 1985 edition, London: HMSO.

Department of Health and Social Security (1985), *Social Work Decisions in Child Care*, London: HMSO.

Dinnage, R. and Pringle, K. (1967), *Residential Child Care: Facts and Fallacies*, London: Longman.

Douglas, R. and Payne, C. (1985), *Developing Residential Practice: A Sourcebook of References and Resources for Staff Development*, London: National Institute for Social Work.

Durkin, R. P. and Durkin, A. B. (1975), 'Evaluating residential treatment programmes for disturbed children', in M. Guttentag and E. L. Strurning (eds), *Handbook of Evaluation Research*, vol. 2, Beverly Hills: Sage.

Firth, B. (1985), 'Practice in residential care' in J. Lishman and E. Horobin (eds), *Developing Services for the Elderly*, Research Highlights in Social Work 3, Aberdeen, University of Aberdeen Department of Social Work: Kogan Page.

Fisher, M., Marsh, P. and Phillips, D. with Sainsbury, E. (1986), *In and Out of Care. The experience of children, parents and social workers*, London: Batsford/BAAF.

Hilgendorf, L. (1981), *Social Workers and Solicitors in Child Care Cases*, London: HMSO.

Kahan, B. (1979), *Growing up in Care*, Oxford: Blackwell.

Lasson, I. (1980), *Where's My Mum? A study of the forgotten children in long term care*, Birmingham: PEPAR publications.

Millham, S., Bullock, R. and Hosie, K. (1980), *Learning to Care*, Farnborough: Gower Publishing Co.

Millham, S., Bullock, R., Hosie, K. and Haak, M. (1985), *Children Lost in Care. The family contact of children in care*, Farnborough: Gower Publishing Co.

Moss, P. (1975), 'Residential care of children: a general view' in J. Tizard, I. Sinclair and R. V. G. Clarke (eds), *Varieties of Residential Experience*, London: Routledge & Kegan Paul.

Packman, J., Randall, J. and Jacques, N. (1986), *Who Needs Care? Social work decisions about children*, Oxford: Blackwell.
Page R. and Clark, G. A. (1977), *Who Cares?*, London: National Children's Bureau.
Payne, C. (1981), 'Research and evaluation' in F. Ainsworth and L. C. Fulcher (eds), *Group Care for Children*.
Prosser, H. (1976), *Perspectives on Child Care*, Windsor: National Foundation for Educational Research/National Children's Bureau.
Reinach, E. and Roberts, G. (1979), *Consequences – the Progress of 65 Children after a Period of Observation and Assessment*, Portsmouth Polytechnic/Hants Social Services Department: Social Services and Research Unit.
Rowe, J., Cain, H., Hundleby, M. and Kean, A. (1984), *Long Term Foster Care*, Batsford/BAAF.
Rutter, M., Quinton, D. and Liddle, C. (1983), 'Parenting in two generations: Looking backwards and looking forwards' in N. Madge (ed.), *Families at Risk*, DHSS and Heinemann Educational Books.
Sinclair, R. (1984), *Decision Making in Statutory Reviews on Children in Care*, Farnborough: Gower Publishing Co.
Stein, M. and Carey, K. (1986), *Leaving Care*, Oxford: Basil Blackwell.
Stevenson, O. and Smith, J., *The Implementation of Section 56 of the Children Act 1975*, Unpublished research report.
Vernon, J. and Fruin, D. (1985), *In Care: A Study of Social Work Decision Making*, London National Children's Bureau.
Whittaker, J. (1979), *Caring for Troubled Children, Residential Treatment in a Community Context*. London: Jossey-Bass.
Wolins, M. (1974), *Successful Group Care. Explorations in the Powerful Environment*, Chicago: Aldine.

24

Research concerning child abuse and child sexual abuse

Consultant:* *Raymond Castle, Child Abuse Consultant, National Society for the Prevention of Cruelty to Children, London.

1 A categorization and a definition

1.1 A broad categorization

1 Physical or emotional violence to children.
2 Physical or emotional neglect of children.
3 Child sexual abuse.

1.2 A definition of physical abuse of children

Gil (1970) defined this as,

> the intentional, nonaccidental use of force on the part of the parent or other caretaker interacting with a child in his care aimed at hurting, injuring or destroying that child.

1.3 A definition of child sexual abuse

Kempe and Kempe (1978) suggested:

> Sexual abuse is defined as the involvement of dependent, developmentally immature children and adolescents in sexual activities they do not truly comprehend, to which they are unable to give informed consent, or that violate the social taboos of family roles.

The British Association for the Study and Prevention of Child Abuse and Neglect included within the definition the following:

a) Incest.
b) Sexual intercourse with children in other relationships not covered by current incest legislation, including adopted children and step-children.
c) Other forms of sexual activity, including fondling, mutual masturbation and involving children in pornographic activity.

2 Prevalence

Figures are available from different sources:

2.1 Official statistics: selected data

		Age Under 1 yr	Age 1–4	Age 5–9	Age 10–14	Total
Homicide and injury, purposely inflicted	1982	13	19	11	7	50
	1983	15	22	3	5	45
Injury undetermined whether accidentally or purposely inflicted	1982	23	15	9	15	62
	1983	16	19	6	6	47

TABLE 24.1 Deaths of children in England and Wales, 1982 and 1983 (*Mortality Statistics*, OPCS, 1983, 1984)

2.2 Data from the NSPCC Special Unit Registers

The NSPCC maintains a number of Special Units concerned with child abuse, and children brought to the attention of unit officers, and who meet specific criteria, are registered there. Creighton (1984), reporting the data for 1977–1982, has written:

> 6532 children were placed on registers of child abuse maintained by NSPCC Special Units during 1977 to 1982. Of these, 4679 (71.6%) had been abused and 1810 (27.7%) were thought to be at serious risk of abuse.

Selected data is shown in Table 24.2.

	1982		1983		1984	
	No.	%	No.	%	No.	%
Physically injured	661	84.4	672	80.9	707	78.2
Fatal	3	0.4	3	0.4	3	0.3
Serious	64	8.2	54	6.5	56	6.2
Moderate	594	75.9	615	74.0	648	71.7
Other abuse	122	15.6	159	19.1	200	22.1
Failure to thrive	21	2.7	15	1.8	34	3.8
Sexual abuse	40	5.1	51	6.1	98	10.8
Neglect	44	5.6	62	7.5	50	5.5
Emotional abuse	17	2.2	31	3.7	18	2.0
Total	783	100	831	100	904	100
Physically injured rate per 1,000 under 15s	0.63		0.70		0.73	
Physically injured rate per 1,000 under 5s	1.20		1.15		1.19	

TABLE 24.2 Number of registered children by year and type and severity of abuse (Creighton, 1984, NSPCC, 1985)

N.B. Creighton noted:

> Child abuse continues to increase. . . . Over the six-year period 1979–1984 the physical abuse of children has increased by 70% from 0.43 per thousand children under 15 in 1979 to 0.73 in 1984.

2.3 Data concerning incest

Official figures of incest offenders are shown in Table 24.3

	1981	1982	1983	1984
Incest	143	133	152	162

TABLE 24.3 Offenders found guilty at all courts or sentenced for indictable sexual offences by offence. (Number of offenders.) (Home Office, *Criminal Statistics*, England and Wales, 1984, HMSO)

2.4 Particular studies of prevalence in the UK

1 **An early study of prevalence** Baldwin and Oliver (1975) examined prevalence in a county in southern England. Only children under four years of age, who met one or more of the following criteria were included:

> Prolonged assaults of such severity that death ensued.
> Skull or facial bone fractures.
> Bleeding into or around the brain, or damage to the central nervous system.
> To or more instances of mutilation requiring medical attention.
> Three or more separate instances of fracture.
> Multiple fractures and/or severe internal injuries.

Using these criteria, Baldwin and Oliver found an incidence of one per thousand children suffering severe abuse, while 0.1 per thousand suffered death (i.e. one per ten thousand).

2 **An overview of British data** Gardner and Gray (1982) report the evidence to the Select Committee on Violence in the Family given by Scott (1977) who 'reports data from several British studies indicating that between one and 12 children per thousand are abused by their parents or guardians.'

Gardner and Gray noted, however, the variability among definitions of 'abuse'.

2.5 A summary statement on prevalence in the USA

Gardner and Gray (1982) reported:

> In the United States, Gil (1970) estimated that there were between 2.5 and 4.1 million cases of child abuse per year. Later investigators

> suggested lower figures of 1.5 million . . . to 50 000 . . . while Gelles (1977) reported that approximately 500 000 American children were either threatened with a gun or a knife or actually attacked by their parents in 1975.

2.6 Prevalence of child sexual abuse in the UK

1 **Data gathered via a postal survey** The British Association for the Study and Prevention of Child Abuse and Neglect report a study by Beezley Mrazek, Lynch and Bentovim (1981) who conducted a postal survey with relevant professionals and reported on 1,065 cases:

		%
Type I	A battered child whose injuries are primarily in the genital area;	4
Type II	A child who has experienced attempted or actual intercourse, or other inappropriate genital contact with an adult;	69
Type III	A child who has been inappropriately involved with an adult in sexual activities, not covered by I and II.	16

TABLE 24.4 Prevalence of child sexual abuse in the U.K. (Beezley Mrazek, Lynch and Bentovim, 1981)

The authors added:

> It should be noted that a further 11% of cases in Type II and Type III were associated with physical abuse as well as those reported in Type I abuse.

2 **Projected figures for the country based on Table 24.3** The same authors suggested:

> A projection of the incidence figures to the whole country suggests an absolute minimum of 1,500 cases per year, an incidence of one in 6,000 children per year or 3 in 1,000 children over the whole of childhood.

3 Child physical abuse: research which contributes to an understanding

3.1 The emergence of a multi-variate model

1. Research findings are far from being integrated. Since the early research of the phenomenon of child abuse by Kempe and colleagues (1962), who took a psychiatric perspective, other researchers have shown that a multiplicity of variables is involved.
2. Increasingly, a framework has been developed for beginning to

understand child abuse as a circumstance to which many variables – sociological, psychological and sometimes psychiatric – contribute. Such a model, devised by Gelles (1972) and concerning family violence in general, is shown in Figure 24.1.

3 Further, Gardner and Gray (1982) highlighted the importance of cognitive factors in child abuse, particularly how the abusers *perceive* the child's behaviour, and the precipitating events which led to the violent incident.

3.2 Research indicating sociological-psychological variables associated with child physical abuse

1 **Some American findings** A summary by Solomon (1980) noted the following characteristics:

A The Abused Child

1 Average age under 4 years, most under 2.
2 Average death rate: 5% to 25%.
3 Average age at death: slightly under 3 years.
4 Average duration of exposure to battering: 1 to 3 years.
5 Sex differentiation: none.

B The Abusive Parent

1 Marital status: overwhelming majority were married and living together at the time of the abuse.
2 Average age of abusive mother: 26 years.
3 Average age of abusive father: 30 years.
4 Abusive parent: father slightly more often than mother.
5 Most serious abuse: mother more often than father.
6 Most common instrument for abuse: hairbrush.

C Family Dynamics

1 Thirty to sixty per cent of abusing parents claim to have been abused as children themselves.
2 High proportion of premarital conceptions.
3 Youthful marriage.
4 Unwanted pregnancies.
5 Illegitimacies.
6 Forced marriages.
7 Social and kinship isolation.
8 Emotional problems in marriage.
9 Financial difficulty.

2 **A further American review of key variables associated with violence at home** In his overview of the research literature, Gelles (1982) suggests that,

> Current research indicates that a number of factors are associated with child abuse, wife abuse and family violence.

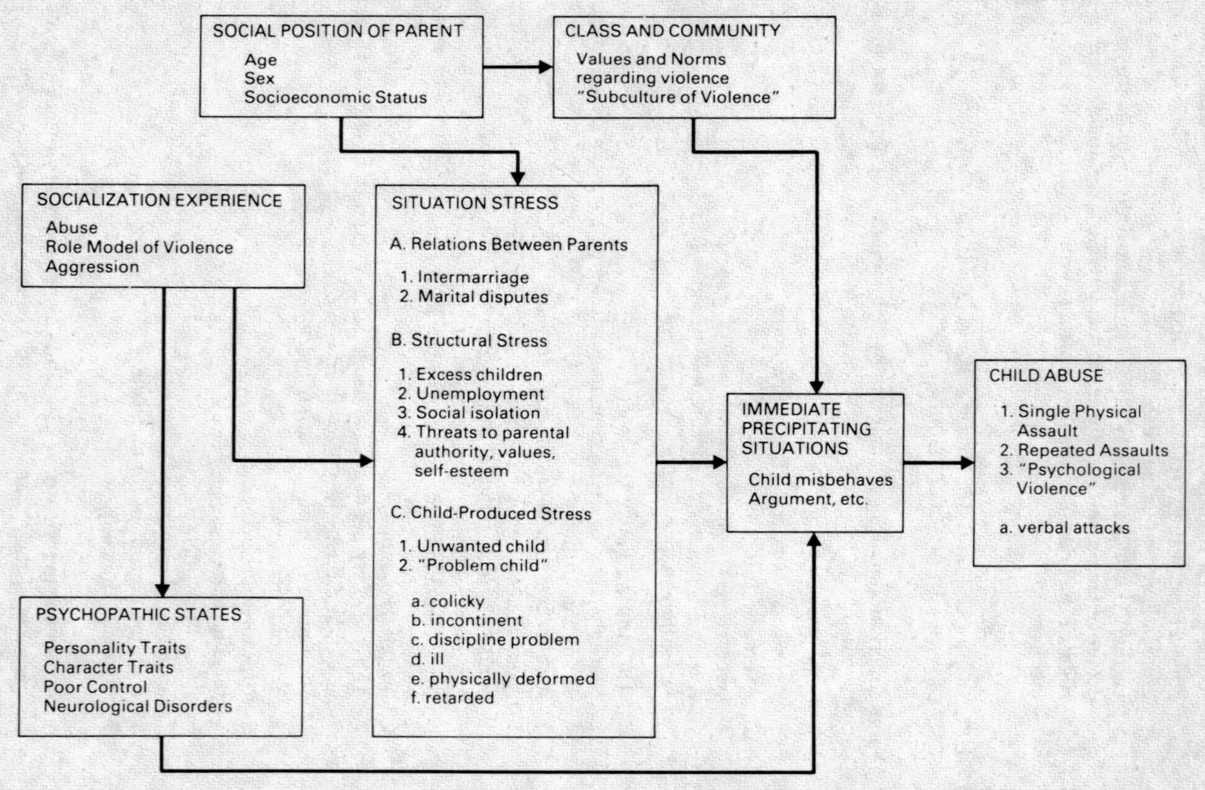

FIGURE 24.1 A social psychological model of the causes of child abuse. Gelles (1979)

1 *The cycle of violence* One of the consistent conclusions of research on child abuse and domestic violence is that individuals who have experienced violent and abusive households are more likely to grow up to becime child and spouse abusers than individuals who experienced little or no violence in their childhood years.
2 *Socioeconomic status* Current research on family violence supports the hypothesis that abuse is more prevalent among those with low economic status. . . . This conclusion, however, does not mean that domestic violence is *confined* to lower-class households. Investigators reporting the differential distribution of violence are frequently careful to point out that child and spouse abuse can be found in families across the spectrum of socio-economic status.
3 *Stress* A third consistent finding of most domestic violence research is that rates of family violence are directly related to social stress in families . . . investigators report associations between various forms of family violence and specific stressful situations and conditions, such as (1) unemployment or part-time employment of males . . . (2) financial problems . . . (3) pregnancy, in the case of wife abuse . . . and (4) single-parent families, in the case of child abuse.
4 *Social isolation* A fourth major finding in the study of both child and spouse abuse is that social isolation raises the risk of severe violence directed at children or between spouses. . .

Gelles noted, however, the need to exercise caution in accepting these findings uncritically: the above factors are *associations* not causes, and are themselves of differing weightings. Further, the research in this field is of very great complexity, and often with small samples.

3 **Some additional British research** Gardner and Gray (1982), writing from the perspective of social learning theory, suggest the following antecedents are involved in child abuse

Historical and social	Isolated from family and friends
	Marital conflict
	Wanted child of the opposite sex
	Deprived social conditions
Immediate	Crying; refusal of food
Overt	Close proximity to child
	Demanding child
	Family conflict of interests
Cognitive	Perception of child's behaviour (e.g. refusal to smile)
	Unrealistic expectations of child
	Unrealistic expectations of parenthood.

TABLE 24.5 Possible antecedents to child abuse (Gardner and Gray, 1982)

4 Research which contributes to understanding how to prevent child physical abuse

4.1 Possible symptoms and signs of physical abuse

Cooper (1978) has drawn up the following list of injuries in children which need careful attention and scrutiny so that child abuse can be ruled out:

bruises, lacerations, wheals and scars;
burns and scalds;
fractures and joint injuries;
brain and eye injuries;
internal injuries to abdomen and chest;
poisoning;
sudden infant death ('cot death syndrome');
drowning;
sexual abuse

Cooper highlights the evidence that '*Skin signs are present in over 90 per cent of all abused children.*'

4.2 Research which attempts to detect children and families at risk of child abuse

A number of different check lists have been devised as pointers of risk of child abuse. Several are quoted in Pringle (1980). Table 24.6 shows that devised by Greenland (1979), quoted because it encompasses variables relating both to parents and children. No special method of scoring is given.

4.3 Child physical abuse: increasing recognition of its multi-variate causation

In view of this increasing recognition among researchers, e.g. Gelles (1982), and Gambrill (1983), efforts towards prevention and intervention are aimed both at taking account of as many variables as possible, such as stress, isolation, and child management problems, and at integrating services.

4.4 Approaches from a sociological/community perspective

1 **In the USA** Kempe and Helfer (1978) described a number of innovative approaches whereby parents considered to be at risk of battering their children are encouraged to make use of a range of community facilities organized both by professionals and by volunteers. These include:

(a) Parent aides: people from all walks of life who offer positive and non-judgmental support in a friendly and practical way.
(b) Foster grandparents: people over sixty-five who take the role of grandparent and visit and play with children in hospital.

Parents	Child
Previously having abused, neglected a child.	Was previously abused or neglected.
Age 20 or less at age of first child.	Under five years of age at the time of abuse or neglect.
Single parent or separated	Premature or low birth-weight.
Partner not biological parent.	Now under-weight.
History of abuse, neglect or deprivation.	Birth defect, chronic illness, developmental lag.
Socially isolated, frequent moves, poor housing.	Prolonged separation from mother.
Poverty, unemployed or unskilled worker.	Cries frequently, difficult to comfort.
Inadequate education.	Difficulties in feeding and elimination.
Abuses alcohol and/or drugs.	Adopted, foster or step-child.
History of criminal assaultive behaviour and/or suicide attempts.	
Pregnancy, post-partum or chronic illness.	

TABLE 24.6 Child abuse: high risk rating check list. Greenland (1979). Revised 1986.

(c) Mothers anonymous: a self-help group offering support and understanding among members.

2 In the UK

(a) Voluntary visiting schemes A number of helping organizations have been established in many towns and cities, through which volunteers offer support and friendship to isolated and demoralized parents, and are able to liaise with the statutory services. Homestart is a well-known organization of this kind.

(b) Voluntary telephone support schemes A number of places also have Parents Anonymous telephone services, whereby distressed and frightened parents can receive supportive help from other parents or from volunteers.

4.5 Approaches from a psychological/social learning theory perspective

1 Research in teaching child management skills Encouraging results have been reported in a survey of the literature by Gambrill (1983) upon behavioural intervention with child abuse and neglect. Acknowledging the need for a multi-variate conceptualization, however, she wrote, 'The literature clearly calls for an ecological approach in which individual, family, community and societal factors are considered.'

She summarized,

> Reports suggest that a behavioural approach is promising. Attention to enhancement of child management skills is supported by research that shows that most abuse occurs as an extension of parental discipline attempts. . . . If applied faithfully, a behavioural approach offers come unique advantages, such as identification of clear outcomes, on-going evaluation of progress, and clear description of procedures. . . . The emphasis on an educational approach involves clients as responsible participants, and encourages them to learn new skills that can help them to exert greater influence on their environment in a more efficient way.

2 **Social learning theory and failure to thrive children** Encouraging progress in teaching the parents of children who fail to thrive has been reported by Iwaniec, Herbert and McNeish (1985); these researchers employed a social learning theory behavioural framework.

5 Research concerning child sexual abuse

5.1 Incestuous relationships

Bluglass (1979) reported the research thus,

> Sibling relationships are probably the most frequent form of incest . . ., although father–daughter incest is the most commonly reported type. Stepfather–stepdaughter relationships (although not legally incest), are equally common. . . .

5.2 Social class and background

Bluglass (1979) reported, 'Incest occurs in all social class groups although it tends, like non-accidental injury to children, to be more easily concealed in the high socioeconomic categories.'

Nelson (1982) reported the work of Forward and Buck (1981) who worked with 300 incest cases,

> (the families) came from every economic, cultural, racial, educational, religious and geographical background. They are doctors, policemen, prostitutes, secretaries, artists and merchants. They are heterosexual, bisexual and homosexual. They are happily married and four times divorced . . . they are emotionally stable and they have multiple personalities. . . .

5.3 Personality characteristics

Maisch (1973) studied sixty-seven paternal offenders, and Bluglass (1979) reported that while about 50 per cent had one or more of the features of alcoholism, tendencies to violence or a previous criminal record, the other 50 per cent appeared to be a relatively 'normal' group without distinguishing characteristics.

6 Research concerning responses to child sexual abuse

6.1 How child sexual abuse comes to light

The authors of *Child Sexual Abuse* (1981) suggested that the majority of cases coming to light do so via a relative, friend or parent or occasionally by the children themselves; some come via anonymous telephone calls to agencies or the police. They reported:

> Other cases present in a more veiled manner, either through behavioural disturbances in children of varying ages, such as running away, hysterical behaviour, or the sudden onset of learning difficulties in school, psychosomatic complaints such as persistent abdominal pains, headaches, sleeplessness or physical symptoms such as cystitis or gonococcal infections (e.g. vaginal discharge, lesions of the anus and pharyngitis).

6.2 Research concerning imprisonment/treatment responses

There is tension between those who favour a response based upon a primarily legal perspective and those who favour a treatment approach. Research in this area is exceedingly difficult and sparse.

1 **Imprisonment** Bluglass (1979) has reported that about half of cases sent for trial received a sentence of imprisonment, usually one to three years, although longer sentences, of up to six to seven years, were given for offences involving daughters under the age of sixteen years.

2 **Treatment, and its critics**

1. The best-known treatment approach is that developed in California by Giarretto (1978). This involves individual and family counselling, communication training and support from former participants in the programme. Giarretto claims only 0.6% recidivism rate, and Renvoize (1982) has commented that: 'in spite of the police being aware of every reported case, over half of the known offenders were not sent to jail.' She added that such an approach has led to much more frequent reporting of the offence, and that over half the child victims never left home at all.
2. Kempe and Kempe (1978) have criticized Giarretto's claims, and the criteria for 'successful outcome': i.e. the reunification of the family. They have also pointed to the need for very long-term follow-up studies.

6.3 A response from the Women's movement

Some feminists have responded very sharply to what they see as assumptions made by some researchers. For example Nelson (1982) has highlighted what she regards as some myths about incest:

(a) Incest is an accepted part of some sub-cultures.
(b) The notion of 'child collusion' or 'victim blame'.
(c) Incest reflects a caring relationship.
(d) Mothers collude with incest.
(e) The man is a deviant.
(f) Incest is a sign of a disorganized family.

Many members of the Women's movement see incest primarily as an abuse of power and a crime.

References

Adcock, M. and White, R. (eds) (1985), *Good-enough parenting. A framework for assessment*, London: British Agencies for Adoption and Fostering.

Baldwin, J. A. and Oliver, J. E. (1975), 'Epidemiology and family characteristics of severely-abused children', *British Journal of Preventive and Social Medicine*, vol. 29, pp. 205–21.

Beezley Mrazek, P., Lynch, M. and Bentovim, A. (1981), 'Sexual Abuse of Children in the United Kingdom', *Journal of Child Abuse and Neglect*, vol. 7, no. 2, pp. 147–53.

Bluglass, R. (1979), 'Incest', *British Journal of Hospital Medicine*, vol. 22, pp. 152–7.

British Association for the Study and Prevention of Child Abuse and Neglect (1981), *Child Sexual Abuse*, London: BASPCAN.

British Association of Social Workers (1985), *Report on the Management of Child Abuse*, Birmingham: BASW.

Ciba Foundation, *Child sexual abuse within the family*, Ruth Porter (ed.), London: Tavistock.

Cooper, C. (1978), 'Symptoms, signs and diagnosis of physical abuse' in V. Carver (ed.), *Child Abuse: A Study Text*, Milton Keynes: Open University.

Creighton, S. (1984), *Trends in Child Abuse. 1977–1981*, The fourth report on the children placed on NSPCC Special Unit Registers, London: NSPCC.

Fontana, V. (1973), *Somewhere a Child is Crying: Maltreatment – its Causes and Prevention*, New York: Macmillan.

Forward, S. and Buck, C. (1981), *Betrayal of Innocence: Incest and its Devastation*, London: Pelican Books.

Gambrill, E. (1983), 'Behavioural intervention with child abuse and neglect' in *Progress in Behavior Modification*, vol. 15, New York: Academic Press, Inc.

Gardner, J. and Gray, M. (1982), 'Violence towards children' in P. Feldman (ed.), *Developments in the Study of Criminal Behaviour*, vol. 2, Chichester: John Wiley and Sons.

Gelles, R. J. (1972), *The Violent Home*, Beverly Hills: Sage Publications.

Gelles, R. J. (1977), 'Violence towards children in the United States', Paper presented at the annual meeting of the American Association for the Advancement of Science.

Gelles, R. J. (1979), *Family Violence*, Beverly Hills: Sage Publications.

Gelles, R. J. (1982), 'Child abuse and family violence: Implications for medical professionals' in E. Newberger (ed.), *Child Abuse*, Boston: Little, Brown & Co.

Giarretto, H. (1978), 'Humanistic treatment of father-daughter incest', *Child Abuse and Neglect*, vol. 1, pp. 411–26.

Gil, D. G. (1970), *Violence Against Children*, Cambridge, Mass.: Harvard University Press.

Greenland, C. (1979), 'A checklist to recognise a possible situation for child abuse', *Contact*, vol. 10, p. 23, McMaster University.

Iwaniec, D., Herbert, M. and McNeish, A. S. (1985), 'Social work with failure-to-thrive children and their families', *British Journal of Social Work*, vol. 15, pp. 243–59.

Kempe, C. H., Silverman, F. N., Steele, B. B., Droegemueller, N. and Silver, H. K. (1962), 'The battered child syndrome', *Journal of the American Medical Association*, vol. 181, pp. 17–24.

Kempe, C. H. and Helfer, R. E. (1978), 'Innovative therapeutic approaches' in C. Lee (ed.), *Child Abuse: a Reader and Sourcebook*, Milton Keynes: Open University.

Kempe, R. S. and Kempe, C. H. (1978), *Child Abuse*, London: Fontana/Open Books.

Maisch, H. (1973), *Incest*, London: Andre Deutsch.

NSPCC (1985), *Child Abuse in 1983 and 1984. Initial Findings from N.S.P.C.C. Register Research. Research Briefing No. 6*, London: National Society for the Prevention of Cruelty to Children.

Nelson, S. (1982), *Incest, Fact and Myth*, Stramullion.

OPCS (1983, 1984), *Mortality Statistics* 1984, London: HMSO.

Pringle, M. Kellmer (1980), 'Towards the prediction of child abuse' in N. Frude (ed.), *Psychological Approaches to Child Abuse*, London: Batsford Academic and Educational Ltd.

Renvoize, J. (1982), *Incest*, London: Routledge & Kegan Paul.

Scott, P. D. (1977), 'Non-accidental injury to children', *British Journal of Psychiatry*, vol. 131, pp. 366–80.

Solomon, T. (1980), 'History and demography of child abuse' in J. Cook and R. T. Bowles (eds), *Child Abuse: Commission and Omission*, Butterworth and Company (Canada), Ltd.

25 Research concerning fostering

Consultant: Tony Hall, Director, Central Council for Education and Training in Social Work, London; formerly Director, British Agencies for Adoption and Fostering, London.

1 A definition and a classification

1.1 A definition

The following is suggested by British Agencies for Adoption and Fostering (1983): 'Fostering is a way of providing family life for children who for various reasons cannot live with their own parents.'

1.2 Types of foster placement

The following classification has been suggested by the British Association of Social Workers (1982):

(i) *Relief care* to assist parents who may have a handicapped child or who may themselves suffer from handicapping conditions. . . .
(ii) *Holiday fostering*. . . .
(iii) *Pre-adoptive fostering* the fostering of babies for a short period prior to placing with adoptive parents. . . .
(iv) *Short-term fostering* the legal term would be eight weeks or a maximum of ten, but in practice is considered to be up to six or eight months. . . .
(v) *Task-related fostering* the foster parents are employed to achieve a task – preparation for adoption of an older child, treatment of maladjustment, rehabilitation of delinquents etc.
(vi) *Medium-term fostering* i.e. longer than short-term but not having permanence as the objective. . . .
(vii) *Long-term fostering* where permanence is intended but legal adoption is either not desired or cannot be achieved. . . .
(viii) *Fostering with the hope of adoption* where adoption is seen to be the best plan for a child but may not yet be legally obtainable. . . .
(ix) *Adoption* legally quite distinct. . . .

2 Statistics

2.1 Official statistics: selected data

The number of children in care and their differing forms of accommodation, including those boarded out, i.e. fostered, is shown in Table 25.1.

England and Wales at 31 March each year					Percentages
	1976	1978	1980	1982	1983
Boarded out	33	34	37	42	44
Community homes	35	32	30	27	24
Voluntary homes and hostels	5	4	4	3	2
Under care of parent, guardian, relative or friend	18	19	18	18	18
Other	10	11	11	10	10
Number of children in care	100,600	100,700	100,200	93,200	86,600

TABLE 25.1 Accommodation of children in care (*Children in Care in England and Wales*. DHSS, March, 1981; March, 1982; March, 1983. Quoted in *Annual Review of British Agencies for Adoption and Fostering*, 1985.)

2.2 Points to be noted from the above figures

1 The decreasing total number of children in care.
2 The increase in fostering by comparison with other forms of care.
3 The decreasing number of children in local authority or voluntary homes: i.e. 26 per cent in 1983 compared with 40 per cent in 1976.

3 Research concerning children who are fostered

3.1 A major study of children waiting in care

Rowe and Lambert (1973) studied 2,812 children under the age of eleven in thirty-three voluntary and statutory agencies throughout the UK. All had been in care for at least six months. Some of their findings, published in *Children Who Wait*, were that,

1 22% (626 children) were thought by their social worker to need a substitute family: i.e. fostering or adoption.
2 61% were expected by their social worker to remain in care until they were 18 years old; restoration to their families was expected for only 25%.
3 55% of the school age children had already been in care for more than 4 years, and most for the greater part of their lives.
4 41% had no parental contact at all; 35% saw one or both parents occasionally; the longer the children remained in care, the less parental contact they had.
5 2 out of 3 of the children were boys; 2 out of 3 were school age children, and 1 in 4 was black, most often full or part Afro-Caribbean.
6 Behaviour problems were noted more frequently than any other difficulty.
7 More than half the children needing placement were living with siblings for whom homes were also required.
8 Perceived difficulties in finding substitute homes included
   (a) Problems of finding places for more than one child at a time or else splitting family groups.
   (b) Doubts about foster parents' abilities to cope with the children's problems.
   (c) The natural parents' attitudes to the children's being placed.
   (d) The colour, behaviour problems and deprivation of the children.

3.2 A further study in the U.K.

Thorpe (1974) interviewed a sample of 121 children aged five to seventeen in long-term foster care in a Midlands local authority. Natural parents and social workers were also interviewed. Findings included:

1 39 per cent of the children scored a rating indicating 'seriously disturbed' on the Rutter Behaviour Questionnaire, compared with 23 per cent of a sample of children of similar social mix not in care.
2 Those children who entered care at age five or older were less disturbed than those who experienced separation before five. The most vulnerable children were those placed between two and four.
3 The mean length of stay of the children was six years; 87 per cent of the children were expected to remain in the foster home until eighteen.
4 26 per cent had a good understanding of their family background and why they were being fostered.
   50 per cent had some, but an inadequate, understanding.
   22 per cent had no understanding.
   Those with a better understanding were better adjusted.

3.3 Outcomes of fostering and other forms of care

Triseliotis (1980) compared outcomes of children growing up in a number of forms of care. Rowe (1983) has summarized these two studies:

The first looked at growing up in foster care; the second dealt with issues of identity and security in long-term fostering and adoption and pointed out some of the problems foster children face. Triseliotis found that young adults who had grown up in long-term foster care were generally less secure and confident than those who had been adopted. He concludes that the ambiguous nature of fostering relationships seemed to have had a qualitative impact on the foster child's sense of identity.

3.4 A study of long-term foster care

Rowe, Cain, Hundleby and Keane (1984) reported their study of 145 children in successful (i.e. enduring) long-term foster care of between four and eighteen years. They concluded that,

(a) these long-term foster placements could be considered very successful in that these children 'did not just live with their foster families, they became part of them'.
(b) the families did not match well to the criteria of 'inclusive fostering' put forward by Holman (1980): see 4.4, below.
(c) such placements can, but do not always manage to, give to children a sense of permanence and security.

4 Research concerning the natural parents of foster children

4.1 Early studies

1 George (1970) studied how far natural parents felt themselves actively encouraged to maintain contact with their children by the social workers concerned.

    03.8 per cent felt actively encouraged to maintain contact.
    40.6 per cent felt actively discouraged.
    44.3 per cent felt the social workers showed a complete passivity.

2 Shaw and Lebens (1976) found that social workers in the county which they studied thought that the amount of parental visiting was satisfactory for 60 per cent of the foster children whom they supervised, although only 9 per cent saw their parents as often as once a month.

4.2 A study of factors influencing length of stay in care, including foster care

Aldgate (1980) studied length of stay of nearly 200 children, almost all of whom had been received voluntarily into care, in two local authorities in Scotland. She found:

1 Children seemed to have most chance of return when they were received into care from two-parent families living in stable accommodation, or

from one-parent families headed by their mother following marital breakdown.

2 Most at risk of remaining in long-term care were children of young, one-parent families.
3 Eviction counted for over one third of the receptions into care; where the main cause of the eviction was financial hardship, some parents were able, with practical support, to find new accommodation, and to have the child back.
4 Children received into care because of their mother's death, desertion or long-term psychiatric illness were much more likely to experience long-term care.
5 Parents' involvement with their children during the placement was closely related to the probability of the children's returning to them.
6 Social work activity, in terms of encouragement to parents, practical support or intensive help with personal difficulties, had a significant effect upon the likelihood of return from care. Practical help, in cash or kind, was seen as the most useful form of intervention by both social workers and parents.
7 Many social workers had a passive attitude towards any planning for the restoration of the children with their parents.

4.3 A major American study

1 Stein, Gambrill and Wiltse (1978), in a major study of important factors within fostering, conducted an inquiry now known as the Almeida project.
2 This concluded e.g., that the involvement of natural and foster parents, via a planned agreement, was an approach likely to lead to constructive continuity of care for the children.

4.4 Convergence of evidence upon variables associated with returning home from care

1 The importance of the length of time in care Aldgate (1980) found that the length of time children were in care influenced their chance of return. After two years, social workers' efforts to encourage contact between natural parents and children declined, and caretakers became more enthusiastic about permanent placement. Thus, the longer a child remained in care, the less likely was he or she to return home.

2 The centrality of parental visiting in the outcome of care In Aldgate's study, where children returned home, there had been some contact between the child and at least one parent in 90 per cent of cases. Fanshel and Shinn (1978), in a major American study, demonstrated conclusively the importance of parental visiting.

3 **Frequency of contact between social worker and natural parents** Both Shapiro (1972) and Aldgate (1980) found that frequent contact between social workers and natural parents was related to the likelihood of the child's returning home. Over half the families in Aldgate's study whose children had returned home had seen their social worker at least once a month – compared with just over one sixth of those whose children were currently in care.

4.5 Research concerning 'exclusive/inclusive' fostering

1 **A summary of the evidence on contact with natural parents** Holman (1980) has summarized this evidence which includes:

1 Weinstein's (1960) finding from interviewing sixty-one foster children that their 'well-being', as rated by social workers, was enhanced if the child:
(a) had a clear understanding of the foster situation
(b) identified predominantly with the natural parents
(c) was in contact with his or her natural parents

2 Holman's own finding (1973) that in general the less the contact between foster child and natural parent, the higher the incidence of events such as soiling and ill-health.

3 Thorpe's (1974) findings that there was a trend suggesting a relationship between satisfactory adjustment and contact between foster child and natural parent; this was not statistically significant, however, except for eleven to thirteen-year-olds.

2 **The concepts of 'inclusive/exclusive' fostering**

1 On the basis of these and other findings, Holman (1980) has developed the concepts of 'exclusive' and 'inclusive' fostering.

2 The former refers to situations where links between foster parents and natural parents are not actively promoted by the foster parents themselves, or by the social workers concerned: by contrast, 'inclusive fostering' refers to situations where natural parents are clearly involved in planning for the future of the child.

3 **A study of 'inclusive/exclusive' fostering** Holman found that in his sample of 122 local authority foster parents, 64 per cent could be described as 'exclusive', in that they regarded the foster child as 'their own', and would have liked to adopt him or her: 36 per cent could be described as 'inclusive' in that, while accepting the foster child fully into their family, they recognized that s/he was not 'theirs', and accepted that the natural parents should have contact with him or her.

5 Research concerning foster parents

5.1 Research concerning success or failure in fostering

1 Attempts to pinpoint predictive factors

1 An early study by Parker (1966) sought to identify particular variables contributing to success or failure in a large sample of long-term foster placements. However, the 'prediction table' of variables associated with success was not generally validated in the study by George (1970).

2 Jobling (1973) summarized research in this field, and concluded that success was more likely where,

(a) The foster parents are 'older' rather than 'younger'.
(b) There is no 'rival' child of the same age and sex as the foster child.
(c) The foster child is under twelve months of age

and that failure is more likely where,

(a) The child has previously had a long stay (two years or more in a residential institution).
(b) The foster parents have high expectations and standards, or are hostile to the natural parents.
(c) The foster child is disturbed prior to placement.

2 Breakdown in fostering There are indications, e.g. Parker (1966) and George (1970), which suggest a high breakdown rate for long-term fostering – of about 50 per cent. There are also some suggestions, though not from national data, that a high proportion of foster parents give up fostering within less than a year.

3 The need for support for foster parents

1 Fogarty (1981) from her study, however, reported the lack of preparation by social workers of both foster parents and child before the placement, as well as the lack of firm support from the social worker for them all during placement.

2 Hampson and Tavormina (1980) compared the effects of offering twenty-one foster mothers reflective group counselling with the effects of offering another twenty-one training in behavioural child-rearing skills. The former group improved primarily in attitudes, and the latter in the use of appropriate behavioural skills – reporting reductions in problem behaviour by foster children and improvements in overall family functioning. The authors suggested an approach integrating both methods of working with foster parents.

6 Research findings concerning specialist fostering

6.1 Early studies

Results in this field are encouraging:

1 An American study (Cox and James, 1970) followed the progress of

sixty-five physically handicapped children placed in foster homes and found very few breakdowns, while another by Shearer (1974) of seven American agencies which placed mentally handicapped children in foster homes found that most of the children showed dramatic improvements, especially where they were the only foster child in the family.

2 A Swedish study by Kalveston (1973) traced the progress of very disturbed and delinquent children aged between five and eighteen placed with forty families: all but one placement was judged successful, with the children and young people demonstrating improved behaviour and adjustment.

6.2 The Kent Family Placement Project

The success of this scheme for fostering children with special need is reported by Hazel (1980). She reports how in five years almost 200 disturbed and delinquent adolescents were placed in foster homes, and that over 70 per cent improved there. She wrote:

> Contracts were central to the project's concept of . . . placements, providing both an agreed statement of objectives for all concerned (adolescent, family of origin, foster-family and social workers), and at the same time providing the foster parents with a job description.

6.3 Survey by Shaw and Hipgrave, 1983

1 Building upon their own pilot project of monitoring the progress of a small number of adolescents in foster care, the authors conducted a national survey of social services departments outside London and some of the large voluntary agencies in the UK. Information was gathered in all from forty-five specialist schemes.

2 Readers are referred to the text for full details, but information included details of provision. This was available:
   1 For mentally handicapped children in 12 schemes
   2 For physically handicapped children in 9 schemes
   3 For disturbed adolescents in 42 schemes
   4 For ethnic minority children in 3 schemes
   5 For 'hard to place' children in 22 schemes

3 76.5 per cent of schemes reported their success as ranks four or five on a five point scale (one = low, five = high).

References

Aldgate, J. (1980), 'Identification of factors influencing children's length of stay in care' in J. Tresiliotis (ed.), *New Developments in Foster Care and Adoption*, London: Routledge & Kegan Paul.

British Agencies for Adoption and Fostering (1982), *Adoption and Fostering Panels*, London: BAAF.

British Association of Social Workers (1982), *Guidelines for Practice in Family Placement*, Birmingham: BASW.

Cox, R. W. and James, M. H. (1970), 'Rescue from limbo; foster home placement for hospitalised, physically disabled children' in H. Prosser (1978), *Perspectives on Foster Care*, Windsor: National Children's Bureau/NFER.

Fanshel, D. and Shinn, E. (1978), *Children in Foster Care*, New York: Columbia.

Fogarty, M. (1981), 'More than just a bed, roof and clothing', *Social Work Today*, 10 February 1981, pp. 10–13.

George, V. (1970), *Foster Care: Theory and Practice*, London: Routledge & Kegan Paul.

Haimes, E. and Timms, N. (1985), *Adoption, Identity and Social Policy: The Search for Distant Relatives*, Aldershot, Hants: Gower.

Hampson, R. B. and Tavormina, J. B. (1980), 'Relative effectiveness of behavioural and reflective group training with foster mothers', *Journal of Consulting and Clinical Psychology*, vol. 48, pp. 294–5.

Hazel, N. (1980), '*A Bridge to Independence*', Oxford: Blackwell.

Holman, R. (1973), *Trading in Children: A Study of Private Fostering*, London: Routledge & Kegan Paul.

Holman, R. (1980), 'Exclusive and inclusive concepts of fostering' in J. Tresiliotis (ed.), *New Developments in Foster Care and Adoption*, London: Routledge & Kegan Paul.

Jobling, M. (1973), 'Success and failure in fostering', National Children's Bureau, Highlight No. 6.

Kalveston, A-L. (1973), *Caring for Children with Special Needs*, Institut Européen Inter-Universitaire de l'Action Sociale.

Parker, R. A. (1966), *Decision in Child Care: A Study of Prediction in Fostering*, London: Allen & Unwin.

Prosser, H. (1978), *Perspectives on Foster Care*, London: National Children's Bureau/NFER.

Rowe, J. (1983), *Fostering in the Eighties*, London: British Agencies for Adoption and Fostering.

Rowe, J. and Lambert, L. (1973), *Children Who Wait*, Association of British Adoption Agencies.

Rowe, J., Cain, H., Hundleby, M. and Keane, A. (1984), *Long-Term Foster Care*, London: Batsford Academic and Educational.

Shapiro, D. (1972), 'Agency investment in foster care: a study', *Social Work*, vol. 17, pp. 20–8.

Shaw, M. and Hipgrave, T. (1983), *Specialist Fostering*, London: Batsford Academic and Educational.

Shaw, M. and Lebens, K. (1976), 'Children between families', *Adoption and Fostering*, no. 84.

Shearer, A. (1974), 'Fostering mentally handicapped children. Is it feasible?' in H. Prosser (ed.), *Perspectives on Foster Care*.

Stein, T. J., Gambrill, E. O. and Wiltse, T. (1978), *Children in Foster Homes: Achieving Permanency of Care*, New York: Praeger.

Thorpe, R. (1974), 'The social and psychological situation of the long-term foster child with regard to his natural parents', Unpublished Ph.D. thesis, University of Nottingham.
Triseliotis, J. (1980), *New Developments in Foster Care and Adoption*, London: Routledge & Kegan Paul.
Triseliotis, J. (1980), 'Growing up in foster care' in J. Triseliotis (ed.), *New Developments in Foster Care and Adoption.*
Triseliotis, J. (1983), 'Identity and security in adoption and long-term fostering', *Adoption and Fostering*, vol. 7, pp. 22–31.
Weinstein, E. (1960), *The Self-Image of the Foster Child*, Russell Sage Foundation.

Research concerning adoption

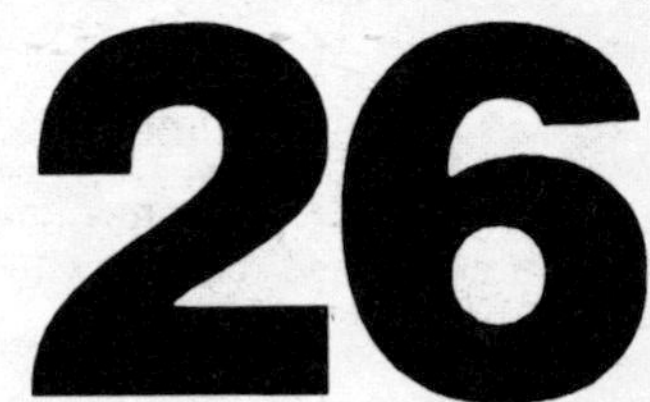

26

Consultant:* *Tony Hall, Director Central Council for Education and Training in Social Work, London; formerly Director, British Agencies for Adoption and Fostering, London.

1 A definition

Hall (1985) has suggested that,

> Adoption is a way of enabling children to grow up in a permanent family if, for any reason, they cannot be brought up by the family into which they were born. It is a formal legal procedure by which all the rights and duties of the natural parents are permanently transferred to the adoptive parents by a court. The adopted child takes the adoptive parents' surname, inherits from them and loses all legal ties to his or her family of birth.

2 Statistics

2.1 The official figures

	One or both a parent	Neither a parent	Sole adopter	Total adoptions
1973	13,677	8,459	111	22,247
1974	14,835	7,508	159	22,502
1975	14,567	6,580	152	21,299
1976	11,827	5,661	133	17,621
1977	7,783	4,867	98	12,748
1978	7,444	4,590	87	12,121
1979	6,534	4,254	82	10,870
1980	6,150	4,364	95	10,609
1981	5,057	4,153	74	9,284
1982	5,807	4,343	90	10,240
1983	4,939	4,008	82	9,029
1984	4,189	3,683	67	7,939

TABLE 26.1 Children adopted under orders registered in England and Wales, 1973–84. (Houghton Report; and Monitors issued by the Office of Population Censuses and Statistics)

2.2 Changes in numbers and patterns of adoption

Hall (1985) commenting on the changing scene shown in Table 26.1 has highlighted the following factors which contribute to this:

(a) the decline in the number of healthy white babies available for adoption as a result of changes in abortion law, contraception and changing social attitudes to single mothers.

(b) the initial growth, and later decline (following the Children Act 1975) of 'step-parent adoptions' – where adoption is used to formalize arrangements in reconstituted families following divorce, and to a lesser extent, for illegitimate children when their single mothers marry for the first time.

(c) the changing focus of adoptions which do occur, from healthy white babies in the late 1960s to children with 'special needs' today. A majority of 'stranger adoptions' today are of 'special needs' children i.e. mentally and/or physically handicapped children of all ages; older children (over ten); black children and sibling groups.

(d) the changing ratio of 'stranger adoptions', where one of the adopters is a natural parent to the child, and single adopters.

3 Research concerning children who are adopted

3.1 Two early American studies

1 **The New York Charities Association study** Theis (1924) traced 910 of the children placed in foster homes by the New York Charities Association who had reached the age of eighteen years. Of these 269 had been adopted. A range of assessments suggested:

   1 Adopted children had fared better than children who remained fostered in terms of
      (a) Social adjustment
      (b) Educational achievement
   2 Almost all adopted children had been placed when under five; children placed under five who were still fostered did rather better than older children. Many children placed after five had also made very good progress.

2 **The Yale study** Wittenborn (1957) compared two samples of 114 and 81 adopted infants with thirty-five children brought up by their own parents. Findings suggested that:

   1 Older, more educationally ambitious adoptive parents had contributed to the higher I.Q. levels of adopted children by comparison with controls.
   2 Early experience of one or even several temporary settings had not affected the child's later development.
   3 It is conducive to healthy development that the child is fully aware that he or she is adopted from as early an age as possible.

3.2 British studies

1 **A comparative study**

   1 Tizard (1977) followed the progress of sixty-five children who remained in a residential nursery run by three large voluntary societies from the age of four months to at least two years. Between the ages of two and seven, thirty children were adopted and twenty-three returned to their natural parents. Tizard compared twenty-five of the former and thirteen of the latter when they were aged eight. She found the majority of the adopted children well adjusted, only three having been referred to a child psychiatrist: eight of the latter group had been so referred. Tizard considered many of the 'restorations' had been actually unhappy and wrote: 'All the mothers had been indecisive about claiming the child, or definitely reluctant – in only one case was there a straightforward housing problem.'
   2 Others, however, particularly the Family Rights Group and the Dartington Social Research Unit, have defended the rights of natural parents and called for much more active encouragement by social workers of links between them and their children.

2 Evidence from the National Child Development Study

1 A number of reports based on this major study have been published. Shaw (1984) has reported:

> The NCDS, following the fortunes of all the children born in England, Scotland and Wales during the first week of March 1958, has been able to draw comparisons between adopted children, those living in one-parent families, and those in 'standard' two-parent families. An early report on the adopted children at the age of seven (Seglow, Pringle and Wedge 1972) not only showed them to be making excellent progress on a broad range of developmental, social and educational measures, but suggested that in some respects they were ahead of the legitimate children living with their birth parents.

2 Lambert (1981) examined the effects of adoption up to the age of sixteen upon a sample of thirty-seven of the total number of children within the NCDS who were adopted. Although some data were missing, Lambert reported that these children were broadly comparable to the total sample of children in the Study in respect of health record, educational attainment and personal and social adjustment.

3.3 An overview of adoption studies and human development

A major overview by Clarke (1981) surveyed a number of earlier studies; among her conclusions were the following:

1 The outcome for very early adopted children is on the whole good; they tend to be of at least average and often above average status intellectually and academically.
2 Studies of early adopted children suggest clearly that they resemble their biological parents more than their adopting relatives, certainly so far as intelligence is concerned and possibly with respect to some personality characteristics.
3 In that adopting families are screened and tend to provide better than average social and educational opportunities for their children, they almost certainly offset some of the risks which the children might otherwise run.
4 Adopted children show on average a heightened risk of childhood maladjustment, the causes of which are likely to be multifactorial. Evidence suggested that this risk declines with age, and that by adolescence it may be little different from that in non-adopted age peers. This finding is in line with the general conclusion that minor childhood disorders do not show continuities in long term: major disorders, however, may well be a different matter.
5 The one large study then available (Scarr and Weinberg, 1976), which reported the adoption of mixed race children, suggested that there was good evidence of a positive outcome.

6 Studies of late adopted children, including some who came to their adoptive parents very late, also give cause for cautious optimism.

4 Some research findings concerning the adoption of children with special needs and in special circumstances

4.1 An American study of the adoption of older children

1 Kadushin (1970) examined the progress of ninety-one families who adopted children aged between five and eleven years in Wisconsin. The forty-two girls and forty-nine boys had experienced an average of 2.3 foster placements before being placed for adoption, and their average age at that placement was seven years, two months.
2 The children had all been 'freed for adoption', and all the children had expressed a clear wish to be adopted.
3 Follow-up was conducted at an average age of thirteen years, nine months. Using the level of satisfaction of parents as the main criterion, the following was found:
   (a) 76 per cent were considered successful
   (b) 15 per cent were considered unsuccessful
   (c) 9 per cent were considered intermediate
   (d) Only two children had been removed from their homes following adoption.

4.2 The adoption, or placing for permanence, of children with special needs

1 **A British study of adoption** Jepson (1981) has described the work of Parents for Children, a specialist adoption agency established to find homes for children with special needs: those with physical, mental and emotional handicaps, older children and sibling groups. Of the first thirty-eight children placed, almost all of whom had been in care all their lives, there were only six placement breakdowns, and four of these children were later successfully placed with new families.

2 **Further studies**

1 Wolkind and Kozaruk (1983) reported the progress of eighty-four children with a range of medical handicaps placed for adoption before the age of three. At three years after placement, 'the vast majority of parents were delighted with their new child, had no regrets and felt well able to cope with any medical or other problems.'
2 Further evidence is offered by a range of studies which have demonstrated clearly that children with conditions such as Down's syndrome, cerebral palsy, spina bifida and hydrocephalus can be successfully adopted.
3 Thoburn (1985) has drawn attention to the wide range of people who

have successfully offered permanence, indicating that they by no means conform to the stereotype of the conventional, middle-class family.

5 Current issues receiving research attention

5.1 Planning for permanence

1 **The nature of the debate** There is disagreement between schools of thought concerning the extent to which permanence should underpin the placing of children on a long-term basis. Hall (1985) has written,

> There is a continuing debate between those who believe that children need a permanent, stable, secure family (through adoption if the natural parents cannot or will not provide it) and those who stress continuing contact with the child's natural family to be the most important issue.

2 **The argument for permanence**

1 Goldstein, Freud and Solnit (1973, 1980) are among those who strongly advocate permanence, suggesting that placement decisions should, above all else, safeguard the child's need for continuity of relationships. While the desirability of such continuity is not questioned as a principle, there are varying views concerning the extent to which natural parents can, in some circumstances, still be associated with the adopted child.
2 This debate affects the issue of adoption and its parameters. Goldstein, Freud and Solnit (1980), in line with their views, advocated, 'that the adoption decree be made final the moment the child is actually placed with an adopting family'.

3 **The position of allowing for continuing contact** Triseliotis (1985) has summarized the impact of social and demographic changes upon the field of adoption and permanance; he reported:

> The main issue about access and contact in present day adoption practice refers mostly to those adolescents who, even though they may be looking for a new family, do not wish to give up existing attachments to members of their original family . . .

The possibility of so-called 'open adoption', formerly uncontemplated, is now a reality: if such arrangements are made, they need very careful research and evaluation.

4 **Some American studies** There have been a number of such studies of planned permanence for children: e.g. Lahti (1982) and Fein, Maluccio, Hamilton and Ward (1983). These have drawn attention to the desirability of working towards the ideal of permanence for children, albeit by a variety of different routes.

5 **Routes into permanence** Thoburn (1985), while recognizing the desirability of

permanence, has questioned, however, the assumption that this is virtually synonymous with adoption. She quoted the comment of the Select Committee on Children in Care:

> The search for permanence, in our view, could be accomplished in many ways including custodianship, long-term fostering, or even in some circumstances a stay in a residential home or, of course, rehabilitation with a child's natural family . . .

6 **Some lessons from research into permanence** Wedge (1986) has summarized these; they include:

1 The recognition that 'the numbers, types and ages of children who might be *considered* for permanent placing is changing';
2 It is likely that arrangements in which families of origin maintain contact with their teenage children will increase;
3 It is likely that increased efforts will be made to place children from ethnic minority groups with families similar to those of origin;
4 The evidence that, '*all* parties should share a common understanding of exactly what "permanent" arrangements are being planned for, worked towards and instituted.'

5.2 Transracial adoption

1 **The issue** There is disagreement concerning the placing of children in need of a home in trans-racial placements. While most parties seem to be agreed that it is desirable for children to be placed in long-term placements with families of the same race, this has not always proved easy to achieve. More energetic efforts are now being made both in the USA and Britain to recruit more parents from minority ethnic groups.

2 **American studies of trans-racial adoption**

1 Simon (1984) reported the American research, including her own: Simon and Altstein, (1977, 1981). It seems that white families can bring up emotionally healthy black children, although there are clear challenges to be met.
2 The two studies by Simon and Altstein constituted a two-stage survey of 204 families who had all adopted a child from an ethnic minority background, first when the children were between three and eight, and then five years later. The earlier study painted a very favourable picture: the later one indicated some difficulties. Simon (1984) summarized,

> For every five families in which there were the usual pleasures and joys, along with sibling rivalries, school-related problems and difficulties in communication between parent and child, there was one family whose difficulties were more profound and *were believed by the* parents to be directly related to the transracial adoption.

3 Concerning school-performance and friendships, 74 per cent of the parents saw the children as having no academic problems or difficulties with teachers. Similarly, 85 per cent of the parents reported their children as having no difficulties in making friends or being part of a group.

3 A British study of trans-racial adoption

1 Harris (1975), in an annotated bibliography on trans-racial adoption (which includes items on inter-country adoption), has reported the study by Gill and Jackson (1983), which is the third follow-up to the British Adoption Project; it involves the families of thirty-six children aged twelve to sixteen.
2 Harris has summarized the main findings of this study:

> (i) no general evidence of children being isolated within families; (ii) large majority were able to relate effectively to peers and adults outside the family; (iii) no evidence of their doing academically worse than their age mates; (iv) most parents made only limited attempts to introduce a sense of racial pride; (v) no general evidence that absence of racial pride or identity was associated with low self-esteem; (vi) distressing racial incidents were reported by most children but were not of central importance to them; (vii) no evidence that experience of racial background differed between black and mixed race children.

3 Harris also reported that the study highlighted the point that the children's 'coping' mechanisms are based on denying their racial background, and concedes the justification for the black community seeing itself as a 'donor' of children for white couples. He quoted a summarizing comment from Gill and Jackson,

> Using conventional measures of adoption success, the children . . . appeared to be doing well. They did not, however, see themselves as black or show any real sign of having developed a sense of racial identity.

6 Research concerning those who become adoptive parents

Pringle (1967), considering such evidence as existed, concluded that the personality of the adopting parents has been found to be crucial to individual success; she reported that warmth, acceptance and stability seem as least as important as age, education and socio-economic status. Findings about the size and structure of the family in which the adopted child best thrives are inconclusive.

7 Research concerning the counselling of those who have been adopted

Since the passing of the 1975 Children Act, those adopted in England and Wales have been able to apply to the Registrar General for a copy of their original birth certificate. In his investigation, Triseliotis (1981) concluded,

(a) Only a minority of people sought access to their birth records.
(b) Of those who did, two out of three were women.
(c) Many did not seek a reunion with their natural parents.

References

Bean, P. (ed.) (1984), *Adoption. Essays in social policy, law and sociology*, London: Tavistock Publications.

Clarke, A. M. (1981), 'Adoption studies and human development', *Adoption and Fostering*, vol. 104.

Fein, E., Maluccio, A. N., Hamilton, V. J. and Ward, D. (1983), 'After foster care: Permanency planning for children', *Child Welfare*, vol. 62.

Freeman, M. D. A. (1984), 'Subsidised adoption' in P. Bend (ed.), *Adoption. Essays in social policy, law and sociology*.

Gill, O. and Jackson, B. (1983), *Adoption and Race: Black, Asian and Mixed Race Children in White Families*, London: Batsford/BAAF.

Goldstein, J., Freud, A. and Solnit, A. (1973), *Beyond the Best Interests of the Child*, New York: The Free Press, Macmillan Publishing Company.

Goldstein, J., Freud, A. and Solnit, A. (1980), *Before the Best Interests of the Child*, New York: The Free Press, Macmillan Publishing Company.

Grow, L. J. and Shapiro, D. (1972). *Black Children, White Parents: A Study of Transracial Adoption*, New York: Child Welfare League of America.

Haimes, E. and Timms, N. (1985), *Adoption, Identity and Social Policy: The Search for Distant Relatives*. Aldershot, Hants: Gower.

Hall, A. (1985), 'Adoption' in *Dictionary of Pastoral Care*, London: SPCK.

Hall, A. (1985), Personal communication.

Harris, K. (1975), *Transracial Adoption*, London: British Agencies for Adoption and Fostering.

Jepson, A. M. (1981), 'Parents for children', *British Medical Journal*, vol. 282.

Jobling, M. (1975), *Adoption: a research abstract*, London: National Children's Bureau, Highlight No. 16.

Kadushin, A. (1970). *Adopting Older Children*, New York: Columbia University Press.

Ladner, J. (1977), *Mixed Families*, New York: Wiley.

Lahti, J. (1982), 'A follow up study of foster children in permanent placements', *Social Service Review*, University of Chicago.

Lambert, L. (1981), 'Adopted from care by the age of seven', *Adoption and Fostering*, vol. 3, pp. 28–36.

Pringle, M. L. (1967), *Adoption: Facts and Fallacies*, London: Longman.

Scarr, S. and Weinberg, R. A. (1976), 'IQ test performance of black children adopted by white families.' *American Psychologist*, vol. 31, pp. 726–39.

Seglow, J., Pringle, M. L. and Wedge, P. (1972), *Growing Up Adopted*, London: NFER.

Shaffer, G. (1981), 'Subsidized adoption in Illinois', *Children and Youth Services Review*, vol. 3, pp. 55–68.

Shaw, M. (1984), 'Growing up adopted' in P. Bean (ed.), *Adoption. Essays in social policy, law and sociology.*

Simon, R. (1984), 'Adoption of black children by white parents in the U.S.A.' in P. Bean (ed.), *Adoption. Essays in social policy, law and sociology.*

Simon, R. and Altstein, H. (1977), *Transracial Adoption*, New York: Wiley.

Simon, R. and Altstein, H. (1981), *Transracial Adoption: A Follow-Up*, Lexington: Lexington Books.

Theis, S. (1924), *How Foster Children Turn Out*, New York: A study by the State Charities Association.

Thoburn, J. (1985), 'What kind of permanence?', *Adoption and Fostering*, vol. 4, pp. 29–33.

Tizard, B. (1977), *Adoption: a Second Chance*, London: Open Books.

Triseliotis, J. (1981), 'Obtaining birth certificates' in P. Bean (ed.), *Adoption. Essays in social policy, law and sociology.*

Triseliotis, J. (1983), 'Identity and security in adoption and long-term fostering', *Adoption and Fostering*, vol. 7, pp. 22–31.

Triseliotis, J. (1985), 'Adoption with contact', *Adoption and Fostering*, vol. 4, pp. 19–24.

Wedge, P. (1986), 'Lessons from research into permanent family placement' in J. Thoburn and P. Wedge (eds), *Quest for Permanence for Children in Care*, London: BAAF.

Wittenborn, J. R. (1957), *The Placement of Adoptive Children*, Springfield, Illinois: Thomas.

Wolkind, S. and Kozaruk, A. (1983), 'The adoption of children with medical handicap', *Adoption and Fostering*, vol. 7, pp. 32–5.

Zastrow, C. H. (1977), *Outcome of Black Children-White Parent Transracial Adoptions*, San Francisco: R. and E. Research Associates.

27

Research concerning residential care of the elderly, the physically handicapped, the mentally handicapped and the mentally ill

***Consultant:* Chris Payne, Lecturer/Consultant in Social Services Development, National Institute for Social Work, London.**

1 The provision of accommodation

1 Legislation concerning the statutory care of persons in the above groups places the main responsibility on local authorities, although with certain reserve powers in central government, other national groups or the National Health Service.

2 Private residential accommodation must be registered with the local authority for the area where the home is located.

1.1 A classification of the range of provision

The classification of forms of care offered by Ainsworth and Fulcher (1981), and shown in Chapter 23 (see p. 216) offers a useful framework for understanding the location of residential care ('residential group living') within the broader range of provision which is now developing for a range of children and adults. However, it should be noted that residential settings for adults and the elderly take some different forms from those for children. For example, homes for the elderly tend to be larger than children's homes; many follow a 'hospital' model, though there has been a trend towards smaller and more specialized units, and group-living arrangements in recent years. Private homes, on average, tend to be smaller than local authority homes.

2 Official statistics

2.1 Accommodation for the elderly

These figures are incorporated into Table 27.1 and Table 27.2

1 People in accommodation provided by or on behalf of local authorities

England		1982	1983	1984
People in accommodation provided by local authorities	Total	108,637	108,569	106,782
	Male	29,360	28,203	27,339
	Female	79,277	80,366	79,443
Aged under 65	Total	4,969	4,971	4,786
Aged 65 and over	Total	103,668	103,598	101,966
Number of homes		2,662	2,669	2,673
People in accommodation provided on behalf of local authorities in voluntary or private homes	Total	17,337	15,993	14,208
	Male	5,263	4,899	4,451
	Female	12,074	11,094	9,757
Aged under 65	Total	4,160	4,053	3,901
Aged 65 and over	Total	13,177	11,940	10,307

TABLE 27.1 Persons in accommodation provided by or on behalf of local authorities. (*Health and Personal Social Services Statistics for England*, 1985)

2 Places and persons in voluntary and private homes for the elderly and physically handicapped

England	1982	1983	1984
Voluntary homes			
Homes	1,119	1,135	1,132
Places	36,743	37,613	38,242
Persons accommodated	31,867	35,543	32,046
Aged under 65	5,751	6,075	6,041
Aged 65 and over	26,116	26,468	26,005
Private homes			
Homes	2,830	3,374	4,090
Places	44,346	51,760	63,072
Persons accommodated	37,791	44,435	55,168
England	**1982**	**1983**	**1984**
Aged under 65	1,952	2,293	2,493
Aged 65 and over	35,839	42,142	52,675

TABLE 27.2 Places and persons in voluntary and private homes for the elderly and the physically handicapped (*Health and Personal Social Services Statistics for England*, 1985)

2.2 Accommodation for the mentally ill and the mentally handicapped

England		1981	1982	1983	1984
Mentally ill					
Local authority homes					
Staffed	Premises	146	149	152	151
	Places	2,467	2,514	2,557	2,523
Unstaffed	Premises	343	351	375	391
	Places	1,514	1,549	1,616	1,723
Voluntary and private homes	Premises	*	*	171	189
	Places	*	*	2,367	2,558
Mentally handicapped					
Local authority homes					
Staffed	Premises	579	593	617	647
	Places	11,494	11,862	12,282	12,800
Unstaffed	Premises	272	290	346	375
	Places	1,218	1,282	1,453	1,550
Voluntary and private homes					
	Premises	*	*	292	363
	Places	*	*	5,046	6,271

* Indicates that data is available but unreliable.

TABLE 27.3 Homes and hostels for the mentally ill and the mentally handicapped (*Health and Personal Social Services Statistics for England*, 1985)

3 Research concerning the residential care of the elderly

The same difficulties of research and evaluation described in Chapter 23 apply also in this and other areas of residential work:

3.1 Overviews of practice

There are several overviews of recent research into the residential care of the elderly, including Goldberg and Connelly (1982), Firth (1985) and Bland and Bland (1983). Among their several surveys a number of issues seem important:

1 **Issues examined by Firth (1985)**

1 Theories of residential care
2 Models of homes for the elderly
3 Criteria and procedures for admission to care
4 Aspects of daily living, activities and health

5 Staff roles, training and management
6 Positive care and natural living

In respect of models of homes, Firth highlighted the work of Clough (1981) and his classification, based on two major variables: 1) the extent to which a resident controls his or her lifestyle and 2) different theories of ageing.

2 Dimensions of the residential social environment

1 Goldberg and Connelly (1982) concluded that the following were of great importance:
   (i) flexibility of management practices
   (ii) individualization and autonomy for residents
   (iii) opportunities for privacy
   (iv) opportunities for social stimulation
   (v) communication and interaction with the outside world
   (vi) social interaction between staff and residents
   (vii) maximum delegation of decision-making to care staff and to residents
   (viii) good communication channels between staff
   (ix) a minimum degree of specialisation of roles and tasks among staff
2 These accord very closely with the views of Clough (1981) that the prime function of an elderly person's home should be: 'to provide a living base in which physical needs are met in a way which allows the individual maximum potential for achieving mastery.'
3 These issues are also examined by Booth (1985), in an examination of old people's homes and the outcome of care.

3.2 A general critique of research into elderly people's homes

1 Bland and Bland (1983) examined a range of research into old people's homes in terms of:
   (a) physical design of homes
   (b) regime and administration
   (c) resident behaviour and attitudes
   (d) the group living concept
2 While recognizing the methodological difficulties of conducting research across establishments, they are very critical of almost all the studies which they examined. They complain of unwarranted conclusions, unwarranted generalizations from limited amounts of data, small sample size, failure to replicate studies and neglect of differences in values, attitudes and expectations among both residents and care staff in such settings.
3 It seems likely that many variables, including home design, regime, mental condition of residents and staff values and attitudes all interact to produce different patterns of behaviour and animation in residents.

3.3 Department of Health and Social Security-sponsored research

1. The DHSS has sponsored a considerable amount of research into the residential care of the elderly in recent years. Studies have included:
   1. Issues related to the costs of care
   2. Measures for admission to care
   3. The physical environment and design of buildings
   4. The use of residential homes for short-stay purposes and the effects on permanent residents
   5. The prescription and administration of drugs
   6. The characteristics of residents and issues relating to the integration of 'confused' and 'lucid' residents.
   7. The use and role of volunteers
   8. Factors associated with the quality of life
   9. Staffing
2. Many of these studies are reported and discussed in Judge and Sinclair (1986).

4 Research concerning residential care of people with physical handicaps

This appears to be a relatively under-researched field, although many of the conclusions concerning the need for the opportunities to maximize self-determination highlighted in other fields of research seem just as important here.

4.1 A study highlighting contrasting models of care

An important pilot study by Miller and Gwynne (1972) of residential institutions for the physically handicapped and the young chronic sick distinguished two approaches to their care:

1. The 'warehousing' model, which merely brought people together and ensured that they were fed and looked after.
2. The 'horticultural' model, which focused upon enabling the potentials of the handicapped person to be developed and brought to fruition.

4.2 Attempts to disseminate the 'horticultural' model

Others, including Greengross (1976) and Dartington, Miller and Gwynne (1981) have developed this theme, and have highlighted for example, the sexual needs of disabled people, and how means may be developed of incorporating people living in institutional care into the mainstream of life in the community.

5 Research concerning residential care of people with mental handicaps

5.1 Some principles of researching and evaluating such work

Kushlick (1973) has described some of the innovatory work in this field, and how it involved:

1 Assessing the size and nature of the over-all problem by means of an epidemiological survey which covers people, both in residential care (including hospitals), and at home.
2 Advising service personnel, on the basis of the data generated . . . to set up alternative forms of care ('experimental') which could be predicted to achieve the defined service aims more simply and effectively than existing ('control') services. . . . This phase involves defining:
   (a) Service aims which can be measured.
   (b) Testable hypotheses on how and why the aims are more or less likely to be achieved.
   (c) Measurable criteria of the quality of care.
   All measures must be reliable (i.e. replicable), valid (i.e. they measure the phenomena that they claim to measure) and relevant. . . .
3 It involves collecting baseline data on 'experimental' and 'control' people and their families before the service begins so that subsequent changes can be measured.

5.2 On-going evaluation of provision

Kushlick (1973) has reported on-going work in small units for the mentally handicapped. Their effectiveness has been measured by their multi-dimensional impact – for example:

1 Changes in client-centred aspects

(a) Measures of change in the cognitive and social abilities of participants.
(b) Measures of change in the family problems arising from the impact of the retarded person on the family.
(c) Measures of change in the families' experience with the relevant services and their satisfaction therewith.

2 Changes in quality of care

(a) Measures of administrative, e.g. staffing, aspects.
(b) Costs, and cost effectiveness.

Such models of multi-dimensional evaluation seem to be among the best ways of measuring the impact of a new system upon the larger system: in this case, the impact of the new small units upon client, families, services and providers of services. (See also Chapter 36, pages 346–8).

5.3 Early studies of residential care for handicapped children

1 Differences in child management practices

1 Tizard and Grad (1961) reported their survey of practices in sixteen institutions for mentally handicapped children, and noted marked differences in child management practices. Indications were:
(a) that heads of units offered vital role models to junior staff.
(b) that unit heads with high rates of interaction with children had received a child care training, while those with low rates had been trained as nurses with emphasis upon physical health.
(c) children in child-oriented units were significantly more advanced than those in institutionally oriented units . . .

2 The work of King, Raynes and Tizard (1971) broadly confirmed the distinction between 'child-oriented' and 'institution-oriented' regimes, and considerable efforts have since been made to enable children growing up in residential care to experience the former.

5.4 Continuing critiques of policy and practice

1 Shearer (1980) has, however, drawn attention to the failure to meet the needs of handicapped children in ways which had been shown to promote intellectual and social development by the studies described in 6.3, some twenty years earlier.

2 She reiterated the findings of Moss (1975) concerning the size of units for handicapped children,

> the average size of a children's home was 15 places . . . the average size of a special boarding school was 61 places, of an independent school for handicapped children, 49, of a local authority home for mentally handicapped children, 18, and of voluntary and private provision for these children, 27. Hospital provision for mentally handicapped children, however, had an average of 113 places. . . .

3 She also highlighted the continuing need, first emphasized by the Curtis Committee in 1946, to give all handicapped children affection and personal interest, stability, and the opportunities of developing to potential and participating in community living.

4 Oswin (1984) and Pritlove (1985) are among those who have registered continuing concern for mentally handicapped people, children and adults, in a range of hospital and institutional provision, and have called for substantial improvements in their care. They recognize, however, that such improvements depend upon major increases in funding and resources.

5.5 A study of group homes for mentally handicapped people

1 The background to the study

1 Malin (1983) compared the progress of twenty-four residents living in

six group homes, and who received only part-time support from home helps and social workers, with that of twenty-four others who lived with care staff in local authority hostels.

2 Residents in both settings were assessed on a range of measures at the start of the study. Effects of group interaction and informal support networks were also considered.

2 Some findings

1 Results indicated that group home residents scored higher than hostel residents – e.g. in handling money and budgeting, language and concept development and self-care skills. Residents in both settings showed few 'maladaptive' behaviours.

2 Residents living in group homes with higher staff support reached higher-than-average scores on several measures.

3 Previous residential placement did not influence successful group home placement: several residents who made the most progress had spent ten or more years in hospital.

3 Implications of the findings Malin identified several needs:

(a) The 'right grouping' of residents in terms of e.g. skills.
(b) Flexibility in staff deployment.
(c) The identification and organisation of community resources.
(d) Clear management policy and guidance.

6 Research concerning residential care of mentally ill people

6.1 The range of provision

1 Davis (1984) has described some of the types of residential provision made for the recovering mentally ill: she noted:

> Four main residential care approaches to crisis and breakdown can be currently identified within specialist residential units run by local authorities and voluntary organisations: crisis work; therapeutic communities; rehabilitative work; long term care.

2 She went on to describe the key features of each type of provision, and pointed out that the approaches are not mutually exclusive, and that: 'in certain situations a "mix" of approaches can be developed to great effect.'

6.2 The need for the evaluation of a range of provision

1 A study by Mosher, Menn and Matthews (1975) (See Chapter 35, page 337) comparing the effects upon people recovering from schizophrenia of treatment via medication or a stay of five to six months in a

therapeutic community, found the latter far more beneficial, as measured by the peoples' subsequent ability to live independently in the community.

2 There seems, however, to be a great shortage of such evaluative studies, and thus a dearth of information concerning which recovering mentally ill person may fare best in which form of provision. As more people formerly accommodated in psychiatric hospitals move into the community, both adequate provision for them, and means of evaluating its effectiveness are urgently needed.

3 Cassidy (1986) has highlighted the advantages of the 'objectives-setting' model as appropriate to evaluating much of the residential and day-care provision; this does indeed seem much more relevant as a means of evaluation than any of the 'classical' designs.

References

Ainsworth, F. and Fulcher, L. C. (1981), *Group Care for Children: Concepts and Issues*, London: Tavistock Publications.

Bland, R. and Bland, R. E. (1983), 'Recent research in old people's homes: a review of the literature', *Research, Policy and Planning*, vol. 1, pp. 16–24.

Booth, T. (1985), *Home Truths: Old People's Homes and the Outcomes of Care*, Aldershot: Gower.

Cassidy, T. (1986), 'Objective setting and evaluation in residential and day care', *Social Work Education*, vol. 5, pp. 22–4.

Clough, R. (1981), *Old Age Homes*, London: Allen & Unwin.

Dartington, T., Miller, E. and Gwynne, G. (1981), *A Life Together: The Distribution of Attitudes Towards the Disabled*, London: Tavistock Publications.

Davis, A. (1984), 'Residential care', in M. R. Olsen (ed.), *Social Work and Mental Health: A Guide for the Approved Social Worker*, London: Tavistock.

Department of Health and Social Security (1971), *Better Services for the Mentally Handicapped*, Command 4683, London: HMSO.

Department of Health and Social Security (1983), *Group Homes for Mentally Handicapped People*, London: HMSO.

Douglas, R. and Payne, C. (1985), *Developing Residential Practice*, London: National Institute of Social Work.

Firth, B. (1985), 'Practice in residential care' in J. Lishman and E. Horobin (eds), *Developing Services for the Elderly*, Research Highlights in Social Work 3. Aberdeen, University of Aberdeen Department of Social Work: Kogan Page.

Goldberg, E. M. and Connelly, N. (1982), *The Effectiveness of Social Care for the Elderly*, London: Heinemann Educational Books.

Greengross, W. (1976), *Sex for the Disabled. The Sexual and Emotional Needs of the Handicapped*, London: Malaby Press.

Judge, K. and Sinclair, I. (eds.) (1986), *Residential Care for Elderly People.*

Research Contributions to the Development of Policy and Practice. London H.M.S.O.

King, R. D., Raynes, N. V. and Tizard, J. (1971), *Patterns of Residential Care: Sociological Studies in Institutions for Handicapped Children*, London: Routledge & Kegan Paul.

Kushlick, A. (1973), 'Evaluating residential services for mentally retarded children' in J. K. Wing and H. Hafner (eds), *Roots of Evaluation: the Epidemiological Basis for Planning Psychiatric Services. An International Symposium.* Oxford: Oxford University Press.

Malin, N. (1983), *Group Homes for Mentally Handicapped People*, London: HMSO.

Miller, E. J. and Gwynne, G. (1972), *A Life Apart: A Pilot Study of Residential Institutions for the Physically Handicapped and the Young Chronic Sick*, London: Tavistock Publications.

Mosher, L. R., Menn, A. and Matthews, S. (1975), 'Sotaria: evaluation of a home-based treatment for schizophrenia', *American Journal of Orthopsychiatry*, vol. 45, pp. 455–67.

Moss, P. (1975), Residential care of children: a general view' in J. Tizard, I. Sinclair and R. V. G. Clarke (eds), *Varieties of Residential Experience*, London: Routledge & Kegan Paul.

Oswin, M. (1984), *They Keep Going Away*, London: King Edward's Fund.

Payne, C. (1981), 'Research and evaluation' in F. Ainsworth and L. C. Fulcher, *Group Care for Children.*

Pritlove, J. (1985), *Group Homes: An Inside Story*, University of Sheffield.

Shearer, A. (1980), *Handicapped Children in Residential Care*, London: Bedford Press.

Thomas, N. (1981), 'Design, management and resident dependency in old people's homes' in E. M. Goldberg and N. Connelly (eds), *Evaluative Research in Social Care*, London: Heinemann Educational Books.

Tizard, J. (1975), 'Quality of residential care for retarded children' in J. Tizard, I. Sinclair and R. V. G. Clarke (eds), *Varieties of Residential Experience.*

Tizard, J. and Grad, J. C. (1961), *The Mentally Handicapped and their Families*, Maudsley Monograph, Oxford University Press.

PART 8

Research concerning young people and adults in trouble with the law

28 Research concerning young offenders

Consultant: Professor Michael Rutter, Professor of Child Psychiatry, Institute of Psychiatry, University of London.

This chapter draws heavily upon three sources:

1 *Juvenile Delinquency: Trends and Perspectives*, by Michael Rutter and Henri Giller, published in 1983 by Penguin.
2 'Juvenile delinquency: trends and perspectives', by Michael Rutter and Henri Giller (1982) and published in the *Research Bulletin* of the Home Office.
3 *Juvenile Crime*, a briefing paper published in 1985 by the National Association for the Care and Resettlement of Offenders.

1 A general classification

Young offenders Young offenders are those who commit an offence against the law, and who are either 'children' (persons under fourteen) or 'young persons' (fourteen and under seventeen). These distinctions by age are given in the Children and Young Persons Act 1933, s. 107.

2 Statistical information

2.1 The unreliability of available statistics

There is near universal agreement that published figures are beset with errors stemming from methodological and other problems. Other methods of sampling, classifying and grouping data show them to be open to serious question, while self-reporting by offenders and reports of victims suggest much higher rates of offending. Since there is no generally accepted alternative, however, some official figures and trends are shown in Table 28.1.

2.2 Some official figures

Offence	1950	1955	1960	1965	1970	1978	% Increase 1950–78
Larceny	10,073	9,434	15,290	21,587	26,706	37,946[1]	+276%[2]
Breaking & entering	4,219	3,550	7,789	10,800	16,164	21,320	+405%
Robbery	83	69	140	238	516	681	+720%
Violence against the person	190	334	1,238	1,714	2,512	4,738	+2,394%
Fraud/ False pretences	42	74	134	189	389	846	+1,914%
Receiving/ Handling stolen goods	560	515	1,206	2,037	2,911	—[3]	+420%[4]

1. Includes receiving/handling stolen goods.
2. Probably an over-estimate because it includes receiving/handling stolen goods.
3. No separate listing, included with larceny.
4. Based on 1970 figures – hence probably an under-estimate.

TABLE 28.1 14–16-year-old males found guilty 1950–78, by type of offence. (Data provided by Home Office.) (Rutter and Giller, 1983).

2.3 Some later trends. See Figure 28.1

2.4 Evidence of changes in rates of offending

There seems to be evidence of a marked increase in the amount of offending, or of *recorded* offending since the 1950s, among both males and females. Since 1974, however, this trend has levelled.

2.5 NACRO's view of the evidence on rates of offending

In their Summary of Conclusions, the authors of NACRO's *Juvenile Crime* (1985) reported:

> *Most juvenile delinquency is minor and transient*
> Most adolescent males commit criminal offences at one time or another; only a small proportion are ever apprehended. The majority (60 per cent) of 'known' juvenile offenders are cautioned rather than prosecuted, usually for minor property offences.

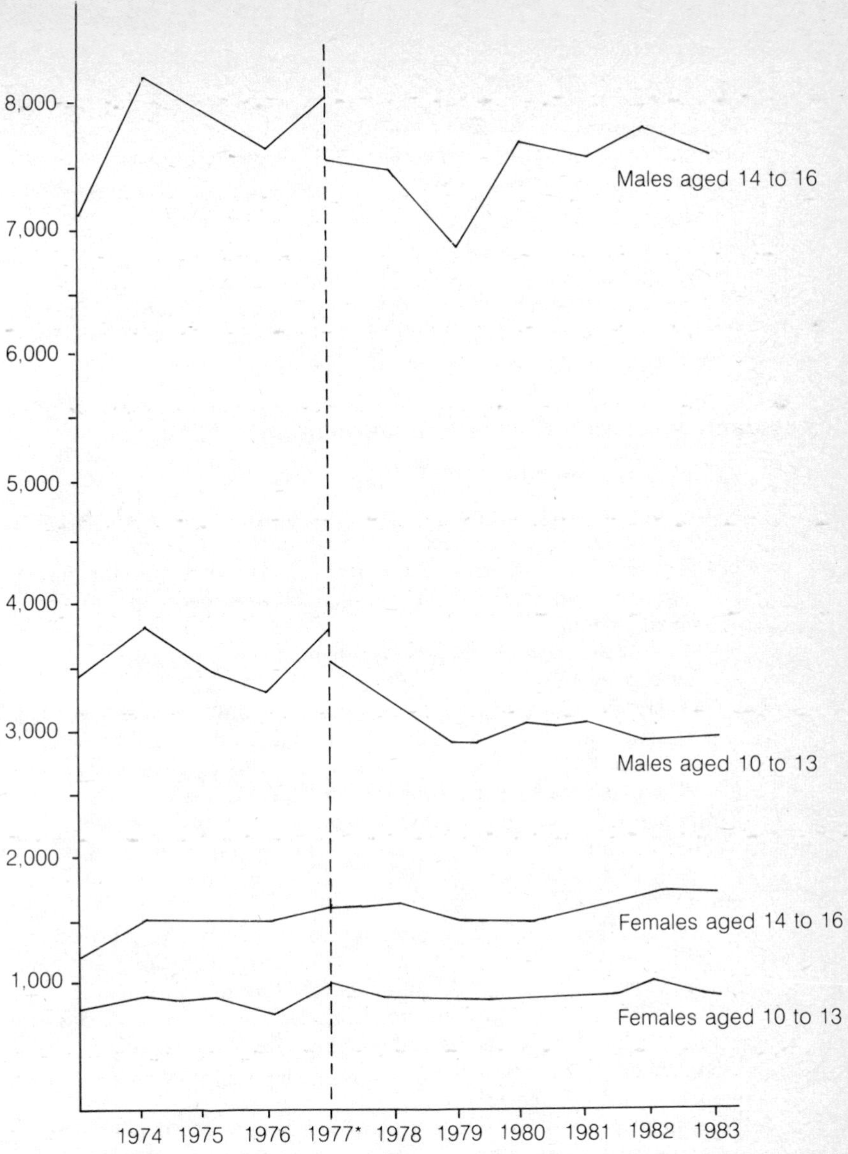

* 1973 to 1976 not adjusted for Criminal Law Act 1977 nor for the change in the counting of proceedings.

FIGURE 28.1 Juveniles found guilty of, or cautioned for, indictable offences per 100,000 population in sex and age groups.
Source: *Juvenile Crime*, (1985), N.A.C.R.O. drawing on *Criminal Statistics in England and Wales*, 1983, H.M.S.O.

The peak age for offending is 15 for males and 14 for females; the rate of offending drops thereafter, with many offenders ceasing to be delinquent in early adulthood.

Offences of theft and handling stolen goods accounted for 66 per cent of juveniles cautioned or sentenced in 1983. Together, offences of violence, sex, and robbery accounted for 8.6 per cent of juveniles dealt with.

Juvenile crime is not on the rise
The number of 'known' juvenile offenders was 10 per cent lower in 1983 than in 1974. The rates of offending (numbers of offenders per 100,000 of that sex and age group) have levelled off or declined since 1980 for all age groups except females aged 14 to 16.

3 Research which contributes to understanding delinquency

3.1 The historical and international context

1 Rutter and Giller (1982) pointed out the following factors which justify questioning the apparent increase in crime among young people:
   (a) The increase has been in delinquent *acts*, rather than in the number of people committing them; that is, there is evidence of an increase in reoffending.
   (b) Part of the apparent increase is attributable to changes in methods of classifying data.
   (c) There are indications that more people are now being brought to court for acts that would formerly have been dealt with informally.
   (d) The public may be reporting more offences to the police.
2 Rutter and Giller saw the rise in the incidence of personal violence as well-documented, however, but as with stealing and other forms of crime, there may be a levelling off, or even a slight reduction since the mid-1970s.
3 Rutter and Giller (1982) drew attention to the parallels in many other western, industrialized societies, where data from American, Canadian, Scandinavian, German and Australian sources all indicated marked increases in crime, and juvenile crime rates. The important exception is Japan, which despite its markedly higher rate of industrialization and urbanization than many western countries, challenges the view that these predispose it to increased crime.
4 They suggested it is possible that increased delinquency may be part of a broader picture of increased distress among young people – since there is evidence of levels of suicide, parasuicide, alcohol and drug dependence all having increased in the same period.

3.2 Investigating developmental trends: can delinquency be predicted?

1 There has been considerable research upon reliable predictors of subsequent delinquency, both in the UK and in the USA. Few studies of continuities of behaviour yet span early childhood, later childhood, adolescence and adulthood, and only slight converging evidence is beginning to emerge.

2 Thus, there is some evidence from Kagan and Moss (1962) and from Richman, Stevenson and Graham (1982) that children who are difficult to manage at age three are also difficult to manage at age eight, but this is *not* clearly borne out by data from the National Child Development Study. (See page 195). Rutter and Giller (1983), however, commenting on the detailed study of Richman, Stevenson and Graham (1982), wrote, 'It is evident that most of the boys with extreme restlessness and/or marked difficulties in management at 3 or 4 were showing conduct disorders at 8.'

3 The major longitudinal studies of older children by West and Farrington (1973, 1977) of a large sample of boys in East London, found that boys regarded as troublesome by teachers and peers at age eight and by peers at age ten, tended to continue to be troublesome in adolescence. Rutter and Giller (1983) summarized:

> Of the most troublesome children, 27 per cent became recividist delinquents, in marked contrast to the rate of 0.7 per cent among the least troublesome children. Expressed in reverse fashion, it is apparent that 68% of recidivists have been in the most troublesome group at primary school compared with 12% of non-delinquents.

4 Rutter and Giller (1983) drew attention to the converging evidence (e.g. Robins, 1966; Rutter, 1977) that: 'Clinic referred children with disorders are more likely than children with emotional disorders (and much more likely than those without disorder) to show persisting psychiatric and social impairment.'

5 The American follow-up studies, notably by Robins (1966, 1978), have supported the notion that children at high risk of delinquency and anti-social behaviour can be detected from early indicators. Rutter and Giller (1983) quoted Robins's summary:

   1 Adult antisocial behaviour virtually requires childhood antisocial behaviour.
   2 Most antisocial children do not become antisocial adults.
   3 The variety of antisocial behaviour in childhood is a better predictor of adult antisocial behaviour than is any particular behaviour.
   4 Adult antisocial behaviour is better predicted by childhood behaviour than by family background or social class of rearing.
   5 Social background makes little contribution to the prediction of serious adult antisocial behaviour.

6 Loeber and Dishion (1983) conducted a major review of the research concerning early predictors of male delinquency. Their data suggested

that the best single predictor was a measure of child and family management techniques.

4 Research concerning specific variables

Rutter and Giller (1983) have summarized research relating to several major variables:

4.1 Sex

1 Whether employing official statistics, self-report data or information from parents or teachers, a consistent finding is that there is a markedly higher incidence of offending by young males than by young females. This is also true for Scandinavian countries, and for the United States. The higher sex ratio of boys to girls is, however, diminishing.
2 Rutter and Giller (1983) noted the evidence of greater aggression, both verbal and physical, among boys than among girls, particularly when interacting with other boys; this may have a biological basis, and be related to hormonal factors.
3 Boys are also known to be more vulnerable to a range of physical stresses, and several studies, though not all, have shown that boys may also be more likely than girls to develop conduct disorders when exposed to family discord.

4.2 Social class

1 While several American studies, using the official statistics and self-report data, have questioned the often-assumed association between delinquency and socio-economic grouping, other British ones, notably Belson (1968) and Farrington (1979) have found such an association, although a modest one. Belson, for example, found 15 per cent of boys from professional or managerial background reported having stolen, compared with 25 per cent of those from an unskilled manual background; McDonald (1969), however, found no social class difference for serious theft or breaking and entering.
2 Concerning differentials in judicial responses to delinquency, Rutter and Giller (1983) considered that despite the shortage of data, there 'probably is some social class differentiation in the detection and processing of delinquents which accounts in part for differences in delinquency rates.'
3 Rutter and Giller concluded from the evidence that there is a modest association between low social status and delinquency, which is due partly to social class differentials in detection and prosecution, and that the association is mainly found with the more serious delinquencies. They drew attention to two particular findings:
(a) There is a stronger association between delinquency and parental

unemployment or reliance on welfare than between delinquency and occupation or education, and

(b) There is a considerable overlap between social status measures and measures of parental behaviour or family relationships which relate to delinquency in all social groups.

4.3 Race

1 Reviewing the many studies in this area, Rutter and Giller (1983) concluded that:

> Firstly, the delinquency rate for Asians has been equal to or lower than that for the white population at all times when it has been studied. Secondly, in sharp contrast to the situation in the 1950s and 1960s, the arrest rates for blacks is now substantially above that for whites, especially for violent crimes (although the degree of 'violence' involved is often minimal). Thirdly, most violent crimes occur between two people who are of the *same* skin colour.

2 These writers considered that the much higher rate of arrests for blacks, mainly Afro-Caribbeans, is partly attributable to the psycho-social factors known to make delinquency more probable, unemployment, poor housing, social disadvantage, etc., and partly attributable to variation of practice in policing, reporting and arresting.

5 Research concerning individual characteristics and psycho-social factors relating to delinquency

5.1 Individual characteristics

In a paper summarizing their review of the evidence concerning this area, Rutter and Giller (1982) concluded that findings on the importance of individual factors are mixed, but that there is evidence that such factors as educational handicaps, hyperactivity and difficulties in maintaining attention can all contribute to delinquent behaviour, particularly among those who reoffend.

5.2 Psycho-social factors

In the same paper, they concluded that there was reasonably good evidence of several psycho-social factors contributing to the causation of delinquency. They noted:

i The most strongly associated family characteristics are parental criminality, ineffective supervision and discipline, family discord, weak parent–child relationships and large family size . . .

ii From a wide range of research into films and television it would seem that prolonged viewing of violent programmes may have *some* effect in increasing a predisposition to behave in a violent and anti-social way among children who are already aggressive or delinquent . . .

iii Whatever the official purposes of judicial action, court appearance has the effect of 'labelling' a delinquent and may influence an individual's view of himself and how he behaves. A first court appearance tends to be followed by an increase in delinquency . . .

iv There is limited evidence on the influence of the school but results suggest there *is* an influence and that pupil intake in terms of intellectual ability and social status (probably in terms of peer group influences) and school ethos and organisation do affect delinquency . . .

v Differences between cities, towns and rural areas in rates of delinquency are marked . . .

vi Research confirms that situational effects, such as physical design features of housing estates, do to some extent affect delinquent activity . . .

vii One area of investigation which . . . may turn out to be important is that of factors which reduce the risk of delinquency among children from high risk backgrounds.

6 The contribution of different theories of delinquency to a multi-variate, systems model

6.1 The contribution of some sociological theories

1 Merton (1957) and Cohen (1956) highlighted the difficulties which working-class young people have in gaining economic success and in acquiring social prestige. Cloward and Ohlin (1961) emphasized the notion of 'differential association', or the grouping of some young people into gangs likely to engage in offending, as well as Cohen's pinpointing the school as a mainly middle-class institution where working-class children find difficulties in achieving success.

Rutter and Giller (1983) reported the testing of the notion of 'differential association' by Elliott and Voss (1974) who broadly confirmed its validity, and noted the link with educational retardation.

2 'Differential association' seems to be implicated in the probability of a young person's becoming delinquent (West and Farrington, 1973). Furthermore, Wilson (1980) found the level of parental supervision exercised to be a key variable in the probability of a young person's becoming delinquent.

6.2 The contribution of some psychological theories

Clarke and Mayhew (1980) and Clarke (1982) have drawn attention to cognitive (i.e. perceptual and decision-making) factors and to situational ones. That is, they highlight the 'person-in-a-situation' phenomenon, and see people as conducting an implicit cost-benefit analysis concerning the anticipated consequences of an action: e.g. of taking part in a burglary.

6.3 The possible contribution of genetic factors

Some researchers, on the basis of twin studies, have concluded that certain individuals are likely to be predisposed to criminality as a result of genetic variables. This evidence, however, is much disputed.

6.4 The development of a multi-factorial model: Clarke (1977)

Amid this diversity, there is a move to devising models which accommodate discrete but interacting levels of probability which all contribute to e.g. the occurrence of a criminal event. See Figure 28.2.

References

Belson, W. A. (1968), 'The extent of stealing by London boys', *Advancement of Science*, vol. 25, pp. 171–84.

Clarke, R. V. G. (1977), 'Psychology and crime', *Bulletin of the British Psychological Society*, vol. 30, pp. 280–3.

Clarke, R. V. G. (1982), 'Crime prevention through environmental management and design', in J. Gunn and D. P. Farrington (eds), *Abnormal Offenders: Delinquency and the Criminal Justice System*, Chichester: Wiley.

Clarke, R. V. G. and Mayhew, P. (eds) (1980), *Designing out Crime*, London: HMSO.

Cloward, R. A. and Ohlin, L. E. (1960), *Delinquency and Opportunity*, Chicago: Free Press.

Cohen, A. K. (1956), *Delinquent Boys: the Culture of the Gang*, London: Routledge & Kegan Paul.

Elliott, D. S. and Voss, H. L. (1974), *Delinquency and Drop Out*, Toronto and London: Lexington Books.

Farrington, D. P. (1979), 'Longitudinal research on crime and delinquency' in N. Morris and M. Tonry (eds), *Criminal Justice: an Annual Review of Research*, Chicago and London: University of Chicago Press, vol. 1, pp. 289–348.

Farrington, D. P. and Bennett, T. (1981), 'Police cautioning of juveniles in London', *British Journal of Criminology*, vol. 21, pp. 123–35.

Kagan, J. and Moss, M. A. (1962), *Birth to Maturity*, New York: Wiley.

Loeber, R. and Dishion, T. (1983), 'Early predictors of male delinquency: a review', *Psychological Bulletin*, vol. 94, No. 1, pp. 68–99.

McDonald, L. (1969), *Social Class and Delinquency*, London: Faber & Faber.

Merton, R. K. (1957), *Social Theory and Social Structure*, New York: Free Press.

NACRO (1985), *Juvenile Crime*, Juvenile Crime Briefing, London: National Council for the Care and Resettlement of Offenders.

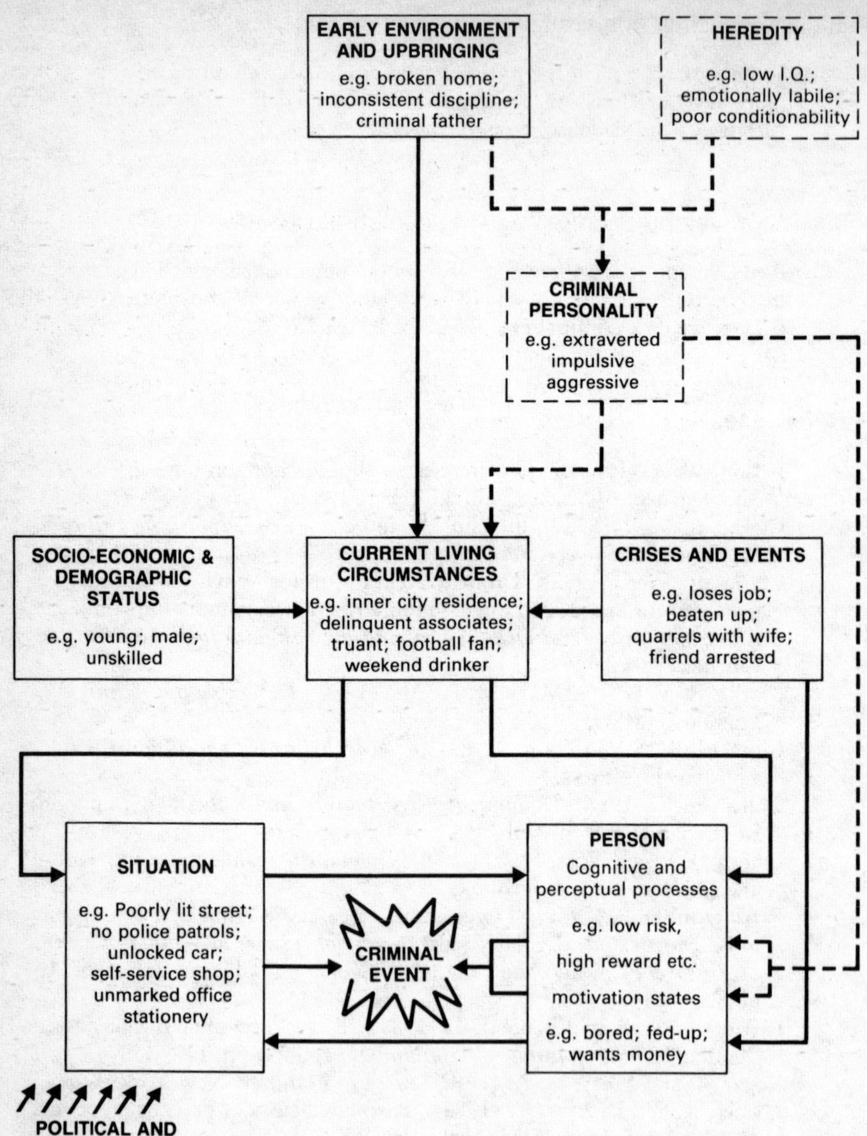

***The examples given within each box will have significance only in respect of particular types of crime**

FIGURE 28.2 Elements contributing to the occurrence of a criminal event. From Clarke, R. V. G. (1977), Psychology and crime. *Bulletin of the British Psychological Society*, vol. 30.

Richman, N., Stevenson, J. and Graham, P. J. (1982), *Pre-school to School: a Behavioural Study*, London: Academic Press.

Robins, L. (1966), *Deviant Chidren Grown Up*, Baltimore: Williams & Wilkins.

Robins, L. (1978), 'Sturdy childhood predictors of adult anti-social behaviour: replications from longitudinal studies', *Psychological Medicine*, vol. 8, pp. 611–12.

Rutter, M. (1977), 'Separation, loss and family influences' in M. Rutter and L. Hersov (eds), *Child Psychiatry: Modern Approaches*, Oxford: Blackwell Scientific.

Rutter, M. (1977), 'Other family influences' in M. Rutter and L. Hersov (eds), *Child Psychiatry: Modern Approaches*, Oxford: Blackwell Scientific.

Rutter, M. and Giller, H. (1982), 'Juvenile delinquency: trends and perspectives', *Research Bulletin*, Home Office Research and Planning Unit, no. 13, pp. 26–9.

Rutter, M. and Giller, H. (1983), *Juvenile Delinquency: Trends and Perspectives*, Harmondsworth: Penguin.

West, D. J. and Farrington, D. P. (1973), *Who Becomes Delinquent?*, London: Heinemann Educational.

West, D. J. and Farrington, D. P. (1977), *The Delinquent Way of Life*, London: Heinemann Educational.

Wilson, H. (1980), 'Parental supervision: a neglected aspect of delinquency', *British Journal of Criminology*, vol. 20, pp. 203–35.

29 Research on differing approaches to young offenders, including intermediate treatment

Consultant: Professor Norman Tutt, Department of Social Administration, University of Lancaster.

1 Some of the differing approaches, and descriptions thereof

The approaches to be considered separately below include:

1 General diversion from the criminal justice system
2 Intermediate treatment
3 Community based projects
4 Family placements

1.1 Diversion from the criminal justice system

This refers to a *range* of strategies aimed at reducing the probability of young offenders' becoming categorized and confirmed as 'criminals' at a young age. Tutt (1983) has reported some antecedents of the approach, noting that the Home Office White Paper, *The Child, the Family and the Young Offender*, 1965, made the case for children being 'spared the stigma of criminality', while the White Paper, *Young Offenders* 1980, stated:

> All the available evidence suggests that juvenile offenders who can be diverted from the criminal justice system at an early stage in their offending are less likely to reoffend than those who become involved in judicial proceedings.

1.2 Intermediate treatment

1 Thorpe (1978) has written of this:

> The term 'intermediate treatment' first appeared in a United Kingdom government White Paper in 1968 ('Children in Trouble', 1968, p. 9) and was used to define a range of services for juvenile offenders to be provided by a projected new Act of Parliament intended to alter substantially the methods used to control juvenile offenders in England and Wales. Both that White Paper and the legislation which followed it – the 1969 Children and Young Persons Act (CYPA) – offered only very vague and broad definitions of intermediate treatment.

2 Thorpe continued that a key principle of the approach is that it makes it possible for the offending 'child to remain in his own home', and he wrote, 'This phrase firmly places intermediate treatment as a community-based service for those offenders who would, in all probability, normally receive a sentence involving custodial care.'
3 Thorpe also drew attention to the DHSS publication, *Intermediate Treatment*, in 1971, which indicated that such provision should 'normally be of a kind in which other children can also participate, and not confined to children under supervision through court orders'.
4 These and other descriptions make it clear that there is no single, unified, body of practice or theory which constitutes Intermediate Treatment. Such research as has been conducted has thus examined a wide variety of activity practised in a variety of ways, by a variety of practitioners, in a variety of settings.

2 Official statistics

It is difficult to obtain precise figures for these means of intervention with young offenders, but the National Association for the Care and Resettlement of Offenders (1985) noted of supervision orders and intermediate treatment:

> *Supervision orders* were imposed on 12,700 juveniles in 1983. The use of the supervision order has declined throughout the last decade. . .
>
> *Intermediate treatment (IT) requirements* were attached to nearly a quarter of supervision orders made in the year ending March 1982.

3 Research into the complexity of factors to be considered when devising strategies of intervention

3.1 Factors contributing to offending in groups

These are also described by Rutter and Giller (1983). (See Chapter 28, page 276). Thorpe, Smith, Green and Paley (1980) in *Out of Care*, which examines community responses to young offenders, summarized the factors, similar to those highlighted by Hirschi (1968), which they consider the evidence implicates in offending – particularly in groups:

(1) Social and emotional deprivation causes children to have few stakes in society, and relatively little to gain from conforming to social norms.
(2) One of the possible responses to this is to become associated with others in a similar position (selection of delinquent peers).
(3) The company of delinquent peers can potentially offer status denied by the adult world.
(4) The central dynamic of the delinquent peer group is a testing-out process which leads to delinquent acts in order to maintain status.
(5) Delinquent acts give status, excitement and sometimes material gain.

(6) The response of the juvenile justice system reinforces dependence on delinquent peers and the rejection of conventional values.

4 Background research findings concerning effective and ineffective strategies of intervention

4.1 A review of the American literature

Antedating the review by Rutter and Giller (1983) (See Chapter 28), Romig (1978), on the basis of his review of 170 studies of a range of American responses to young offenders, having a matched or randomly assigned control group, devised the following lists:

Summary of approaches found to be ineffective

1 Casework.
2 Direct services.
3 Diagnosis and recommendations only.
4 Discussion groups.
5 Use of behavioural approaches for performance of complex behaviours.
6 Manipulating what teachers expect of their pupils.
7 School attendance alone.
8 Job placement.
9 Vocational training.
10 Occupational orientation and work programmes.
11 Field trips; camping.
12 Group counselling.
13 Individual psychotherapy.
14 Family therapy.

Summary of approaches found to be effective

1 Use of behavioural approaches for simple behaviours.
2 Involving young people in setting their own goals.
3 Differential reinforcement.
4 Specificity for rehabilitation goals.
5 Education, when it utilized:
   Individualized diagnosis
   Specific learning goal
   Individualized programme based on relevant material
   Basic academic skills
   Breaking complex behaviour into simpler ones
   Rewarding attention and persistence initially
   Differential reinforcement of learning performance.
6 Job training with supportive educational training.
7 Training in job advancement skills.
8 Training in career decision making skills.
9 Educational programmes that culminate in a qualification.
10 Follow-up help after job placement.
11 Group therapy with a teaching focus.

12 Individual counselling with the following ingredients:
   Getting input from young people on their views
   Diagnosis of a specific difficulty and its setting
   Setting a behavioural goal
   Practising new behaviour in the problem setting
   The staff member who provided the counselling directly observing the young people in its setting
   The evaluation and setting of future goals.
13 Family intervention . . . upon improving . . . communication.
14 Parent training in . . . problem solving and disciplining.

5 Research concerning the outcomes of diversion

There is as yet little firm research in this area, but Thorpe (1983) has reported the evidence from Northamptonshire where a Juvenile Liaison Bureau is staffed by an interdisciplinary team from the police, social services, probation, youth service and education. Thorpe (1983), describing the evidence for the effectiveness of the diversionary approach for the two-year period July 1980 to June 1982, included the following data:

1 An increase of police use of the 'caution' from 56% to 73%.
2 A reduction in police prosecutions from 40% to 19%.
3 Among sentences, an increase of deferred sentence from 1% to 19%.
4 Among sentences, an increase of supervision order or intermediate treatment from 26% to 35%.
5 Among sentences, a reduction of care orders from 5 to 0, a reduction of detention centre sentences from 3 to 0 and a reduction of Crown Court sentences from 4 to 0.

6 Research concerning intermediate treatment

6.1 Intermediate Treatment schemes in the UK

1 The shortage of research

1 A number of initiatives have taken place in reporting the means of working and outcomes of short term IT projects, notably by the National Youth Bureau. These, however, have been constrained by e.g. funding limitations, to consider only short-term outcomes.
2 Preston (1982), has written of some of the general problems of researching Intermediate Treatment (IT) thus:

> The target population is not clearly defined, and the treatment methods and aims of intervention in IT are vague and open to broad interpretation. Even where treatment techniques are specified, these do not appear to be based on any recent research or results of similar intervention.

3 Preston reports a number of projects throughout the country, and writes, 'All have reported a variety of schemes and individual approaches which on the surface would appear excellent, but unfortunately overall evaluation of the projects has been very limited.' She does, however, report one carefully evaluated project:

2 **The Birmingham Action for Youth (BAY) Centre**

1 This Centre was set up as an alternative to residential care. Contracts were written, with short- and long-term goals worked out between offenders, parents and Centre staff. Evaluation at six months compared the progress of twenty-four participants in the goal-setting approach with the progress of twenty-six earlier attenders who had not developed goals.

2 Results from both groups were equally encouraging; only five from the goal-setting group and six from the earlier group were known to have committed a single further offence – although two from each group were in residential establishments as a result. Costs were 50 per cent of those of custodial care. Preston suggests that the results indicate the need for on-going support for participants from the Centre, rather than a 'one-off' intervention, as well as the desirability of closer involvement of families.

3 **A study in Portsmouth** Lupton and Roberts (1982) reported that of the 100 juveniles undergoing IT from 1974 to 1980, only three were charged with new offences in 1980, and of the twenty-one IT requirements made in 1980 only 16 per cent reappeared in court within two years.

7 Research concerning community-based projects

7.1 Community-based behavioural projects in the USA

Preston (1982) reports a number of these, of which features are clear goal-setting, the devising of contracts and active planning for success by the participants. They include:

1 **Kentfields Rehabilitation Program** This scheme in Michigan, reported by Davidson and Robinson (1975), is a community-based programme for relatively serious male offenders who would otherwise have received custodial sentences. Results were very encouraging, but Preston (1982) noted the absence of a control group.

2 **Achievement Place** This is a community-based group home, in which the programme is directed by members of the community, and where the primary focus is upon enabling the boys to achieve. Several studies have noted early successes, and Kirigin *et al.* (1979), for example, reported two-year follow-up data, with fewer Achievement Place boys in custody than from a comparison group who had originally been in custody.

7.2 Community-based behavioural projects in the UK

1 The Shape Project

1 This project is reported by Ostapiuk (1982), and provides accommodation, work experience and training in 'survival' skills for young adult offenders. Ostapiuk reports the outcomes for thirty-six participants, median age eighteen, who took part in the project for an average of twenty-six weeks, and almost all of whom had a previous history of offending and of custodial institutions.

2 At follow-up, minimum length six months, there was evidence of only eight offences among the thirty-six participants, and Ostapiuk has written:

> The data clearly show that most of the clients who re-offend do so within 6 months of leaving the project, and suggest that the longer a client remains out of the programme without offending the better his chances in the long term. . . . Nevertheless the overall figure of 78 per cent success for all clients taken together is impressive.

8 Research concerning family placements

8.1 The Kent Family Placement Project

1 This scheme, initiated by Hazel and reported by her in 1980, has received considerable attention. In five years, almost 200 disturbed and delinquent adolescents were fostered by families who had volunteered for what they knew would be a demanding task, and who received considerable financial and other support.

2 Hazel reported that over 70 per cent of the young people placed met criteria for 'success', and wrote,

> Contracts were central to the project's concept of . . . placements, providing both an agreed statement of objectives for all concerned (adolescent, family of origin, foster-family and social workers) and at the same time providing the foster parents with a job description.

References

Davidson, W. S. and Robinson, M. J. (1975), 'Community psychology and behavior modification: a community-based program for the prevention of delinquency', *Journal of Corrective Psychiatry and Behaviour Therapy*, vol. 21, pp. 1–12.

DHSS (1971), *Intermediate Treatment: a Guide for the Regional Planning for New Forms of Treatment for Children in Trouble*, London: HMSO.

Hazel, N. (1980), *A Bridge to Independence*, Oxford: Basil Blackwell.

Hirschi, T. (1968), *Causes of Delinquency*, Berkeley: University of California Press.

Home Office (1965), *The Child, the Family and the Young Offender*, Cmnd. 2742, London: HMSO.

Home Office (1968), *Children in Trouble*, Cmnd. 3601, London: HMSO.

Home Office, Department of Health and Social Security, and Welsh Office (1980), *Young Offenders*, Cmnd. 8045, London: HMSO.

Kirigin, K. A., Wolf, M. M., Braukman, C. J., Fixsen, D. L. and Phillips, E. L. (1979), 'Achievement Place: A preliminary outcome evaluation' in J. S. Stumphauzer (ed.), *Progress in Behaviour Therapy with Delinquents*, Springfield, Illinois: Thomas.

Lupton, C. and Roberts, G. (1982), *On Record . . . Young People Appearing Before a Juvenile Court*, Portsmouth Social Services Research and Intelligence Unit.

Morris, A. (1978), 'Diversion of juvenile offenders from the criminal justice system' in N. Tutt (ed.) (1978), *Alternative Strategies for Coping with Crime*, Oxford: Basil Blackwell and Martin Robertson.

National Association for the Care and Resettlement of Offenders (1985), *Juvenile Crime*, London: N.A.C.R.O. May, 1985.

Ostapiuk, E. (1982), 'Strategies for community intervention in offender rehabilitation: an overview' in M. P. Feldman (ed.), *Developments in the Study of Criminal Behaviour, vol. 1: The Prevention and Control of Offending* (1982), Chichester: Wiley.

Preston, M. A. (1982), 'Intermediate treatment: a new approach to community care' in M. P. Feldman (ed.), *Developments in the Study of Criminal Behaviour vol. 1: The Prevention and Control of Offending.*

Romig, D. A. (1978), *Justice for our Children*, Lexington, Massachusetts: Lexington Books.

Rutter, M. and Giller, H. (1983), *Juvenile Delinquency: Trends and Perspectives*, Harmondsworth: Penguin.

Thorpe, D. (1978), 'Intermediate treatment' in N. Tutt (ed.) (1978), *Alternative Strategies for Coping with Crime*, Oxford: Basil Blackwell and Martin Robertson.

Thorpe, D. H., Smith, D., Green, C. J. and Paley, J. H. (1980), *Out of Care: The Community Support of Juvenile Offenders*, London: Allen & Unwin.

Thorpe, D. H. (1983), 'Does the Northamptonshire model work? The Wellingborough study – some preliminary results' in *Crime Prevention: Diversion – Corporate Action with Juveniles*, Proceedings of a Conference, 4–6 December 1983, Centre of Youth, Crime and Community, University of Lancaster.

Tutt, N. (ed.) (1978), *Alternative Strategies for Coping with Crime*, Oxford: Basil Blackwell and Martin Robertson.

Tutt, N. (1983), 'Diversion – What is it?' in *Crime Prevention: Diversion – Corporate Action with Juveniles.*

Research concerning probation

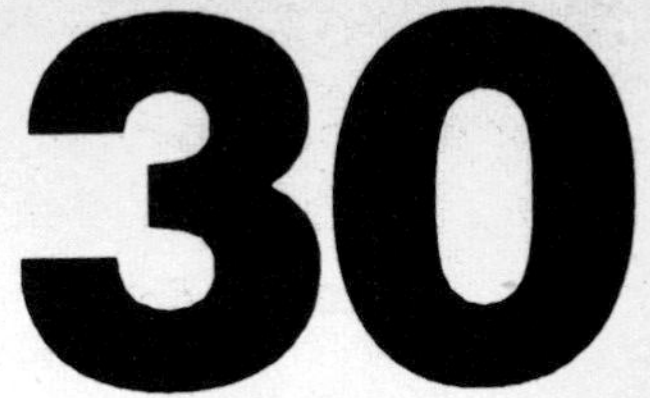

Consultant:* *Professor Martin Davies, School of Economic and Social Studies, University of East Anglia, Norwich.

1 A general definition

Jarvis (1980) reported that the Morison Committee defined probation as,

> the submission of an offender while at liberty to a specified period of supervision by a social caseworker who is an officer of the court: during this period the offender remains liable, if not of good conduct, to be otherwise dealt with by the court (Report of the Departmental Committee on the Probation Service (1962) Cmnd. 1650, para. 9).
>
> The probationer must give his consent to the making of the probation order and to any requirements contained in it.

and he continued:

> Probation is not confined to first offenders nor to trivial offences. There is no restriction on the type of person who may be placed on probation except that he must be aged 17 or over.

2 Statistics

2.1 Number of probation orders

	England and Wales					
	Males			Females		
	17–20	21 or over	All ages	17–20	21 or over	All ages
Type of sentence						
Probation order	10.8	13.3	24.1	3.1	6.8	9.8

TABLE 30.1 Probation orders in England and Wales, 1983. Thousands. (*Social Trends*, 1985)

2.2 After care

Those receiving after-care on 31 December 1985 numbered just over 51 thousand (*Social Trends* 1987).

3 A way of considering the research

Bottoms and McWilliams have written,

> In relation to the criminal side of probation practice, there have been four basic aims of the service, under which all other objectives could be subsumed as second order ones. These four primary aims are and have been:
> 1 The provision of appropriate help for offenders.
> 2 The statutory supervision of offenders.
> 3 Diverting appropriate offenders from custodial sentences.
> 4 The reduction of crime.

These 'four basic aims' have thus been chosen as the headings under which the research findings are grouped – though not in the order shown above.

4 Research concerning the reduction of crime

4.1 The review by Brody (1976)

An early review of the effects of different types of sentence, as measured by subsequent offending, was conducted by Brody in 1976. Those studies involving probation are summarized below.

1 **Custodial versus non-custodial sentences** Brody surveyed nine studies in which the outcomes of custodial sentences were compared with the effects of probation, or comparable intensive supervision, measured by subsequent rates of reoffending.

(a) *Outcomes with juveniles and early adults* Of those five in this group, Empey and Erickson (1972) in the American PROVO study, and Kraus (1974) in an Australian study, both found probation to be more effective than custody. Pond (1970), however, found no differences in outcome, while Palmer in two consecutive Community Treatment Projects in 1971 and 1974, found that anxious, neurotic boys did better than rebellious and manipulative ones.

(b) *Outcomes with adults*

1 Of those four studies concerning adults, Wilkins (1958) found no different effects in terms of subsequent reoffending between two courts giving different numbers of custodial or non-custodial sentences, and Davis (1964) correlated the frequency with which probation was given in two counties with the revoking of parole, and found minimal results.
2 Two other studies, Hammond (1964) and Babst and Mannering (1965), gave conflicting results: the former found probation less effective than prison for first offenders: the latter found it more. The study by Conbose (1966) found probation slightly more effective in terms of reoffending rates.

(c) Summary comment by Brody (1976)

The major implication of research findings in this aspect of sentencing is again that different types of offenders respond in different ways to the various treatments applied to them.

4.2 More recent evidence of the 'holding' effect of probation

Ashworth (1983) drew attention to the evidence in the Probation and After Care statistics of 1981 that the following percentages of orders were terminated without reconviction or revocation for other reasons:

88% of orders for 1 year
73% of orders for 2 years
67% of orders for 3 years

Ashworth noted that, by comparison, the figures show that 57 per cent of those receiving sentences of six months' imprisonment are reconvicted within two years of release.

4.3 Methodology

There is a fundamental problem with most of the statistical comparisons in this area: almost no studies cope with the criticism that those placed on probation may be inherently better risks than those sent to prison, and therefore that any comparisons made are entirely spurious.

5 Research concerning models of statutory supervision

5.1 The review by Brody (1976)

Brody reviewed nine studies in this field, eight American and one British.

1 Studies showing no effect of treatment

1. Of the ten, six demonstrated no effects, in terms of rates of reoffending, of differential forms of non-custodial treatment. Powers and Witmer (1951) compared 'special' supervision of 325 young offenders with 'ordinary' supervision of 325 matched other young offenders, but found no differences of outcome. Johnson (1962), comparing sizes of caseload, found no effect of size. Lohman (1967), working in the San Francisco Project, similarly found no differential effect of caseload size. Empey and Erickson (1972), already mentioned, found no effects of intensive or ordinary supervision in their PROVO study.
2. The British study, by Folkard and colleagues (1974), found first, no effects of type of offender matched to type of probation officer; second, there were no differential effects of 'intensive' or 'ordinary' supervision by probation officers working with both male and female probationers.

2 Studies showing an effect of treatment

1 Four other studies did, however, show some differential effect. The Los Angeles Probation study (1959) showed that intensive supervision gave a better outcome than conventional supervision, and Johnson, in a second study in 1962, found that 'adequate' probation officers had more effects than 'inadequate'.
2 Adams and Hopkinson (1964) found that a smaller probation caseload proved more effective than a larger one; and Palmer (1971, 1974) found varying effectiveness of different types of supervision according to the personality type of the offender.

3 **Commentary by Brody (1976)** Brody noted that because of methodological and other problems in conducting such research, only tentative conclusions were possible, such as: 'the falling off of crime with increasing age is a well established fact. . . . Generally, the younger the offender, the higher the risk.'

He also concluded:

> the usefulness of probationary sentences, in particular, seems to be dependent to some extent on whether the offender has a record of previous convictions or not. . . . The strongest evidence . . . seems to indicate that an intermediate group of offenders, who are neither first offenders nor yet confirmed recidivists, are possibly the best targets for experimental measures.

6 Research concerning work to divert offenders from custodial sentences

1 The numbers of those potentially 'divertible'

1 Bottoms and McWilliams (1979) quote the Home Office Research Unit's review of the prison population of the SE Region as indicating that, on certain given criteria, about one third of the 771 men imprisoned were potentially 'divertible'.
2 In exploring the desirability, in their view, of far more offenders' being diverted from custody, Bottoms and McWilliams drew attention to the clear evidence, e.g. from the Home Office Circular 195 (1974) that probation officers have, on occasion, recommended both custodial and suspended sentences. They questioned the appropriateness of this.

7 The provision of help for offenders

7.1 Studies of after-care and multi-facility schemes

1 Silberman and Chapman's (1971) study of after-care units in London, Liverpool and Manchester, showed that over a third of the clients came for one interview only, and only one in five kept contact with the probation service for more than three months. Bottoms and McWilliams

report similar findings by Morris and Beverly (1975) in their study of parolees on compulsory supervision.

2 Crow, Pease and Hillary (1980), in their study of the Manchester and Wiltshire multi-facility schemes for offenders and other users, found inconclusive evidence of the usefulness of such provision.

3 On the basis of such admittedly limited evidence, Bottoms and McWilliams and others questioned whether the probation service could be said to be providing appropriate help for offenders; and Davies (1969) identified a further paradox when he found that probation officers were 'best able to make a good relationship with those who appear to need least help'.

8 Indications of an increasing consensus among criminologists

8.1 The limitations of the 'treatment model'

1 There seems to be evidence of an increasing convergence of opinion among commentators upon the research concerning aspects of probation work; Brody (1976), Bottoms and McWilliams (1979) and Jones (1981) all consider that the 'treatment model' has been found wanting.

2 Some commentators recommend a more community-oriented response to offending, drawing upon concepts being pioneered, among others, by the National Association for the Care and Resettlement of Offenders. It is early days for much of this type of work to have been evaluated.

8.2 Recent developments within the service

1 Partly as a result of the evidence above, and of the clear value of the practical *help* which probation officers are able to give, further ways of offering this help are developing. These include the provision of services of the kind described by Haxby (1978):

   1 The provision of better accommodation: further hostels.
   2 Day centres.
   3 Supportive work with the families of those on probation.
   4 Work towards clear and specific goals, using 'short-term contracts'.
   5 Help with specific difficulties: e.g. debts, legal problems, welfare rights entitlement and the search for employment.

2 There is also a developing involvement in some localities of probation officers in community development work, but there is as yet no substantial research literature in this area.

8.3 The trend to notions of reparation and restitution

Schemes are being initiated in several parts of the UK in which offenders and their victims are brought face to face in the presence of a probation officer or a volunteer mediator. Such victim–offender mediation schemes are now successfully established in the USA, but are still in the process of being implemented and evaluated in the UK.

9 Some research upon probation hostels

9.1 A study of wardens and matrons and their influence

1. Sinclair (1975) reported a study involving 4,343 boys who entered probation hostels between January 1954 and January 1963. The difference in failure rate, (i.e. absconding or committing further offences) among forty-six regimes ranged from 14.5 per cent to 78.1 per cent.
2. Preliminary indications were that:

   > failure rates were characteristic of wardens, not of hostels. The differences between successive wardens in the same hostel were as wide as those between wardens in different hostels, and there was no association between failure rate, and the size, age range, or location of hostels. . . . Some wardens had better success with older boys, others with younger ones.

3. Further investigations based upon fourteen hostels suggested 'that "successful" wardens were likely to be strict, warm and – in disciplinary matters at least – in agreement with their wives.'

References

Adams, S. and Hopkinson, C. C. (1964), *Evaluation of the Intensive Supervision Case-load Project*, Los Angeles County Probation Department, Research Report, no. 12.

Ashworth, A. (1983), *Sentencing and Penal Policy*, London: Weidenfeld & Nicolson.

Babst, D. V. and Mannering, J. W. (1965), 'Probation versus imprisonment for similar types of offenders – a comparison by subsequent violations', *Journal of Research in Crime and Delinquency*, vol. 2, pp. 60–8.

Bottoms, A. E. and McWilliams, W. (1979), 'A non-treatment paradigm for probation practice', *British Journal of Social Work*, vol. 9, pp. 159–202.

Brody, S. R. (1976), *The Effectiveness of Sentencing*, Home Office Research Study, No. 35.

Conbose, E. (1966), *Final report of the San Francisco Rehabilitation Project for Offenders*, North California Service League.

Crow, I., Pease, K. and Hillary, J. (1980), *The Manchester and Wiltshire Multifacility Schemes*, National Association for the Care and Resettlement of Offenders.

Davies, M. (1969), *Probationers in their Social Environment. A Study of Male Probationers Aged 17–20, together with an Analysis of those Reconvicted within Twelve Months*, Home Office Research Study, No. 2, London: HMSO.

Davis, G. F. (1964), 'A study of adult probation violation rates by means of the cohort approach', *Journal of Criminal Law, Criminology and Police Science*, vol. 55, p. 70–6.

Empey, L. T. and Erickson, M. L. (1972), *The Provo Experiment*, Boston: Heath.

Folkard, M. S., Fowles, A. J., McWilliams, B. C., McWilliams, W., Smith, D. D., Smith, D. E. and Walmsley, G. R. (1974), *IMPACT. Intensive Matched Probation and After-Care Treatment. Vol. I. The Design of the Experiment and an Interim Evaluation*, Home Office Research Studies, No. 24, London: HMSO.

Folkard, M. S., Smith, D. E. and Smith, D. D. (1976), *IMPACT: Intensive Matched Probation and After-Care Treatment. Vol. II. The Results of the Experiment*, Home Office Research Study, No. 36, London: HMSO.

Hammond, W. H. (1974), *The Sentence of the Court. A handbook for courts on the treatment of offenders*, Home Office Circular, 195, London: HMSO.

Haxby, D. (1978), *Probation: A Changing Service*, London: Constable.

Jarvis, F. (1980), *Probation Officer's Manual*, London: Butterworth.

Johnson, B. M. (1962), *Parole Research Project: evaluation of reduced caseloads*, California Youth Authority, Research Report No. 27.

Johnson, B. M. (1962), *An analysis of parole performance and judgments of supervision in the Parole Research Project*, Research Report No. 32, California Youth and Adult Corrections Agency, Sacramento, California.

Jones, H. (1981), 'Old and new ways in probation' in H. Jones (ed.), *Society Against Crime*, Harmondsworth: Penguin.

Kraus, J. (1974), 'A comparison of correction effects of probation and detention on male juvenile offenders', *British Journal of Criminology*, vol. 14, no. 1, pp. 49–54.

Lohman, J. D., Wahl, A. and Carter, R. M. (1967), *The San Francisco Project*, Research Report No. 11, Berkeley, California, School of Criminology, University of California.

Los Angeles County Probation Department (1959), *The effectiveness of reduced case-loads for juvenile probation officers.*

Morris, P. and Beverly, F. (1975), *On Licence: A Study of Parole*, Chichester: Wiley.

Palmer, T. B. (1971), 'California's Community Treatment Project for Delinquents', *Journal of Research in Crime and Delinquency*, vol. 8, pp. 74–9.

Palmer, T. B. (1974), 'The Youth Authority's Community Treatment Project', *Federal Probation*, vol. 38, pp. 3–12.

Pond, E. (1970), *The Los Angeles Delinquency Control Project*, State of California, Department of the Youth Authority.

Powers, E. and Witmer, H. (1951), *An Experiment in the Prevention of Delinquency: The Cambridge-Somerville Youth Study*, New York: Columbia University Press.

Report of the Departmental Committee on the Probation Service (1962), Cmnd. 1650, London: HMSO.

Silberman, M. and Chapman, B. (1971), 'After-care units in London, Liverpool and Manchester' in *Explorations in After-Care*, Home Office Research Study, No. 9, HMSO.
Sinclair, I. A. (1975), 'The influence of wardens and matrons on probation hostels' in J. Tizard, I. Sinclair and R. V. G. Clarke (eds), *Varieties of Residential Experience*, London: Routledge & Kegan Paul.
Wilkins, L. T. (1958), 'A small comparative study of the effects of probation', *British Journal of Delinquency*, vol. 3, pp. 201–5.

31 Research concerning custodial and other responses to offenders

Consultant: Dr Ken Pease, Lecturer in Social Administration, Dept. of Social Administration, University of Manchester.

1 The complexity of the field

Research in this field is in a state of considerable flux. The material below illustrates a few of the major issues and of the research studies.

2 Statistics

2.1 Official figures

	Percentages				
	1981	1982	1983	1984	1985
Males					
Total number of offenders (thousands) = 100 per cent	399.2	409.6	399.2	387.8	382.9
Sentence or order					
Absolute discharge	0.6	0.6	0.6	0.5	0.5
Conditional discharge	9.9	10.2	10.5	11.2	11.0
Probation order	5.4	5.5	6.0	6.7	7.1
Supervision order	3.3	3.1	2.8	2.8	2.7
Fine	45.0	44.0	42.8	41.2	39.7
Community service order	5.9	6.5	7.5	8.2	8.4
Attendance centre order	3.4	3.5	3.6	3.4	3.3

	Percentages				
	1981	1982	1983	1984	1985
Detention centre order	3.2	3.1	2.9	2.8	2.8
Care order	0.8	0.7	0.5	0.4	0.3
Borstal training/Youth custody	2.1	2.0	3.6	4.9	5.1
Imprisonment					
Fully suspended	7.6	7.7	6.7	6.0	6.4
Partly suspended		0.3	0.9	0.9	0.9
Unsuspended	11.3	11.7	10.4	9.7	10.7
Other sentence or order	1.1	1.2	1.2	1.2	1.2
Females					
Total number of offenders (thousands) = 100 per cent	65.4	66.0	62.7	59.9	59.1
Sentence or order					
Absolute discharge	0.8	0.8	0.8	0.8	0.7
Conditional discharge	20.8	21.7	22.3	23.5	25.2
Probation order	14.9	15.2	15.8	16.4	16.7
Supervision order	3.5	3.2	2.5	2.4	2.1
Fine	46.2	45.0	44.0	41.7	40.0
Community service order	1.9	2.3	2.6	3.0	3.0
Attendance centre order	0.7	0.8	0.8	0.7	0.6
Detention centre order	–	–	–	–	–
Care order	0.9	0.6	0.5	0.3	0.3
Borstal training/Youth custody	0.4	0.3	0.9	1.4	1.5
Imprisonment					
Fully suspended	5.3	5.7	5.0	4.9	5.3
Partly suspended		0.2	0.6	0.7	0.6
Unsuspended	3.4	3.5	3.2	3.3	3.7
Other sentence or order	0.9	0.9	1.0	1.1	1.0

TABLE 31.1 Sentence or order passed on offenders sentenced for indictable offences: by sex. Magistrates' courts and the Crown Court. England and Wales. (*Annual Abstract of Statistics*, No. 121, 1985, HMSO)

3 Issues arising from research into custodial sentencing

3.1 The criterion used to evaluate a penal sanction

Ashworth (1983) has summarized the position:

> The effectiveness of a penal sanction has generally been measured by examining the rate of re-convictions in the two years after sentence, and, despite the drawbacks of this approach, there is not a more satisfactory approach in general penological use.

The two-year period conventionally runs from release in the case of custodial sentences.

3.2 The increasing acceptance of the principle of 'parsimony'

Ashworth (1983) has written: 'There is now widespread support for applying the principle of parsimony to custodial sentences . . . that custodial sentences should be used as sparingly as possible.'

He suggests three main reasons for this:

1 Doubts about the reformative potential of penal institutions.
2 Belief in the actively damaging effects of such institutions.
3 Doubts about the deterrent effect of custodial sentences.

3.3 The disproportionate number of black people in prison

N.A.C.R.O. (1986) noted with concern that at 30 June 1985 the proportion of all ethnic minority groups in the prison population was substantially higher than in the general population. NACRO concluded that the overall picture was disturbing, and would justify an official enquiry into ethnic minorities and the criminal justice system.

4 Research concerning the outcome of custodial and other responses to offenders

4.1 Probation: See Chapter 30, page 287

4.2 Supervision orders

The authors of *Juvenile Crime*, published by NACRO (1985) wrote of this,

> *Supervision orders* were imposed on 12,700 juveniles in 1983. The use of the supervision order has declined throughout the last decade. In 1969, 26 per cent of juveniles sentenced received probation orders (supervision orders replaced probation orders for those aged under 17 in 1971); by 1973 that had dropped to 20 per cent, and by 1983 to 17 per cent. . . .
>
> Forty-seven per cent of those commencing supervision by the probation service following criminal proceedings in the first half of 1983 were known to have had no previous convictions. . . .

4.3 Community service orders

1 Pease (1985) quoted the definition of community service programs given by Harris (1980):

> A community service program is a program through which convicted offenders are placed in unpaid positions with non-profit or tax-supported agencies to serve a specified number of hours performing work or service within a given time limit as a sentencing option or condition.

2 Community service is supervised by the Probation service, though it is often carried out under the supervision of non-probation staff. Pease (1985) has reviewed a number of studies and highlighted the following:
   (a) The anomaly that Community service is advocated and justified as an alternative to custody, but only about half of those sentenced to it would have been likely to incur a custodial sentence.
   (b) Disparities in the extent of the making of orders, in the lengths of orders and in the use of sanctions against offenders who do not comply with orders.
   (c) Reconviction studies are inconclusive. A Home Office study (1983) found that of 2,468 people given such orders:
   36% were reconvicted within 1 year
   51% were reconvicted within 2 years
   59% were reconvicted within 3 years

   There is no reason to suppose that the imposition of a community service order influences the probability of reconviction.

4.4 Detention centre

1 Banks (1964) compared the outcome, in terms of reoffending rates, of sentencing 300 men of seventeen to twenty years to each of the following: detention centre, borstal and prison. At follow-up there were no differences in reoffending rates between groups.
2 Thornton, Curran, Grayson and Holloway (1984) undertook a pilot evaluation of the 'tougher regimes in detention centres' policy. A centre for seniors, aged seventeen and under twenty-one, which implemented the 'tougher regimes' policy, was compared with two others which did not; a centre for juniors, aged fourteen and under seventeen, which implemented the policy, was compared with two others which did not. At one year follow-up there were no significant effects of the 'tougher regimes' policy in terms of reoffending rates: between 50 per cent and 57 per cent in all junior centres and between 43 per cent and 52 per cent in all senior centres had reoffended.

4.5 Borstal training/youth custody

Mannheim and Wilkins (1955) compared the length of time spent in Borstal by 385 boys, but found inconclusive results in terms of reoffending. They then compared outcomes between open and closed borstals, and concluded that open borstals led to less probability of reoffending. Benson (1959), comparing the effects of borstals and prisons, found no differences of outcome among young male offenders. Cockett (1967), comparing 110 boys in each of seven different borstals, found no differences of outcome. Williams (1970), however, considering 610 offenders randomly allocated to three different borstals, did find slight differences. Certainly no dramatic effect of borstal (or its successor, youth custody) can be assumed.

4.6 Imprisonment

The many fields of research concerning aspects of custody include:

1 **Length of sentence**

1 Many studies have examined differential time spent in prison and the associated outcomes: e.g. in an American study, Garrity (1961) compared lengths of sentence of 1,265 adult males and concluded that longer sentences led to worse outcomes for recidivists and unstable men.

2 In a major study in 1963, Hammond and Chayen compared the outcomes of preventive detention and differing lengths of long-term imprisonment, using samples ranging between 77 and 429: no differences in reoffending rates were found. Two other studies in the mid-1960s: Hammond (1964) and Banks (1964) both found no effect of differential lengths of sentence, while two American studies, the Florida Division of Corrections (1966) and Jaman (1968), both found that prisoners with longer sentences were more likely to reoffend than those with shorter sentences.

2 **Reconviction following a first offence** A major Home Office study, by Phillpots and Lancucki (1979), found that only 29 per cent of first offenders were reconvicted within six years whatever the sentence passed upon them. (One implication of this is that the mildest sentence may be as much of a deterrent as the most severe for this 29 per cent.)

3 **Imprisonment as a deterrent to offending** Pease (1985) has summarized the position as he sees it: 'I know of no evidence that imprisonment serves as a specific deterrent to offending, although it has an obvious *incapacitation* effect.'

4 **Provision of social/welfare help** Clarke and Cornish (1983) reported that Berntsen and Christiansen (1965) had found in Sweden that increased social/welfare work contributed to reduced reconviction. Two British studies found somewhat conflicting results from making the same provision: Shaw and colleagues (1974) found that seventy-five adult male prisoners, given such help, were less likely to re-offend than seventy-five controls not offered this help, but Fowles (1978) found no such effect in his broadly comparable study.

5 **Parole** Nuttall and colleagues (1977) suggested a possible effect of parole in reducing the likelihood of reconviction.

6 **'Rehabilitation'** Despite the generally negative tone of much of the work in this area, there are enough straws in the wind to encourage social workers and others in the hope that more sophisticated techniques might yield reductions in the probability of further convictions.

7 **Review of the results of social research** Mott (1985), in a Home Office Research Study of adult prisons and prisoners in England and Wales from 1970–1982, reviewed published or accessible research. After highlighting the serious shortage of *recent* research, she summarised some of the results thus:

i. none of the special regimes, or the adjuncts to regimes, that were studied were found to have significant effects in reducing the post-release reconviction rates of the prisoners;

ii. around a third of the male prison population between 1966 and 1977, particularly those serving short sentences, were found to have considerably impaired social functioning or to be mentally disordered, or both, before reaching prison;

iii. no evidence was found of intellectual impairment or deterioration amongst long-term prisoners experiencing the quality of life and regimes operating in the prisons at the time; . . .

Mott echoed the report of the Control Review Committee (1984) concerning the need for a new approach to research, concentrated on prisons, rather than prisoners:

> We think that the time has come for the actual running of the prison system to be given much higher research priority, and that the control dimension should be specifically addressed in studies of areas where it may not be the main target.

5 Differing perspectives upon offending and responses thereto

5.1 The view of radical sociologists

Many radical sociologists, such as Taylor, Walton and Young (1974) who make a Marxist analysis of crime, consider this is a reflection of the gross inequalities generated in capitalist societies and until these are rectified crime is inevitable.

5.2 The 'prevention is better than cure' perspective

Martinson (1974) has questioned the validity of the 'treatment' approach, together with many other commentators, e.g. Bottoms and McWilliams (1979) (see Chapter 30, page 288) and has called for a fresh look at the 'deterrent effect of prison'. The data are consistent with the view that attempting to prevent criminal behaviour in the first place may be a more effective approach than seeking to reform offenders after the event – which is, in any case, obviously sensible.

5.3 The 'crime as opportunity' perspective

1 There is a large body of opinion, shared by some sociologists, psychologists, other social scientists and at least some burglars, e.g.

Bennett and Wright (1984), that crime can usefully be understood in multi-variate/systems, terms. This implies that crime is an event to which many variables contribute, including economic, situational, individual, cognitive, thrill-seeking and cost/benefit analysis factors.

2 This view has contributed to the approach whereby efforts are made to reduce the opportunities for crime within a community e.g., by fitting strong locks to doors and windows and by making shop-lifting and burglary more difficult to get away with. Research upon this approach has yet to be evaluated, although there are some hopeful signs. (See Laycock, 1983).

6 Some principles which social workers and probation officers might bear in mind when compiling reports

The following are suggested by Pease (1985):

1 An understanding of the way in which criminal careers can be intensified by, e.g., patterns of sentencing, is crucial.
2 The way in which court reports and social inquiry reports can project people too far up the tariff of sentences is vital.
3 It is clear that the effect of a criminal conviction is, on balance, to *increase* the likelihood of further offending.
4 The likelihood of a further conviction within two years of a first conviction is less than 50% for all offence types.
5 Equally importantly, if a second conviction occurs, it is likely to be for a *different* offence type.
6 There is no evidence that imprisonment serves as a specific deterrent.
7 There is therefore a strong case for 'parsimony' – i.e. that custodial sentences should be used as sparingly as possible.
8 If people are, however, imprisoned, on a 'justice model', then every opportunity should be taken of offering them practical *help*: e.g. sorting out debts and personal difficulties, teaching literacy and other skills, maintaining relationships with families and giving on-going support upon discharge. This must *not* be a justification of imprisonment, but should be an opportunity *during* imprisonment.

References

Annual Abstract of Statistics No. 121 (1985), London: HMSO.

Ashworth, A. (1983), *Sentencing and Penal Policy*, London: Weidenfeld & Nicolson.

Banks, C. (1964), 'Reconviction of young offenders' in K. W. Keaton and E. N. Schwarzenberger (eds), *Current Legal Problems*, vol. 17, pp. 61–5.

Bennett, T. and Wright, R. (1984), *Burglars on Burglary*, Hampshire: Gower.

Benson, G. (1959), 'Prediction methods and young prisoners', *British Journal of Delinquency*, 1959, vol. 9, pp. 192–7.

Berntsen, K. and Christiansen, K. O. (1965), 'A resocialisation experiment with short-term offenders' in K. O. Christiansen *et al.* (eds), *Scandinavian Studies in Criminology*, London: Tavistock.

Bottoms, A. E. and McWilliams, W. (1979), 'A non-treatment paradigm for probation practice', *British Journal of Social Work*, vol. 9, pp. 159–202.

Clarke, R. V. G. and Cornish, D. B. (1983), *Crime Control in Britain: A Review of Policy Research*, Albany: State University of New York Press.

Cockett, R. (1967), 'Borstal training: a follow-up study', *British Journal of Criminology*, 1967, vol. 7, pp. 150–8.

Florida Division of Corrections (1966), *Impact of the Gideon decision upon crime and sentencing in Florida: a study of recidivism and socio-cultural change*, Research and Statistics Division, Research Monograph no. 2.

Fowles, A. J. (1978), 'Prison welfare: An account of an experiment at Liverpool' in R. V. G. Clarke and D. B. Cornish (eds) (1983), *Crime Control in Britain: A Review of Policy Research*.

Garrity, D. C. (1961), 'The prison as a rehabilitative agency', in D. R. Cressey (ed.), *Studies in Institutional Organisation and Change*, New York: Holt, Rinehart & Winston.

Hammond, W. H. (1964), *The Sentence of the Court. A handbook for courts on the treatment of offenders*, London: HMSO.

Hammond, W. H. and Chayen, E. (1963), *Persistent Criminals*. Home Office Studies in the Causes of Delinquency and the Treatment of Offenders, No. 5. London: HMSO.

Harris, M. J. (1980), *Community Service by Offenders*, Washington, D. C.: American Bar Association, Basic Program.

Home Office (1983), Reconvictions of those given community service orders. *Home Office Statistical Bulletin* 18/83. Surbiton, Surrey: Home Office Statistical Department.

Home Office (1984) *Managing the Long-term Prison System* (The Report of the Control Review Committee) London: HMSO.

Hood, R. G. (1966), *Homeless Borstal Boys*, London: Bell & Sons.

Jaman, D. (1968), *Parole outcome and Time Served by First Releases Convicted for Robbery and Burglary: 1975 Releases*. California Department of Corrections, Measurement Unit.

Laycock, G. K. (1983), *Crime Prevention Unit Paper 1*, London: HMSO.

Mannheim, M. and Wilkins, L. T. (1955), *Prediction Methods in Relation to Borstal Training*, London: HMSO.

Martinson, R. (1974), 'What works? – questions and answers about prison reform', *The Public Interest*, vol. 25, pp. 22–54.

Mott, J. (1985), *Adult Prisons & Prisoners in England and Wales 1970–1982*, Home Office Research Study No. 84. London: HMSO.

National Association for the Care and Resettlement of Offenders (1985), *Juvenile Crime*, London: NACRO.

Nuttall, C. P. (1977), *Parole in England and Wales*, Home Office Research Study, No. 38, London: HMSO.

Pease, K. (1975), *Community service orders*, Home Office Research Study, No. 29, London: HMSO.

Pease, K. (1978), 'Community service and the tariff', *Criminal Law Review*, pp. 269–75.

Pease, K. (1978), 'Community service and the tariff – a reply to the critics', *Criminal Law Review*, pp. 546–8.

Pease, K. (1985), 'Community service orders' in *Crime and Justice: An Annual Review of Research*, vol. 6, Chicago: University of Chicago Press.

Pease, K. (1985), Personal communication.

Pease, K. and McWilliams, B. (1980), *Community Service by Order*, Edinburgh: Scottish Academic Press.

Persons, R. W. (1966), 'Psychological and behaviour change in delinquents following psychotherapy', *Journal of Clinical Psychology*, vol. 22, no. 3, p. 337.

Phillpotts, G. J. O. and Lancucki, L. B. (1979), *Previous Convictions, Sentence and Reconviction*, Home Office Research Study, No. 53, London: HMSO.

Seckel, J. P. (1965), *Experiments in group counselling at two Youth Authority institutions*, Research Report, No. 46, State of California, Department of Youth Authority.

Seckel, J. P. (1967), *The Fremont Experiment: an assessment of residential treatment at a Youth Authority reception centre*, Research Report No. 50. State of California, Department of Youth Authority.

Show, M. (1974), *Social Work in Prison: An Experiment in the Use of Extended Contact with Prisoners*, Home Office Research Study No. 22, London: HMSO.

Taylor, A. J. (1967), 'An evaluation of group psychotherapy in a girls' borstal', *International Journal of Group Psychotherapy*, no. 17, pp. 168–72.

Taylor, L., Walton, P. and Young, J. (1974), *The New Criminology*, New York: Harper & Row.

Thornton, D., Curran, L., Grayson, D. and Holloway, V. (1984), *Tougher Regimes in Detention Centres*, HMSO, Crown Copyright.

Williams, M. (1970), *A Study of Some Aspects of Borstal Allocation*, Report No. 33, Office of the Chief Psychologist, Prison Department, Home Office.

PART 9

Research concerning aspects of mental health and mental handicap

32 Research concerning anxiety and forms of anxiety: phobias and obsessive disorders

Consultant: Dr Anthony T. Carr, Head of the Clinical Teaching Unit, Department of Psychology, The Polytechnic, Plymouth.

1 Definitions of anxiety

1.1 A broad definition

A condition varying along a continuum from a state of arousal, which may be facilitatory, to one of agitation which is unquestionably immobilizing. The condition arises in essence from a subjective appraisal by the person concerned that there is a threat to the physical or psychological self.

1.2 The nature of anxiety

1 **Anxiety is multi-variate** It is now commonly accepted, since the work of Lang (1968) and Rachman and Hodgson (1974), that there are four separate systems which comprise the anxiety response:

(a) the physiological: the person's response via the autonomic nervous system
(b) the subjective: the person's experience
(c) the cognitive: the person's self-statements and thoughts
(d) the behavioural: the person's observable behaviours

It is also accepted that these channels are not all synchronized one with another: i.e. changes in one are not necessarily immediately reflected by changes in the others.

2 **Anxiety is idiosyncratic** Disabling anxiety in a person can be thought of as the outcome of the interaction of many variables: those internal to the person, e.g., his or her values, attitudes, expectations and history, and those pertaining to the situation and its meaning for that person.

3 **Anxiety lies on a continuum with fear** Carr (1979) has suggested that fear and anxiety can usefully be regarded as synonymous, the differences being those of degree. Anxiety can be understood as lesser, and fear as greater, forms of the same phenomenon.

4 **Normal and abnormal anxiety** Anxiety is sometimes a normal and appropriate response to a situation, and sometimes an abnormal and inappropriate one. Carr (1979) has suggested that many fears are reasonable, but where fears are pathological, this 'lies in the degree to which the fear disrupts, directly or indirectly, behaviours or other processes which are functionally important to the individual'. It is these disruptive responses which constitute the anxiety disorders when they persist.

1.3 Psychiatric definitions

Relevant passages of the section on Anxiety Disorders in the Diagnostic and Statistical Manual III (1980) of the American Psychiatric Association are given below:

PHOBIC DISORDERS (OR PHOBIC NEUROSES)

The essential feature is persistent and irrational fear of a specific object, activity or situation that results in a compelling desire to avoid the dreaded object, activity or situation. . .

300.21 *Agoraphobia with panic attacks*

300.22 *Agoraphobia without panic attacks*

The essential feature is a marked fear of being alone, or being in public places from which escape might be difficult. . . .

300.23 *Social phobia*

The essential feature is a persistent, irrational fear of, and compelling desire to avoid, situations in which the individual might be exposed to scrutiny by others. . . .

300.29 *Simple phobia*

ANXIETY STATES (OR ANXIETY NEUROSES)

300.01 *Panic disorder*

The essential features are recurrent panic (anxiety) attacks that occur at times unpredictably, though certain situations, e.g. driving a car, may become associated with a panic attack. . . .

The panic attacks are manifested by the sudden onset of intense apprehension, fear, or terror, often associated with feelings of impending doom. . . .

300.02 *Generalized anxiety disorder*

. . . Although the specific manifestations of the anxiety vary from individual to individual, generally there are signs of. . . .

(1) *Motor tension* Shakiness, jitteriness, jumpiness, tension, muscle aches, fatigability, and inability to relax. . . .

(2) *Autonomic hyperactivity* There may be sweating, heart pounding or racing, cold, clammy hands, dry mouth, dizziness, light-headedness . . . upset stomach, hot or cold spells. . . .

(3) *Apprehensive expectation* The individual is generally apprehensive and continually feels anxious. . . .

(4) *Vigilance and scanning* Apprehensive expectation may cause hyper-attentiveness. . . .

300.30 *Obsessive compulsive disorder* (or Obsessive compulsive neurosis)

The essential features are recurrent obsessions or compulsions. *Obsessions* are recurrent, persistent ideas, thoughts, images, or impulses . . . that are not experienced as voluntarily produced. . . . *Compulsions* are repetitive and seemingly purposeful behaviours that are performed according to certain rules or in a stereotyped fashion.

2 Prevalence

The authors of the Diagnostic and Statistical Manual of Mental Disorders III (1980) have suggested, 'that from 2% to 4% of the general population has at some time had a disorder that this manual would classify as an Anxiety Disorder'.

3 Some findings or theories which contribute to understanding anxiety

3.1 A multi-variate model of anxiety

While there is as yet no unified theory of anxiety, it seems likely that the ultimate model will be one which can accommodate many interacting variables and systems.

3.2 Some processes by which anxiety is elicited or learned

1 **Via the appraisal of threat: separation in young children** Anxiety in young children between about six months and four years upon separation from the care-taker (often the mother), to whom they have become attached, is a well-documented phenomenon. (Bowlby, 1969). The stages e.g. upon unaccompanied hospital admission, are often:

(a) Protest: marked by acute distress and crying
(b) Despair: marked by misery and apathy
(c) Detachment: marked by apparent resignation and contentment

2 **Via the appraisal of threat: other situations**

1 The human being is equipped via the autonomic nervous system to

respond to perceived danger and threat. This alerts the person to react effectively in the event of any stimulus *perceived* to be threatening. Responses characteristically take the form of:
(a) fight: an aggressive response, to combat potential threat
(b) flight: a retreating response, to avoid potential threat
(c) freeze: an alert, but immobile response, in the hope of escaping the notice of the potential threat.

2 Such appraisals of threat are essentially idiosyncratic: e.g. a ride on a roller coaster, or a cut and thrust debate, may be stimulating events to one person, and terrifying ordeals to another.

3 **Via associative learning or conditioning**

1 This, in essence, is the pairing of a state of fear or pain with a previously neutral stimulus event or situation. This takes place within the framework offered by social learning theory.

2 An example of conditioning: people who are consistently anxious about travelling to work (in anticipation of work) may find that their anxiety becomes associated with the vehicle in which they travel: i.e. conditioned to the bus or train.

3.3 Principles from social learning theory which affect anxiety

1 **Modelling** The person *learns* to be anxious by noting the indications of anxiety in others, *whom he or she perceives to be similar to him or herself*. For example, children may acquire anxiety at the doctor or dentist by seeing other children respond fearfully.

2 **Traumatic learning** This is dependent upon an experience of intense fear or pain. For example, a person involved in a road accident, and who suffers serious injury, may experience dread at the prospect of travelling again in a car.

3 **Generalization of learned anxiety to other settings** The extension of anxiety from the setting where it was learned to other settings. For example, the anxiety felt by a child bullied in the school situation may generalize to the entire school setting, so that a reluctance to attend school at all develops.

4 **Cognitive processes** As suggested in 3.2.2, (above), the ways in which people perceive situations and circumstances are crucial; for example, an inexperienced swimmer may become panicky when he *thinks* he is out of his depth (even when he is not): by contrast, an experienced swimmer may be inappropriately non-anxious when deciding to swim in a rough sea because he overestimates his skill in the wish to impress his friends.

5 **'Prepared learning' of certain fears** Seligman (1971) hypothesized that evolutionary processes have 'prepared' us to learn certain fears: e.g. of snakes,

of heights and of the dark. This is because those of our ancestors who possessed the characteristics of ready acquisition of fears to real dangers left more descendants due to the survival value of fear-based avoidance behaviours.

3.4 Principles from psychoanalytic theory which affect anxiety

Freud (1933) postulated anxiety as an unavoidable aspect of the conflict between aspects of the personality – to be resolved by psychoanalysis. His daughter, Anna Freud, in *The Ego and Mechanisms of Defence* (1967), proposed hypotheses concerning ways a person learns to defend him or herself against anxiety: e.g., via denial, repression and projection.

4 Research findings concerning anxiety and its treatment

4.1 Some effects of separation from mother or care-taker

Rutter (1974), in an extensive review of the evidence concerning maternal deprivation, highlighted the subtleties of the variables involved, such as a child's temperament, and short- and long-term effects. He distinguished:

(a) Very brief separations
(b) Transient separations, lasting several weeks
(c) Permanent separations

He concluded:

(a) that there is no substantial evidence indicating adverse effects of very brief separations, e.g. associated with mothers being in employment.
(b) that children who have experienced separation for at least a month in early life have a slightly increased risk of later psychological disturbance.
(c) that in instances of permanent separation, e.g. via death or divorce, it was the *cause* of the separation rather than the separation itself, which led to undesirable long-term effects. Separations accompanied by much stress and discord were unhelpful to the child.

4.2 A range of strategies for helping anxious people

These include:

1 **Medication** It seems likely that most anxiety-related conditions which are reported to doctors are treated with drugs: these directly affect the autonomic nervous system.

2 **Progressive relaxation** Jacobson's (1938) model of relaxation for reducing anxiety has been developed by other researchers. Among these, Wolpe (1958) showed that the fear response could be inhibited by substituting deep muscular relaxation – its opposite. Such deep relaxation, acquired via

repeated practice over a period of time, is widely employed in the management of many forms of anxiety.

3 **Cognitive approaches** Researchers such as Ellis (1970) have shown that the 'self-statements' which people often unwittingly make to themselves, (e.g. 'I can't cope'; 'I'll never manage') are self-defeating. Much research by e.g. Goldfried and Goldfried (1975) suggests that teaching people to make positive, *coping* self-statements, ('I'll manage: I know I can'; 'Take it slowly, and you'll do it'), can markedly reduce anxiety and enhance effectiveness.

4.3 The importance of structuring the help offered

Where a disabling anxiety state is diagnosed, the following model or plan of helping is important:

1 **Assessment** This can profitably be based upon gathering data and information concerning the person's history, and e.g. under the headings suggested by Lazarus (1973):

(a) Behaviour: what the anxious person *does*
(b) Affect: how the anxious person feels emotionally
(c) Sensation: what the anxious person feels physiologically
(d) Imagery: what the anxious person imagines visually
(e) Cognition: what the anxious person thinks or says
(f) Interpersonal situations which may affect the situation
(g) Drugs: medication the person may be taking

2 **Intervention** This is likely to involve

(a) Building trust between the helper and the anxious person.
(b) Reassurance about the *normality* of the anxiety response. i.e. the manifestations of anxiety shown under generalized anxiety disorder, pages 306–7.
(c) Shared goal setting: see 3 below.
(d) Engaging the anxious person in anxiety-reducing exercises, e.g. practising relaxation, substituting images of himself dealing effectively in situations, working towards simple attainable goals and rehearsing positive, coping thoughts.

3 **Goal setting** Agreeing a hierarchy of attainable goals which, with support and encouragement, the anxious person can achieve over time. Very simple tasks and exercises are placed at the bottom of the hierarchy: the hardest at the top.

4 **Evaluation** Involving the helper and the anxious person in reviewing the extent to which progress towards the previously agreed goals has been achieved and, where necessary, setting fresh ones. Follow-up will also be involved, some months later.

4.4 Prognosis

Rachman and Wilson (1980), in a review of treatment effectiveness for specific disorders, have reported 'the demonstrated efficacy of progressive relaxation with anxiety related disorders such as hypertension, insomnia, and general tension states. . . .' Additional strategies, such as those described in 4.2.3, (page 310), are likely to enhance such effectiveness.

5 Research concerning how to help with forms of anxiety: phobias, agoraphobia and obsessive-compulsive conditions

5.1 Preliminary considerations

1 Attempts to relieve such conditions should be conducted under the supervision of an appropriately qualified practitioner.
2 Marks (1978) drew attention to the principle that all treatment of anxiety-related disorder is based upon the concept of enabling the anxious person to experience exposure to the feared stimulus – but in a supportive setting. This enables him or her to learn, over time (often several weeks or months), that the anticipated threat does *not* materialize.

5.2 The treatment of phobias

1 These acute and disabling anxiety states, where fear is centred upon a particular stimulus, e.g. dogs, water, public situations, have been shown to respond well to intervention – particularly to 'desensitization'.
2 Such desensitization enables the anxious person to tolerate first brief exposure to the feared item or situation, then longer exposure and finally prolonged exposure. This has been shown, over time, by e.g. Gelder, Marks and Wolff (1967), to produce clear improvement in many phobic people.
3 Bandura, Adams and Beyer (1977) concluded that the most effective approach in helping with phobic fears was to,
   (a) Provide a model of someone behaving without fear in the situation which the person found fearful, and also to
   (b) Encourage self-sufficiency by coaching the person in mastering the fear-provoking event.
4 Marks (1978) found that an average of eleven sessions of structured help was required for major relief, if not full cure, of phobic fear to occur. At four years' follow-up this improvement was maintained.

5.3 Prognosis

Rachman and Wilson (1980) concluded that desensitization has been demonstrably effective in treating phobic disorders. They also noted that therapist-directed, prolonged exposure to the phobic stimuli (flooding) has been shown to be either more, or equally effective. Such treatments, however, require highly trained therapists.

5.4 Research concerning the treatment of agoraphobia

This disorder was once thought to be linked with open spaces, but there is now evidence that it is more accurately associated with general social anxiety and with public places. While it may best be understood as occurring within a 'systems' framework, e.g. a complex family situation, much valuable help can often be given by implementing the principles of anxiety management described above.

1 Issues relating to treatment

1 Mathews (1978) has summarized findings in this field. He concludes that gradual encounter with the feared situation (cf. desensitization) in the context of supportive encouragement from the helper, has provided the most beneficial and long-lasting outcomes.
2 Rabavilas (1976) found that prolonged exposure to the feared situation was more effective than short; e.g. an outing or a visit to the shops lasting eighty minutes proved more effective than four short outings of twenty minutes.
3 Bandura (1977) coined the idea of 'self-efficacy'; i.e. that the anxious person should perceive the improvement in his or her situation and *his or her part in producing that improvement.*
4 Hafner and Marks (1976) found that trying to help agoraphobic people in groups was more effective than working with them individually.

2 **Prognosis** Rachman and Wilson (1980) concluded from their review that there is sound evidence that desensitization can result in improvement in complex reactions such as agoraphobia, but they emphasized that other approaches, such as assertion training, and active support from family members, are valuable additional strategies.

5.5 Research concerning the treatment of obsessive-compulsive conditions

1 Issues relating to treatment

1 In this field also, relaxation training has been found to be a useful adjunct to other forms of intervention, rather than sufficient in itself. (Rachman, Hodgson and Marks, 1971).
2 Turner, Hersen, Bellack and Wells (1979) endorsed previous indications that an effective procedure for people with obsessive compulsive disorders is 'response prevention'; i.e. gently but firmly preventing the person from carrying out the rituals he or she formerly practised: e.g. those of cleaning or checking.

3 In summary, helpful components of work with compulsive people seem to be:
   (a) Reassurance by the therapist or helper
   (b) Relaxation practice
   (c) The provision of a model performing the feared actions
   (d) Gentle response prevention
   (e) Graduated practice towards a goal
   (f) Encouraging self-efficacy

2 **Prognosis** Rachman and Wilson (1980) reported that, 'It is reasonable to conclude that behavioural treatment is capable of producing significant changes in obsessional problems, and fairly rapidly at that.'

5.6 Summary note on the treatment of anxiety-related disorders

In the light of the above research, it may be said that the outlook for those experiencing disabling anxiety is good. Clearly such people need the skills of qualified practitioners, many of whom will be clinical psychologists.

References

American Psychiatric Association (1980), *Diagnostic and Statistical Manual of Mental Disorders* (D.S.M. III), Washington: APA.

Bandura, A. (1977), 'Self-efficacy. Towards a unifying theory of behavioral change', *Psychological Review*, vol. 84, pp. 191–215.

Bandura, A., Adams, N. E. and Beyer, J. (1977), 'Cognitive processes mediating behaviour change', *Journal of Personality and Social Psychology*, vol. 35, pp. 125–39.

Bowlby, J. (1979), *Attachment and Loss: 1 Attachment*, London: Hogarth Press.

Carr, A. T. (1979), 'The psychopathology of fear' in W. Sluckin (ed.), *Fear in Animals and Man*, New York: Van Nostrand Reinhold.

Carr, A. T. (1984), 'Anxiety and depression' in A. Gale and A. Chapman (eds), *Psychology and Social Problems*, Chichester: John Wiley & Sons.

Ellis, A. (1970), *The Essence of Rational Psychotherapy. A Comprehensive Approach to Treatment*, New York: Institute for Rational Living.

Freud, A. (1967), *The Ego and Mechanisms of Defence*, London: Hogarth Press.

Freud, S. (1933), *New Introductory Lectures on Psychoanalysis*, New York: Norton, 1965 edition.

Gelder, M. G., Marks, I. and Wolff, H. (1967), 'Desensitisation and psychotherapy in phobic states: a controlled enquiry', *British Journal of Psychiatry*, vol. 113, pp. 53–5.

Goldfried, M. R. and Goldfried, A. (1975), 'Cognitive change methods' in F. H. Kanfer and A. P. Goldstein (eds), *Helping People Change*, New York: Pergamon.

Hafner, J. and Marks, I. M. (1976), 'Exposure in vivo of agoraphobics: the contributions of diazepam, group exposure and anxiety evocation', *Psychological Medicine*, vol. 6, pp. 71–88.

Jacobson, E. (1938), *Progressive Relaxation*, Chicago: University of Chicago Press.

Lang, P. J. (1968), 'Fear reduction and fear behaviour. Problems in treating a construct' in J. M. Shlien (ed.), *Research in Psychotherapy* vol. 3, Washington, D.C.: American Psychological Association.

Lazarus, A. A. (1973), 'Multimodal behavior therapy: Treating the "BASIC ID"', *Journal of Nervous and Mental Disease*, vol. 156, pp. 404–11.

Marks, I. (1969), *Fears and Phobias*, New York: Academic Press.

Marks, I. (1978), 'Behavioral psychotherapy of adult neurosis' in S. Garfield and A. E. Bergin (eds), *Handbook of Psychotherapy and Behavior Change*, 2nd edition, New York: Wiley.

Mathews, A. (1978), 'Fear reduction research and clinical phobias', *Psychological Bulletin*, vol. 85, pp. 390–404.

Rabavilas, A. D., Boulougouris, J. C. and Stefanis, C. (1976), 'Duration of flooding session in the treatment of obsessive-compulsive patients', *Behavior Research and Therapy*, vol. 14, pp. 349–55.

Rachman, S. and Hodgson, R. (1974), 'Synchrony and desynchrony in fear and avoidance', *Behavior Research and Therapy*, vol. 12, pp. 311–18.

Rachman, S., Hodgson, R. and Marks, I. (1971), 'Treatment of chronic obsessive-compulsive neurosis', *Behavior Research and Therapy*, vol. 9, pp. 237–47.

Rachman, S. and Wilson, G. (1980), *The Effects of Psychological Therapy*, Oxford: Pergamon Press.

Rutter, M. (1974), *Maternal Deprivation Reassessed*, Harmondsworth: Penguin.

Seligman, M. E. (1971), 'Phobias and preparedness', *Behavior Research and Therapy*, vol. 2, pp. 307–20.

Turner, S., Hersen, M., Bellack, A. S. and Wells, K. (1979), 'Behavioral treatment of obsessive-compulsive neurosis', *Behavior Research and Therapy*, vol. 17, pp. 95–106.

Wolpe, J. (1958), *Psychotherapy by Reciprocal Inhibition*, Stanford: Stanford University Press.

33

Research concerning depression

Consultant: Dr J. Dominian, Consultant Psychiatrist, Central Middlesex Hospital, London.

1 A general definition

A condition characterized by disturbance of:

1 Affect (emotions) of sadness and misery
2 Behaviour marked by slowness and lethargy
3 Cognitions (thoughts) of hopelessness and sometimes suicide.

2 Further classifications and definitions

2.1 A commonly used classification

1 **Endogenous depression** This term is used when the depression is not obviously linked to any clear precipitating event, but seems to have arisen spontaneously. It can take two forms:

a) *Bipolar depression*: here the person swings between moods of deep sadness or misery to a manic condition marked by elation, talkativeness and over-inflated confidence.
b) *Unipolar depression*: here the person suffers only the depressive symptoms without experiencing mania.

2 **Reactive depression** This term is used when the depression can be reasonably understood as *reactive to* a particular depressing event: a bereavement, a broken relationship, loss of a job, etc.

N.B. There are other specific forms of depression, e.g. post-puerperal depression, i.e. following childbirth, and grief reactions, but the main currently accepted categories are those shown above.

3 Characteristics of depression

These have been classified by Dominian (1984) in Table 33.1; see overleaf.

Characteristics of Depression		
Psychological	*Endogenous*	*Reactive*
Mood	A shift towards depression is marked, continuous and usually worse in the morning.	The mood is less severely depressed, fluctuates and gets worse, if at all, in the evening and when alone.
Psychomotor Retardation	Is marked and expresses itself by a general slowing up in thinking and activity.	Not marked, if at all.
Agitation Anxiety Irritation	Agitation is usually present.	Anxiety and irritability are the principal characteristics. Fears are commonly present.
Feelings of inferiority, uselessness and hopelessness	Markedly present but disappear with the lifting of the depression.	Not so pronounced but often other variations in the personality present.
Delusions of self-reproach and guilt.	May be marked.	Usually not present.
Hallucinations	May be present.	Absent.
Physical		
Insomnia	Marked, characterized by early morning waking.	Marked, characterized by difficulty in going off to sleep and further interruptions.
Appetite and weight	Severely affected.	Usually little change.
Libido	Can be lost completely or partially.	Usually little change.
Energy	Markedly reduced.	Variably reduced.
Bodily pain	Present – clears up with lifting of depression.	Present – may clear up or persist.

TABLE 33.1 Characteristics of depression (Dominian, 1984)

4 Prevalence

4.1 Diversity of diagnosis

It is exceedingly difficult to give accurate figures of the number of people who experience depression in its many forms, in view of the variability of diagnosis and treatment. One source of data, however, is the number of prescriptions written for anti-depressants, and these figures are given in Table 33.2.

	1975	1980
Anti-depressants	7,906,000	6,263,000

TABLE 33.2 Prescriptions for preparations acting on the nervous system in England in 1975 and 1980 (*Health and Personal Social Services Statistics for England*, 1976 and 1982)

5 Research which contributes to understanding depression

5.1 The range of theories or models of depression

Akiskal and McKinney (1975) have drawn together no less than ten major theories of depression into a general classification. This is shown in Table 33.3.

School/theory	*Model*	*Mechanism*
Psychoanalytical Psychodynamic	Aggression turned inward Loss of close object of attachment (e.g. parent) Loss of self esteem	Conversion of aggression into depression Separation: disruption of an attachment bond
	Negative cognitive attitude	Helplessness in attaining goals of ego-ideal Helplessness
Behavioural	Learned helplessness Loss of rewards	Uncontrollable unpleasant events (e.g. loss of job) Some rewards of sick role
Sociological	Sociological	Loss of role status
Existential	Existential	Loss of sense of meaning in life
Biological	Biochemical/genetic Neurophysiological	Impaired biochemical functioning

TABLE 33.3 Ten models of depression (After Akiskal and McKinney, 1975)

5.2 A multi-variate, systems model of depression

Akiskal and McKinney (1975) have integrated these various models, where there is evidence to justify it, into a single, multi-factorial model; the emphasis is upon *interacting variables*, and from these depression flows as the 'final common pathway'. Within this integrated model, depression can be either very severe or less severe. See Table 33.4.

Physiological stressors	*Biological: e.g. genetic predisposition*	*Psychosocial stressors*	*Developmental predisposition*
Biochemical factors: e.g. hyperthyroidism Infection	Malfunctioning of aspects of brain bio-chemistry	Loss of close relationship Stress from poverty, loss of job, status isolation	Loss of close relationship in early childhood: e.g. parent

These interacting factors or variables may converge into a 'final common pathway' which reflect changes in brain biochemistry. These are experienced by the person or patient as depression or 'melancholia'.

TABLE 33.4 Depression as a 'final common pathway' (After Akiskal and McKinney, 1975)

Akiskal and McKinney (1975) summarized: 'In our model depression is simultaneously conceptualised at several levels, rather than having any one to one relationship with a single event – whether defined in chemical, psycho-dynamic or behavioral language.'

1 **Research on the contribution of physiological stresses** There is evidence that the following can contribute to depression:

(a) events such as pre-menstrual hormonal changes (Dalton, 1977)
(b) the major hormonal changes linked with childbirth (Cox, 1986)
(c) stressors such as viral infections

2 **Research on the contribution of genetic factors** Among the recognized genetic contributions are those demonstrated by Frazer, Pandey and Mendels (1973) who have shown an apparent genetic vulnerability to bi-polar (i.e. manic-depressive) disorder. (This means not that any child of a person with manic-depressive illness will automatically inherit it, but that there is a significant genetic contribution to the total, multi-factorial interaction.)

3 **Research on the contribution of psycho-social stresses** There is convergence of the evidence that stress arising from life experience can precipitate depression. (Paykel, 1974; Depue, 1979; Anisman and Zacharko, 1982). Stressful life events such as loss of employment, the impact of accidents, changes in important relationships, particularly bereavement and divorce, all make great demands upon a person's capacity for coping, while Holmes and Rahe (1967) have shown how *cumulative* stresses make it more likely that a person will succumb to illness.

Paykel (1979) has shown how modifying factors may affect the impact of an event upon different individuals. This is illustrated in Figure 33.1.

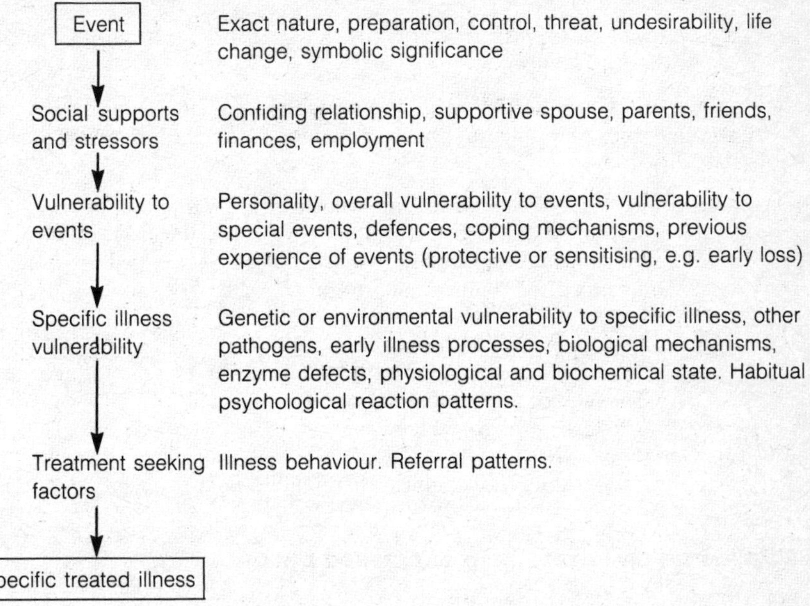

FIGURE 33.1 Modifying factors between stressful event and possible subsequent depressive illness. (Paykel, 1979)

4 **Research on the contribution of developmental predisposition** Akiskal and McKinney (1975) included here the vulnerability to depression which, they suggest, is induced by the *early* loss of important relationships, with the associated feelings of helplessness. They drew particular attention to the concept of 'learned helplessness', proposed by Seligman (1975) who wrote:

> the model suggests that the cause of depression is the belief that action is futile. What kinds of events set off reactive depressions? Failure at work and school, death of loved ones, rejection or separation from friends or loved ones, physical disease, financial difficulty, being faced with insoluble problems, and growing old . . . the depressed person believes or has learned that he cannot control those elements of his life that relieve suffering, bring gratification, or provide nurture – in short he believes he is helpless.

5 **Research on the contribution of cognitive factors** Beck (1976) has demonstrated the clear evidence that depressed people tend to perceive situations selectively and negatively. They tend to 'rehearse negative self-statements'; e.g. 'I can't cope'; 'I'll never manage to sort things out'; 'I am a total failure'.

Such rehearsals tend to intensify and prolong depression. This work endorses that of Ellis (1962).

5.3 An example of research which gives support to a multi-factorial model of depression

Brown and Harris (1978) examined variables associated with depression in a large group of women in an Inner London Borough. Olsen (1984) writes that this study:

> provided . . . evidence of the importance of key-variables, 'provoking agents', in mental disorder. But other psycho-social aspects involving more fundamental aspects of a woman's life, also emerged as vital determinants of her vulnerability to these events. The vulnerability factors are:
>
> 1 Loss of mother before the age of 11 years.
> 2 Three or more children in the family under 14 years of age.
> 3 The lack of a confiding partner.
> 4 The lack of paid employment.
>
> It was found that working-class women were four times more likely to present with a depressive illness than middle-class women.

6 Research on how to help depressed people

6.1 The course of depression

1 **Duration of depressive episodes** Rosenhan and Seligman (1984) have written optimistically of this,

> After the initial attack, which comes on suddenly about three quarters of the time, depression seems to last an average of about three months in outpatients. Among inpatients, who are usually more severely depressed, it lasts about six months on the average. At first, the depression gets progressively worse, eventually reaching the bottom, but then the depressed individual begins to recover gradually to the state that existed before the onset (Beck, 1967. . . .)
>
> Without minimizing the suffering the patient is feeling now, the therapist should tell the patient that complete recovery from the episode occurs in 70 to 95 per cent of the cases.

2 **Subsequent depressive episodes** Rosenhan and Seligman (1984) reported three possible outcomes:

(a) Recovery without recurrence: about 50 per cent of patients do not have another attack within the subsequent ten years.
(b) Recovery with recurrence: about 50 per cent of patients are likely to have an attack similar to the first – but not for a further three years.

(c) Chronic depression: a very small proportion do not fully recover, and continue to be depressed.

6.2 The importance of very careful assessment to pinpoint the specific variables contributing to the depression

As with any disorder, the stage of careful assessment is crucial. Among other variables, it will need to include attention to the following:

1 Early life experiences: loss by death or family separation.
2 Depressive disorders among parents or relatives.
3 Long-term stresses within the person's life: e.g. own disability, care of a sick relative or handicapped child.
4 Recent stresses within the person's life: e.g. marital stress, moving away of friends.
5 Availability of support networks: friends, community, etc.
6 Living circumstances: housing, isolation, poverty, cold.
7 Employment circumstances: redundancy, status of work, etc.
8 The person's own view of what triggered the depression that he or she is experiencing.

7 Research concerning forms of treatment for depression

7.1 Somatic treatments for unipolar depression

1 **Medication** This is by far the commonest form of treatment. The drugs given are usually 'tricyclics', and they have an effect upon centres in the brain which influence mood. Rosenhan and Seligman (1984) write, 'On the average, between 63 and 75 per cent of depressed patients given tricyclics show significant clinical improvement.' A large proportion (80 per cent) of people who experience bi-polar (manic depressive) depression, can be effectively helped by the administration of lithium carbonate.

2 **Electroconvulsive therapy (ECT)** Despite entirely understandable public fears of this, there is consistent evidence of the helpfulness of this approach. (West, 1981). Further, Rosenhan and Seligman (1984) write, 'strong evidence exists that ECT, when given to severely depressed unipolar depressive patients, is a highly effective antidepressant therapy.'

7.2 The provision of social support to depressed people

Studies such as that of Aneshensel and Stone (1982) have indicated that not only does social support, such as that available from social networks of relationships, lessen the adverse effects of stress and depression, but it may itself actively improve the depressive symptoms.

7.3 Cognitive-behavioural approaches in the treatment of depression

There is consistent and increasing evidence that these methods can prove as effective as medication in the management of unipolar depression. For example, Rush, Beck, Kovacs and Hollon (1977) compared cognitive therapy with standard treatment using medication (imipramine). Such cognitive therapy, which is highly structured, includes teaching people to collect instances of their thought patterns, negative self-statements and rehearsals of problems, to question the realistic basis of such negativity and actively to practise mastery behaviour. Cognitive therapy was found to be superior both in the level of response obtained and in fewer people leaving treatment. There is a great deal of continuing research in this area, and very encouraging work continues to appear.

References

Akiskal, H. S. and McKinney, W. T. (1975), 'Overview of recent research in depression', *Archives of General Psychiatry*, vol. 32, pp. 285–305.

Aneshensel, C. S. and Stone, J. D. (1982), 'Stress and depression', *Archives of General Psychiatry*, vol. 39, pp. 1392–6.

Anisman, H. and Zacharko, R. M. (1982), 'Depression: The pre-disposing influence of stress', *The Behavioral and Brain Sciences*, vol. 5, pp. 89–137.

Beck, A. T. (1967), *Depression: Clinical, Experimental and Theoretical Aspects*, New York: Hoeber.

Beck, A. T. (1976), *Cognitive Therapy and the Emotional Disorders*, New York: International Universities Press.

Brown, G. W. and Harris, T. (1978), *The Social Origins of Depression*, London: Tavistock.

Cox, J. (1986), *Postnatal Depression – A Guide for Health Professionals*, Edinburgh: Churchill Livingstone.

Dalton, K. (1977), *The Premenstrual Syndrome and Progesterone Therapy*, London: Heinemann Medical Books.

Depue, R. (ed.) (1979), *Psychobiology of Depressive Disorders. Implications for the Effect of Stress*, New York: Academic Press.

Dominian, J. (1984), *Depression*, London: Fontana/Collins.

Ellis, A. (1962), *Reason and Emotion in Psychotherapy*, New York: Lyle Stuart.

Frazer, A., Pandey, G. and Mendels, J. (1973), 'Metabolism of tryptophan in depressive disease', *Archives of General Psychiatry*, vol. 29, pp. 528–35.

Holmes, T. H. and Rahe, R. (1967), 'The social readjustment rating scale', *Journal of Psychosomatic Research*, vol. 11, pp. 213–18.

Olsen, M. R. (ed.) (1984), *Social Work and Mental Health*, London: Tavistock.

Paykel, E. S. (1974), 'Recent life events and clinical depression' in E. K.

Gunderson and R. H. Rahe (eds), *Life Stress and Illness*, Springfield, Illinois: Thomas.

Paykel, E. S. (1979), 'Recent life events in the development of the depressive disorders' in R. Depue (ed.), *Psychobiology of Depressive Disorders. Implications for the Effect of Stress.*

Rosenhan, D. L. and Seligman, M. E. (1984), *Abnormal Psychology*, New York: Norton and Co.

Rush, A., Beck, A., Kovacs, M. and Hollon, G. (1977), 'Comparative efficacy of cognitive therapy and pharmacotherapy in the treatment of depressed outpatients', *Cognitive Therapy and Research*, vol. 1, pp. 17–37.

Seligman, M. L. P. (1975), *Helplessness: On Depression, Development and Death*, San Francisco: Freeman.

West, E. D. (1981), 'Electric convulsion therapy in depression: a double-blind controlled trial', *British Medical Journal*, vol. 282, pp. 355–7.

World Health Organization (1980), *Glossary of Mental Disorders and Guide to their Classification*, Geneva: WHO.

Research concerning suicide and parasuicide

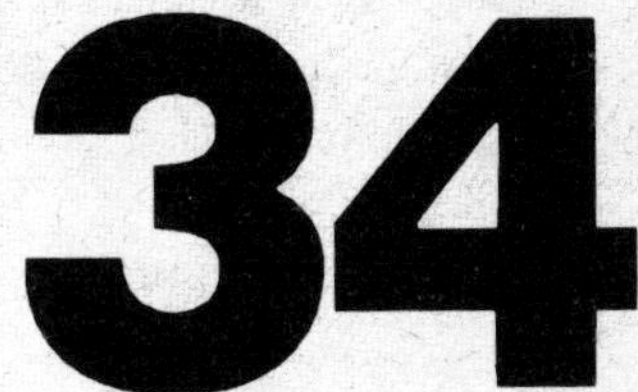

***Consultant:* Dr Norman Kreitman, MRC Unit for Epidemiological Studies in Psychiatry, University Department of Psychiatry, Royal Edinburgh Hospital, Edinburgh.**

1 Definitions

1.1 Definition of suicide

The definition of suicide contains two components: that the person brought about his own death, and that he did so knowingly.

1.2 Definition of parasuicide (deliberate self-harm, or DSH)

Any non-fatal act of self-injury or taking of a substance in excess of the generally recognized or prescribed therapeutic dose. By convention, alcohol intoxication alone is excluded. (Kreitman, 1977)

2 Frequency of suicide and parasuicide

2.1 Frequency of suicide: England and Wales

Official statistics

		Age 15–24	Age 25–44	Age 45–64	Age 65+	All 15+
1974						
Numbers	Male	203	684	883	509	2,279
	Female	97	371	668	482	1,618
Rate per 100,000	Male	5.8	11.0	15.7	19.1	12.6
	Female	2.9	6.1	11.2	11.5	10.5
1983						
Numbers	Male	275	1,003	965	567	2,810
	Female	89	319	561	492	1,461
Rate per 100,000	Male	6.7	15.0	17.7	19.2	14.6
	Female	2.3	4.8	9.8	10.8	7.0

TABLE 34.1 Frequency of suicide in England and Wales, by age and sex. Figures supplied by Kreitman (1985).

N.B. It will be noted that men have higher rates of suicide than women, and the old have higher rates than the young.

2.2 Frequency of parasuicide: Edinburgh

		Age 15–24	Age 25–44	Age 45–64	Age 65+	All 15+
1983						
Numbers	Male	133	210	93	22	458
	Female	267	251	100	40	658
Rate per 100,000	Male	172.5	358.2	192.2	86.6	220.4
	Female	355.9	428.7	189.9	85.2	282.2

TABLE 34.2 Frequency of parasuicide in Edinburgh. Figures provided by Kreitman (1985).

N.B. Here it will be noted that men have lower rates of parasuicide than women, and the old have lower rates than the young.

3 Research concerning the causation of suicide

3.1 Pioneer sociological study

In 1897 Durkheim published his major study, *Le Suicide*, in which he divided acts of suicide into three principal groups:

1 The 'egoists': those people whose social groupings were losing, or had lost, cohesion and integration. Durkheim noted: 'The suicide rate varies inversely with the degree of integration of the social group.'
2 The 'altruists': those people whose attachment to their social groups was too strong, and who died as an act of duty, piety or devotion to a cause.
3 Those who killed themselves in situations of 'anomie' or 'normlessness': that is, during periods of crisis or social upheaval, national or personal, when there were no adequate guides to behaviour.

3.2 Characteristics of those who do, and of those who do not, commit suicide

Stengel (1970) reported the situation at the time of writing:

> No one single cause or group of causes can account for the level of suicide rates. Many factors are at work at the same time. Suicide rates, for example, have been found to be positively correlated with the following factors: *male sex, increasing age, widowhood, single and divorced state, childlessness, high density of population, residence in big towns, a high standard of living, economic crisis, alcohol and addictive drug consumption, a broken home in childhood, mental disorder and physical illness.*
>
> Among factors inversely related to the suicide rate are *female sex, youth, low density of population (though it must not be too low), rural occupation, religious devoutness, the married state, a large number of children, membership of the lower socio-economic classes, war.*
>
> These correlations have been found in most Western communities and possibly do not obtain in other types of society.

3.3 Evidence of two groups among those who complete suicide

Ovenstone and Kreitman (1974), from their work in Edinburgh, suggested two main groups, to be considered separately below:

1 The chronically disorganized.
2 The acutely disrupted.

1 **The chronically disorganized** These were characterized by:

(a) Psychological instability and social disruption over at least the five years preceding the suicide.
(b) At least 80 per cent had consulted their GPs over the last three months of their lives, and many had experienced fairly frequent contact with psychiatrists.
(c) Having told a variety of others that they intended to harm themselves.

2 **The acutely disrupted** These were characterized by:

(a) Much greater stability in their preceding lives – which, however, was sometimes precarious in that it rested on a single emotional attachment, which, when broken, precipitated the suicide.
(b) A marked change in their lives, such as a severe physical disability or the impact of unemployment.

3.4 Aspects of the act of deliberate self-harm suggesting a clear suicidal intent

Beck, Schuyler and Herman (1974) distinguish the following:

1 Isolation: planning so that no one should be nearby.
2 Timing: planning so that intervention is unlikely.
3 Not acting to get help after self harm.
4 Actions in anticipation of death: e.g. making a will.
5 Active preparation for self harm: e.g. obtaining drugs.
6 Writing a suicide note.

4 Research concerning the causation of parasuicide

4.1 Characteristics of parasuicides

1 All studies in developed countries report a ratio of women to men of 2:1.
2 For women, there is a peak in the late teens and early twenties: for men, the rate is highest between twenty and thirty-five.
3 The action is frequently unplanned, impulsive and undertaken in a way which is likely to be discovered.
4 Motivation is often difficult to assess, but commonly includes both a 'cry for help' and the seeking of a period of oblivion to relieve stress. An intent to die is often absent.

4.2 Stressful life events as precipitants of a suicide attempt

Paykel, Prusoff and Myers (1975) compared stressful life events among fifty-three people who attempted suicide, and a matched control group. The former reported four times as many such events as the control group, and many of these events had occurred in the month preceding the attempt.

4.3 Different groups among parasuicides

Paykel and Rassaby (1978), in a study in the USA, distinguished three groups among the 236 people who attempted suicide and who attended an emergency treatment centre:

1 Those who took an overdose of minor drugs, with less risk to life and mainly interpersonal motivations.

2 A smaller group who employed more violent methods, and who were more greatly at risk.
3 A group of recurrent attempters, who had made many previous attempts, and who were overtly hostile.

4.4 Attempting to identify those at risk of suicide after parasuicide

Kreitman (1983) indicates the following risk factors:

1 Age: risk increases with age.
2 Sex: males are more at risk than females.
3 Social isolation: especially after loss of an important relationship.
4 Unemployment.
5 Alcohol and drug abuse – especially with recent loss of job.
6 Sociopathic personality.
7 History of multiple previous suicide attempts.

They also stress the importance of certain features relating to the current parasuicidal episode:

1 Depression, which may be accompanied by suicidal thoughts, persistent insomnia and social withdrawal.
2 Feelings of hopelessness and worthlessness.
3 Use of violent methods of self harm, or serious overdose.

5 The relationship of suicide and parasuicide

5.1 Features of 'overlap' between the two groups

1 In their survey of studies of suicide, Dorpat and Ripley (1967) found that between 8.6 per cent and 33.1 per cent of those who completed suicide had made prior attempts.
2 Ovenstone (1973) found in Edinburgh that an 'overlap' group defined as completed suicides with a history of a previous attempt, were characterized by a high incidence of drug addiction, mental illness, alcoholism and unemployment.

5.2 Comparative data

The table devised by Kreitman (1983) summarized much information.

	Parasuicide	Suicide
Secular trend	Becoming commoner	Slowly increasing among males
Sex	Commoner in females	Commoner in males
Age group	Mostly below 45	Mostly above 45
Marital status	Highest rates in divorced, and single	Highest rates in divorced, single and widowed

continued overleaf

	Parasuicide	Suicide
Social class	Higher in lower classes	No obvious gradient
Urban/rural	Commoner in cities	Commoner in cities
Employment status	Associated with unemployment	Associated with unemployment and retirement
Effects of war	?	Lower in wartime
Seasonal variation	None evident	Spring peak
Broken home in childhood	Common	Common
Physical illness	No obvious association	Probable association
Psychiatric diagnosis	Situational reaction, depression, alcoholism	Depression, alcoholism
Personality type	Psychopathy common	No special type

TABLE 34.3 Summary comparison of parasuicides and suicides in the UK (Kreitman, 1983)

6 Research concerning how to help people at risk of suicide or parasuicide

Kreitman (1983) summarized the major risk factors for suicide and parasuicide among the general population:

6.1 Risk factors for suicide

1. Being an older male
2. Living alone
3. Coincident psychiatric illness
4. Unemployment
5. A past history of parasuicide

6.2 Risk factors for a first ever episode of parasuicide

1. Being a younger female, especially a teenager who is married
2. Domestic conflict
3. Financial stresses, especially those linked with heavy drinking in the husband
4. Living in over-crowded and socially deprived conditions
5. Debt
6. Criminality
7. A background of interpersonal violence

6.3 A further study of parasuicide

A study of ninety-three first ever parasuicides who were admitted to the Edinburgh Regional Poisoning Treatment Centre indicated that:

1 15 per cent were unaware of available sources of help
2 15 per cent could not accept the idea of seeking help for personal problems
3 19 per cent wanted immediate relief from stress
4 19 per cent wanted to die
5 19 per cent wanted to influence other people

6.4 The assessment of the parasuicidal person

1 **The necessity of considering multi-factorial causation** Kreitman (1983) writes: 'The interviewer has to satisfy himself that he can answer the question "Why did this person take an overdose at this particular time?" '

The answer may be found in considering a multi-factorial (interacting 'systems') set of variables, including:

1 Particular events and difficulties preceding the act.
2 The person's particular personality or habitual ways of relating to other people.
3 Symptoms of psychiatric illness.

2 **The risk of repetition** Bluglass and Hawton (1974) also identified a number of factors distinguishing those at risk of further parasuicide:

1 A diagnosis of sociopathy
2 Problems in the use of alcohol
3 Previous history of psychiatric treatment
4 Previous parasuicide
5 Drug dependence
6 Lower social class
7 Unemployment
8 A history of criminal behaviour

6.5 The management of people at risk of suicide

Kreitman (1983) considers that the management of high-risk people is based on three essential ingredients:

1 The prompt treatment of any coexisting mental disorder.
2 The modification of the social context in which the person lives.
3 The maintenance of contact over a long period, so that supportive listening, common sense guidance and the acceptance of the fact that many people fear their own suicidal impulses may be offered.

6.6 Help from supportive agencies

The best known of the agencies which have arisen to help the suicidal is the Samaritans. A study by Greer and Anderson (1979) of the organization and of those who had attempted suicide found:

1 72% of the sample of attempters knew of the organisation
2 1.4% of the sample had sought help from it.
3 20% simply 'did not think of it' before taking an overdose
4 20% were seeking oblivion from their difficulties
5 7% were seeking to influence others by attempting suicide

References

Beck, A. T., Schuyler, D. and Herman, I. (1974), 'Development of suicidal intent scales' in A. T. Beck, H. L. P. Resnick and D. Lettieri (eds), *The Prediction of Suicide*, Maryland: Charles Press.

Bluglass, D. and Hawton, J. (1974), 'The repetition of parasuicide: comparison of three cohorts', *British Journal of Psychiatry*, vol. 125, pp. 168–74.

Dorpat, T. L. and Ripley, H. (1967), 'The relationship between attempted suicide and committed suicide', *Comparative Psychiatry*, vol. 8, pp. 74–5.

Durkheim, E. (1897), *Le suicide*, Nouveau Edition Alcan (1930).

Greer, S. and Anderson, M. (1979), 'Samaritan contact among 325 parasuicide patients', *British Journal of Psychiatry*, vol. 135, pp. 263–8.

Kreitman, N. (1977), *Parasuicide*, Chichester: John Wiley.

Kreitman, N. (1983), 'Suicide and parasuicide' in R. E. Kendall and A. K. Zealley (eds), *Companion to Psychiatric Studies*, 3rd edition, Edinburgh: Churchill Livingstone.

Kreitman, N. (1985), Personal communication.

Ovenstone, I. M. K. (1973), 'Spectrum of suicidal behaviours in Edinburgh', *British Journal of Preventive and Social Medicine*, vol. 27, pp. 27–35.

Ovenstone, I. M. K. and Kreitman, N. (1974), 'Two syndromes of suicide', *British Journal of Psychiatry*, vol. 124, pp. 336–45.

Paykel, E. and Rassaby, E. (1978), 'Classification of suicide attempters by cluster analysis', *British Journal of Psychiatry*, vol. 135, pp. 45–52.

Paykel, E. S., Prusoff, B. A. and Myers, J. K. (1975), 'Suicide attempts and recent life events', *Archives of General Psychiatry*, vol. 32, pp. 327–33.

Stengel, E. (1970), *Suicide and Attempted Suicide*, Harmondsworth: Penguin.

Wells, N. (1981), *Suicide and Deliberate Self Harm*, London: Office of Health Economics.

35 Research concerning schizophrenia

Consultant: Professor John Wing, Institute of Psychiatry, University of London.

1 Definitions

1.1 Psychiatric definition

This definition is according to the World Health Organization's *International Classification of Diseases* (9th edition):

> 295 *Schizophrenic psychoses*: A group of psychoses in which there is a fundamental disturbance of personality, a characteristic distortion of hinking, often a sense of being controlled by alien forces, delusions which may be bizarre, disturbed perception, abnormal affect out of keeping with the real situation, and autism. Nevertheless, clear consciousness and intellectual capacity are usually maintained.

Several subdivisions are also defined but the boundaries between them cannot be precisely drawn.

1.2 A practical working definition

Wing (1978) suggested that schizophrenia is usually a severe and disabling mental illness, with a lifetime expectancy rate of about 1 per cent, on average, in all the populations so far investigated throughout the world. There are two major syndromes:

1 **The acute episode** This is characterized by experiences noted by Schneider (1959), and by delusions and/or hallucinations based upon them. The afflicted person reports that he or she,

   1 Hears his or her thoughts spoken aloud.
   2 Hears voices commenting on his or her behaviour.
   3 Believes that his or her behaviour is influenced by external agents.
   4 Believes that his or her thinking is influenced by external agents.
   5 Believes that his or her bodily functions are so influenced.
   6 Explains these experiences in terms of physical or supernatural forces.

2 **The 'negative' syndrome** This is characterized by features noted by Bleuler (1911).

1 Flattening of affect (loss of emotional liveliness).
2 Loosening of associations in thinking: i.e. making remarks which don't make sense.
3 Slowness, underactivity, lack of motivation.

In about a quarter of cases, the disorder is limited to one or a few acute episodes and the prognosis is good. In about another quarter, the course is marked by severe negative symptoms from the outset and the prognosis is poor. In half or more cases, the course is fluctuating, marked by acute episodes and a moderate degree of 'negative' disability. Much depends on the quality of the social environment.

2 Prevalence

2.1 Difficulties of obtaining accurate figures

Such figures as are available are questionable because it is known that a diagnosis of schizophrenia is made in different countries according to different criteria.

1 **Estimates of frequency, using tight diagnostic criteria** Wing (1978), using such criteria, has suggested,

1 An incidence of 12–15 per 100,000 per year.
2 A fairly even distribution among nationalities.
3 A fairly even distribution among social classes.
4 A prevalence of 3–4 per 1000 in the U.K., higher among unskilled or homeless people.

2 **An American study, using looser diagnostic criteria** A study by Turner and Wagenfeld (1967) of an entire county in New York State found the prevalence of schizophrenia to be highest in people of the lowest occupational group. Other research has confirmed the drift of people with schizophrenia towards a low occupational and social position.

2.2 Admissions to psychiatric hospitals in England

The following figures are given as an *indication* only of the prevalence of schizophrenia.

	1981	1982
Mental illness beds only	18,071	17,125
Mental illness and general beds	10,516	10,208
Mental illness and geriatric beds	401	428
Total	28,988	27,761

TABLE 35.1 Total admissions in England for schizophrenia, paranoia to types of hospital or unit in 1981 and 1982 (*DHSS In-patient Statistics from the Mental Health Enquiry for England, 1981 and 1982*, HMSO.)

3 Research concerning the origins of schizophrenia

3.1 The contribution of genetic factors

This has taken place within three main fields, to be considered separately below:

1 Inheritance studies within families
2 Twin studies
3 Adoption studies

Criticisms of the view that genetic factors contribute to schizophrenia will also be considered.

1 **Inheritance studies within families** Slater (1968) has summarized these, and estimates of the vulnerability to schizophrenia of various degrees of relatives to schizophrenically ill people. Part of his table is shown in Table 35.2.

	% risk of developing schizophrenia
Parents	3.8
Brothers and sisters	8.7
Children	12.0
Uncles and aunts	2.0
First cousins	2.9

TABLE 35.2 Risk among relatives of schizophrenically ill people of developing the disorder (Slater, 1968).

2 **Twin studies: identical and non-identical twins** Shields (1978), surveying the evidence from studies of schizophrenia among identical twins by comparison with non-identical twins, summarized this as follows:

> If forced to make a best estimate of the average morbid risk for twins of schizophrenics, it would probably be wisest to rely on the recent studies. Rates of approximately 50% for MZ (identical) pairs and 17% for DZ (non-identical) pairs may not be far from the mark . . .

3 **Adoption studies** Below are two examples of these:

1 Heston (1966) compared two groups of children: the experimental group was forty-seven children placed for adoption at less than one month old and of whom the mothers had been diagnosed as schizophrenic: the control group was fifty children brought up in the same homes. Psychiatrists who did not know the background of any of the children examined them all. Of the forty-seven children born to schizophrenic mothers, thirty-seven were given some kind of psychiatric diagnosis, including five diagnosed as schizophrenic; only nine of the control group were given any kind of psychiatric diagnosis.

2 Kety and others (1975) compared the prevalence of schizophrenia among the parents of thirty-three children who were adopted, but who later became schizophrenically ill, with its prevalence among the parents of thirty-three control children, also adopted but who did not later become schizophrenically ill. Part of the table compiled by Kety is shown in Table 35.3.

Relatives	No.	% schizophrenic, including latent* schizophrenia
Biological parents of schizophrenic adoptees	66	12.1
Biological parents of control adoptees	65	6.2
Adoptive parents of schizophrenic adoptees	63	1.6
Adoptive parents of control adoptees	68	4.4

TABLE 35.3 Schizophrenic illness in the biological and adoptive families of schizophrenic index cases and controls (Wing, 1978)

*'Latent' schizophrenia refers to a group without typical symptoms.

4 **Criticisms of the 'genetic-contribution' view** The evidence from these three sources of studies seems to suggest a genetic *contribution* to schizophrenia. This view, however, has been vigorously rejected by a number of other researchers, including Rose, Kamin and Lewontin (1984), who disputed both the research designs of studies such as those referred to above, and the provisional findings. Active research in this field continues in many countries.

3.2 Research into theories that families cause schizophrenia

1 **The theory of the 'double-bind' family** Bateson (1956) suggested that some families send conflicting messages to their children which are irresolvable, and which thus precipitate breakdown. No empirical evidence has been found to support this hypothesis.

2 **The theory of 'marital skew' or 'marital schism' within the family** Lidz (1973) suggested that families in which a child has become schizophrenically ill were characterized by parents in conflict with each other and in competition for the child's loyalty. No empirical evidence which so distinguishes such families from others has been found.

3 **The theory of schizophrenia as a therapeutic experience** Laing and Esterson (1964) suggested that people choose to become schizophrenic in order to

preserve their own integrity in a situation of alienation and distress. This hypothesis is so ill-defined as to be incapable of empirical testing.

4 **The theory of the over-critical family** Brown, Birley and Wing (1972) found that once patients had recovered, it was essential that they be offered support. Relapse *was* found to be significantly associated with hostility to the patient, critical comments or emotional over-involvement. Tolerant and uncritical families (half the series) were protective against relapse. These findings were broadly supported by Vaughn and Leff (1976), by Leff and colleagues (1982), and by recent American studies.

The evidence from these studies suggest no specific schizophrenia-provoking family situations: rather, it seems that families need support and help in dealing with stress and with the care of their relatives who have become schizophrenically ill.

3.3 Research into neuro-chemical factors associated with schizophrenia

1 **The theory of the particular importance of dopamine** Dopamine is one of the many important chemicals which transmit impulses across nerve endings in the brain. Several studies, e.g. Snyder (1981), have suggested that there may be an over-production of dopamine in the brains of schizophrenically ill people.

2 **The link with low motivation** Support for the above hypothesis is offered by the well-known phenomenon of low levels of interest and initiative which are frequently a feature of schizophrenia. Goal-directed behaviour seems to depend on specific pathways in the brain which are reliant upon the smooth functioning of an enzyme which converts dopamine into noradrenalin: if there is too much dopamine and too little of the enzyme, then goal-directed behaviour is likely to be undermined.

3 **The link with response to specific medication** Yet further support for the hypothesis seems to come from the observation that people with schizophrenia do seem to benefit from medication containing drugs which interact with dopamine: e.g. chlorpromazine. Further research into this important field continues.

3.4 Increasing consensus upon the origins of schizophrenia

There appears to be increasing consensus among the leading researchers in this field that schizophrenia arises from a genetic predisposition interacting with environmental 'triggers'; frequently the trigger appears to be stress. Recent reports, e.g. Dean and James (1984), have drawn attention to stresses associated with poor quality housing and other pressures of the urban environment.

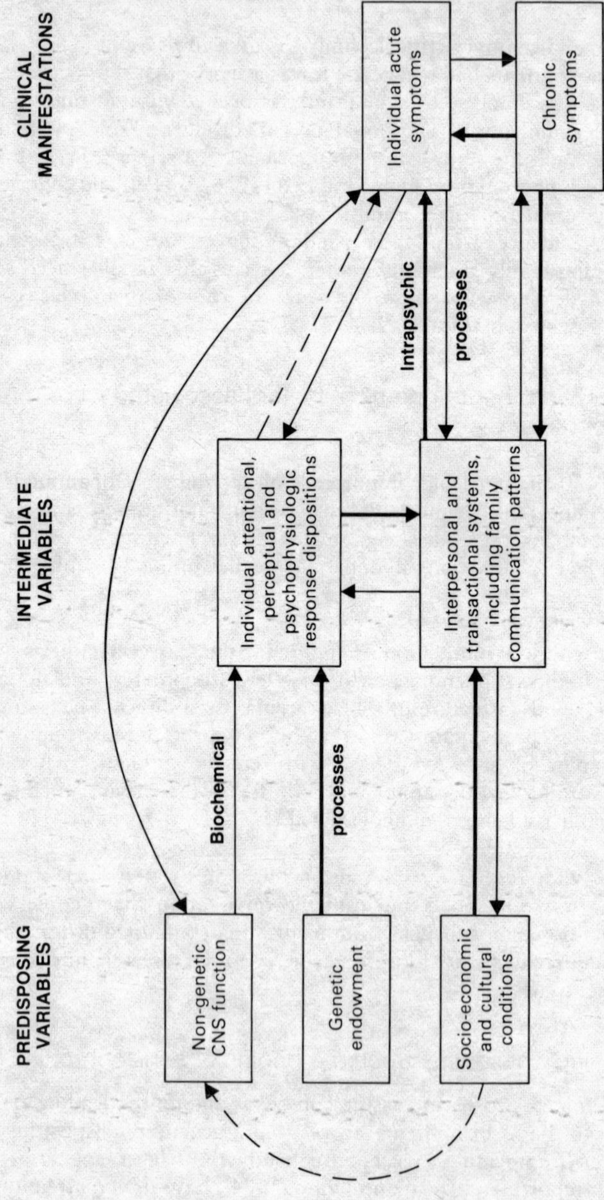

FIGURE 35.1 Simplified schema for studying the origin, development and perpetuation of the schizophrenias and similar disorders. (From Wynne, L. C., 1977, p. 258).

4 Research into the treatment or management of schizophrenia

4.1 The contribution of medication

The major tranquillizers which have helped to cut short acute episodes of schizophrenically ill people are the phenothiazine drugs, such as:

1 Chlorpromazine ('Largactil')
2 Fluphenazine ('Modecate')
3 Flupenthixol ('Depixol')
4 Other drugs with similar effects, e.g. Haloperidol.

Slow-acting forms, given by injection, are convenient for those who tend to forget to take pills.

4.2 Milieu therapy

This broad title refers to a range of support and provision made available to the recovering mentally ill: e.g. the development of life skills, and communication training. A study by Fairweather and his colleagues (1969) compared the progress of seventy-five patients who volunteered to participate in running a pre-discharge unit, where they carried major responsibilities for budgeting and supporting each other, with the progress of seventy-five others who received the routine discharge services offered by the hospital. After six months 65 per cent of the former, experimental, group remained in the community, while only 27 per cent of the control group did so.

4.3 Therapeutic communities

The effects of such settings are hard to evaluate. One study reported by Mosher, Menn and Matthews (1975) compared the effects of giving schizophrenically ill people treatment based upon medication, which required a two months' stay in hospital, with the effects of giving strong, positive support in a therapeutic community over an average of five to six months. Six months after discharge, only 4 per cent of the former were able to live independently, compared with 60 per cent of the latter.

4.4 Longer-term 'management'

Since many of the environmental factors which are beneficial or harmful to people with schizophrenia are now known, it is important that they should remain in contact with health and social services (out-patient clinics, day centres, group homes, etc.) for as long as they remain at risk of breakdown.

References

Bateson, G., Jackson, D., Haley, J. and Weakland, J. (1956), 'Toward a theory of schizophrenia', *Behavioural Science*, vol. 1, pp. 251–64.

Bleuler, E. (1911), *Dementia Praecox or the Group of Schizophrenias*, trans. J. Zinkin (1950), New York: International University Press.

Brown, G. W., Birley, J. L. T. and Wing, J. K. (1972), 'Influences of family life on the course of schizophrenic disorders: A replication', *British Journal of Psychiatry*, vol. 121, pp. 241–58.

Dean, K. and James, H. (1984), 'Depression and schizophrenia in an English city' in H. Freeman (ed.) (1984), *Mental Health and the Environment*, London: Churchill Livingstone.

Fairweather, G. W., Sanders, D. H., Cressler, D. L. and Maynard, H. (1969), *Community Life for the Mentally Ill*, Chicago: Aldine.

Heston, L. L. (1966), 'Psychiatric disorders in foster home reared children of schizophrenic mothers', *British Journal of Psychiatry*, 1966, vol. 112, pp. 819–25.

Kety, S. S., Rosenthal, D., Wender, P. H., Schulsinger, F. and Jacobsen, B. (1975), 'Mental illness in the biological and adoptive families of adopted individuals who have become schizophrenic: a preliminary report based on psychiatric interviews' in R. R. Fieve, D. Rosenthal and H. Brill (eds) (1975), *Genetic Research in Psychiatry*, Baltimore: Johns Hopkins University Press.

Laing, R. D. and Esterson, D. (1964), *Sanity, Madness and the Family*, London: Tavistock.

Leff, J. P. (1976), 'Schizophrenia and sensitivity to the family environment', *Schizophrenia Bulletin*, vol. 2, pp. 566–74.

Leff, J. P., Knipers, L., Berkowitz, R., Eberlau-Vries, R. and Sturgeon, D. (1982), 'A controlled trial of social intervention in the families of schizophrenic patients', *British Journal of Psychiatry*, vol. 141, pp. 121–34.

Lidz, T. (1973), *The Origins and Treatment of the Schizophrenic Disorders*, London: Hutchinson.

Mosher, L. R., Menn, A. and Matthews, S. (1975), 'Soteria: evaluation of a home-based treatment for schizophrenia', *American Journal of Orthopsychiatry*, 1975, vol. 75, pp. 455–67.

Rose, S., Kamin, L. J. and Lewontin, R. C. (1984), *Not in Our Genes*, Harmondsworth: Penguin.

Schneider, K. (1959), *Clinical Psychopathology*, trans. Hamilton, M. W. (1959), New York: Grune & Stratton. (Translation of the 1946 edition.)

Shields, J. (1978), 'Genetics' in J. Wing (ed.), *Schizophrenia: Towards a New Synthesis*, London: Academic Press.

Slater, E. (1968), 'A review of earlier evidence on genetic factors in schizophrenia' in D. Rosenthal and S. Kety (eds), *The Transmission of Schizophrenia*, Oxford: Pergamon Press.

Snyder, S. H. (1981), 'Dopamine receptors, neuroleptics and schizophrenia', *American Journal of Psychiatry*, vol. 138, pp. 460–4.

Turner, R. J. and Wagenfeld, M. O. (1967), 'Occupational mobility and schizophrenia', *American Sociological Review*, vol. 32, pp. 104–13.

Vaughn, C. E. and Leff, J. P. (1976), 'The influence of family and social factors on the course of psychiatric illness: A comparison of schizophrenic and depressive-neurotic patients', *British Journal of Psychiatry*, vol. 129, pp. 127–37.

Wing, J. K. (ed.) (1978), *Schizophrenia: Towards a New Synthesis*, London: Academic Press.

Wynne, L. (1977), 'Schizophrenics and their families: research on parental communication' in J. Tanner (ed.), *Developments in Psychiatric Research*, London: Hodder & Stoughton.

World Health Organization (1980), *Glossary of Mental Disorders and Guide to their Classification*, Geneva: WHO.

Research concerning people with mental handicaps

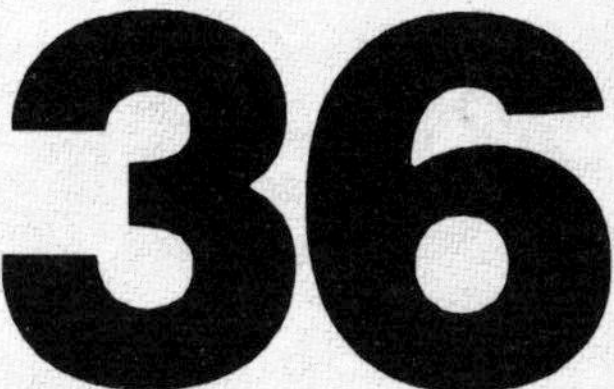

***Consultant:* Professor Peter Mittler, Professor of Special Education, Department of Education, University of Manchester.**

1 Use of terms and diagnostic criteria

1.1 Use of terms

The World Mental Health publication, *Mental Retardation: Meeting the Challenge* (1985), has reported:

> As the term is used today mental retardation involves two essential components a) intellectual functioning that is significantly below average b) marked impairment of the ability of the individual to adapt to the daily demands of the social environment. There is now widespread agreement that both intellectual functioning and adaptive behaviour must be impaired before a person can be considered mentally retarded. Neither low intelligence nor impaired adaptive behaviour alone is sufficient.

1.2 Diagnostic criteria

Russell (1985) noted that the increasingly recognized Diagnostic and Statistical Manual of the American Psychiatric Association (1980) gives the following criteria:

A Significantly subaverage general intellectual functioning: an IQ of 70 or below on an individually administered IQ test.
B Concurrent deficits or impairments in adaptive behaviour taking the person's age into consideration.
C Onset of the intellectual impairment before the age of 18.

2 Prevalence and demographic data

2.1 Categories and approximate prevalence based on IQ tests

Russell (1985) suggested that the formulations above allow for four groupings of mental handicap, according to degree of intellectual impairment. See Table 36.1

Category of mental handicap	Intellectual impairment	Approx. prevalence in the population
Mild	50–70	30/1000
Moderate	35–49)	
Severe	20–34)	3.0/1000
Profound	below 20	0.5/1000

TABLE 36.1 The four categories of mental handicap (Quoted by Russell, 1985)

2.2 Other estimates of prevalence: United Kingdom figures

1 **Estimates using DHSS data** The authors of *Mental Handicap* (Office of Health Economics, 1978), using the categories employed at the time of writing, suggested the following prevalences:

(a) *Mild mental handicap: IQ equivalent 50–69* It was estimated that there were about a million people in this category, but only a proportion came to the attention of the service-providing authorities. Most lived independently in the community.

(b) *Severe mental handicap: IQ equivalent 0–49* It was estimated that there were approximately 160,000 severely mentally handicapped people in the United Kingdom, of whom 60,000 were children. At that time four of every five of the children lived at home with their parents, while about two of every five adults lived with their families.

2 **The Warnock Report** (1978) This Report (1978), which contributed to the Education Act, 1981, noted that 2 per cent of children were educated in special schools and units at that time. It estimated that about one in six of all children would in fact need 'special educational provision' in the future – where possible in ordinary schools.

2.3 Limitations of an exclusively IQ-based categorization

1 Many researchers, e.g. Mittler (1979) and the contributors to the Warnock Report, stress the inadequacy of any classification based solely on intellectual ability, as measured by IQ tests; these are of uncertain validity and reliability and are often lacking in 'culture fairness'.
2 Mittler and Serpell (1985) have discussed their preferred use of the term 'intellectual disability', which conveys that such a feature of an individual is not a static or unchanging one; this term is coming into increasing use in many countries.
3 Such authors emphasize the importance of focusing upon the *potentials for learning and development* of handicapped people, and also the importance of social and physical skills, together with behavioural competencies.

2.4 Demographic differences

There are major differences in the prevalence of mild mental handicap between socio-economic groups. Birch and colleagues (1970), for example, in a study in Aberdeen, found the prevalence of mild mental handicap to be almost nine times greater among the children of unskilled manual workers than among people of non-manual occupations.

3 Some research concerning the causes of mental handicaps

3.1 Mental handicap: a multi-variate model

The authors of *Mental Handicap* (Office of Health Economics, 1978), represent the multi-factorial nature of the causation of mental handicap as an interacting set of variables. This is shown in Figure 36.1.

3.2 Severe mental handicap: further evidence on causation

There are both known and unknown factors associated with the various forms of severe mental handicap; these have been brought together by Weatherall (1983), and are shown in Table 36.2. (see overleaf).

Other researchers have, however, questioned that the prevalence of severe mental handicap attributable to unknown causation is as high as 34 per cent. Such uncertainty highlights the necessity for extremely careful medical investigation of all mentally handicapped children.

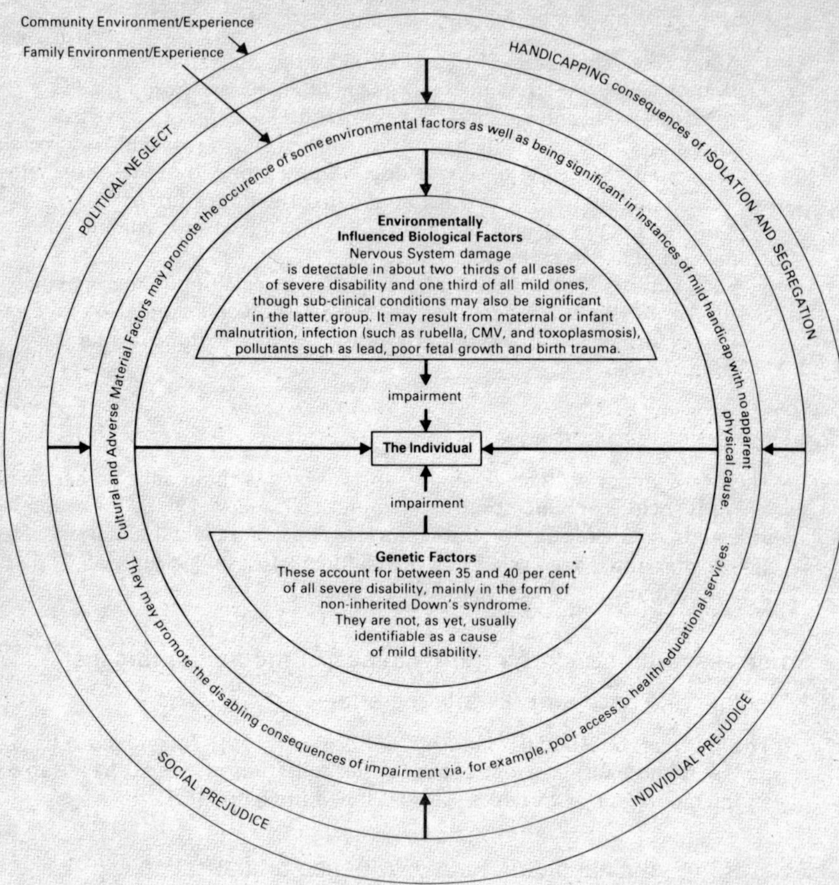

FIGURE 36.1 The causes of mental impairment, disability and handicap. From *Mental Handicap*. (Office of Health Economics/Mencap, 1986)

Cause		%
Prefertilization		
Chromosomal:	Down's syndrome	32
	other autosomal	2
	sex-chromosomal (average both sexes)	6
Monogenic		15
Intrauterine: environmental (maternal infection)		2
Perinatal: asphyxia/cerebral haemorrhage		7
Postnatal: meningitis, encephalitis, etc.		2
Total known		66

Table 36.2 continued

Unknown	
With congenital defect, etc.	14
With additional evidence of brain damage	10
Without other abnormality	10
Total unknown	34

TABLE 36.2 Diagnosis of underlying impairment in children with severe mental handicap (After Weatherall, 1983).

3.3 Mild mental handicap: the contribution of social factors

Mittler (1979) highlighted the evidence from the National Child Development Study concerning social disadvantage, and its impacts on children's development and learning. He wrote, of children with moderate learning difficulties, (see page 340), 'there is general agreement that many of the learning difficulties which they experience are related to environmental factors, including poverty, poor housing and deprivation of experience.'

4 Research concerning the prevention of mental handicap

4.1 Counselling and screening for genetic factors

Genetic counselling can usually be offered to parents thought to be carriers of inherited conditions. In some circumstances, amniocentesis can be offered.

4.2 The link between maternal age and Down's syndrome babies

The authors of *Mental Handicap* (OHE, 1978) have reported,

> Women between aged 15–19 stand less than a 1 in 2,000 chance of giving birth to a Down's syndrome baby. For those over 40 the risk is around 1 in 100. For mothers over 45 it is 1 in 50.

5 Research concerning the education and development of the potential of mentally handicapped people

5.1 The Portage Project

1 **The nature of the Project** This Project, described by Shearer and Shearer (1972), was developed in Portage, Wisconsin, as a home-teaching service for mentally handicapped young children. Wilcock (1981) has written,

> The Portage model is a home intervention programme. It centres on a home teacher who trains parents to be more effective teachers of their own children by instructing them in how to target appropriate teaching tasks, how to present them and how to record and assess their child's performance.

2 **Components of the model** Wilcock (1981) has described these as follows:

1 Identification and referral of appropriate pre-school children
2 Screening
3 Assessment
  (a) Formal assessment using standardised developmental tests.
  (b) Informal assessment, to learn of a child's individuality.
  (c) Assessment of a child's existing repertoire, in terms of five developmental areas: cognition, self-help, motor skills, language and socialisation.
  (d) Ongoing assessment, as parents teach and work with their children, using carefully devised activity charts.
4 The home teaching process. This is based upon the parents teaching the child precisely defined tasks, tuned to his or her developmental stage in the areas given in (c), above, and agreed with the visiting home teacher. Much emphasis is placed upon enabling the parent and child to *succeed.*

3 **Evaluations of the Project** Pugh (1981) has described the evaluations undertaken of the Project, first in America, and then after its implementation in Wales. She reported,

> Evaluation of the Portage project in Wisconsin, USA showed that the service was of positive benefit to pre-school retarded children. Seventy-five multiply handicapped children, with ages ranging from birth to six years and an average IQ of 75, gained on average 13 mental-age months in an eight-month period. On average 128 activity charts were written per child during this period and the children were successful in 91% of these. (Shearer and Shearer, 1974).

Of the experience in Wales, Pugh wrote,

> the children acted as their own controls, and baseline measures were taken before the Portage intervention started. Of 306 different tasks set during the research phase of the project, 270 were learned (88.2%), 206 (or 67.3%) being learned within one week.

5.2 The findings of other studies involving parents

Following the Warnock Report (1978) great efforts have been made in some places to build closer links between professional workers and the families of handicapped children. Some of these are described by Pugh and Russell (1977) and Pugh (1981), and include:

1 The Honeylands home-visiting project in Exeter This scheme involved a multi-disciplinary support team, including a paediatrician, a psychologist, specialist health visitor, a teacher, nurses, a parent, a social worker and occupational and speech therapists. Each family was visited weekly by one team member who could draw on the skills of the whole team. At evaluation, these families were found to be more positive in attitudes, by comparison with an unvisited group of families.

2 **Health Visitor Home Visiting Project, Hester Adrian Research Centre**

1 This scheme is part of a broader research programme with the families of mentally handicapped, mainly Down's syndrome, children at Manchester University. An early study, involving a year of six-weekly visits (Cunningham and Sloper, 1977), indicated gains by the child and a positive response from parents.
2 A second study, involving training special health visitors, enabled them to give information and support, as well as very clear recommendations upon ways in which the child might be stimulated and encouraged. At evaluation, there was evidence of clear gains by the children, and of satisfaction from parents.

3 **Kith and Kids Project, North London** This group, initiated by parents and described by Collins and Collins (1976), focuses upon providing social and community links for families with mentally handicapped children, and enlisting the co-operation of professionals and volunteers to achieve this. The psychologists and parents together devise and work towards precise and attainable goals, social rather than purely academic. Formal evaluation had not been possible at the time of writing, but there appeared to be very clear gains for all concerned.

4 **The Southend-on-Sea group therapy scheme** This scheme is based upon enabling parents of handicapped children to meet regularly, to gain support, to discuss the stresses of living with a handicapped child, to learn aspects of child development and how he or she may be helpfully stimulated. Its continuation and growth are indicators of the group's effectiveness.

6 Research concerning educational developments in special schools

6.1 A new system to replace categorization

1 The Warnock Report (1978) made a number of specific recommendations; the authors wrote: 'We . . . recommend that the statutory categorisation of handicapped pupils be abolished.' The Committee also recommended that terms such as 'educationally sub-normal' be discarded, and reported,

> *We recommend that the term 'children with learning difficulties' should be used in future to describe both those children who are currently categorised as educationally sub-normal and those with educational difficulties who are often at present the concern of remedial services.* Learning difficulties might be described as 'mild', 'moderate' or 'severe'. Children with particular difficulties, such as specific reading difficulties, might be described as having 'specific learning difficulties' . . .

2 These and other recommendations have been implemented in the UK Education Act of 1981, and major moves have occurred towards the integration of children with learning difficulties into ordinary schools.

6.2 Developments in special education

Encouraging developments in the education of handicapped children include:

1 **The Education of the Developmentally Young project** Foxen and McBrien (1978), working from the Hester Adrian Centre at the University of Manchester, have developed a means of training teachers of the handicapped how to foster and enhance in their pupils a wide range of conceptual abilities and other skills. This integrated method of training staff to teach children is highly structured and very precise in both its training and its monitoring of achievement.

2 **The Derbyshire Language Scheme** Masidlover and Knowles (1982) have similarly developed carefully tested resources and strategies for fostering language abilities among the handicapped. Knowledge of such resources is gradually being disseminated and built upon in local authorities.

7 Services for mentally handicapped people in the community

7.1

Services are shown schematically in Figure 36.1.

7.2 Developing a community-based service

There have been major developments in some localities towards developing community-based residential services for mentally handicapped people. The working paper, *An Ordinary Life* (1980), 'aims to provide an overview of the principles which should guide new residential services and the constituent elements of such provision'. The paper then examines a number of specific issues, including:

1 **Principles and practice in a residential service** These principles are:

(a) Mentally handicapped people have the same human value as anyone else and so the same human rights.
(b) Living like others within the community is both a right and a need.
(c) Services must recognize the individuality of mentally handicapped people.

2 **Components of a comprehensive community service**

(a) The range of places needed for people to live in.
(b) An integrated system of housing.
(c) Integration with non-residential services.

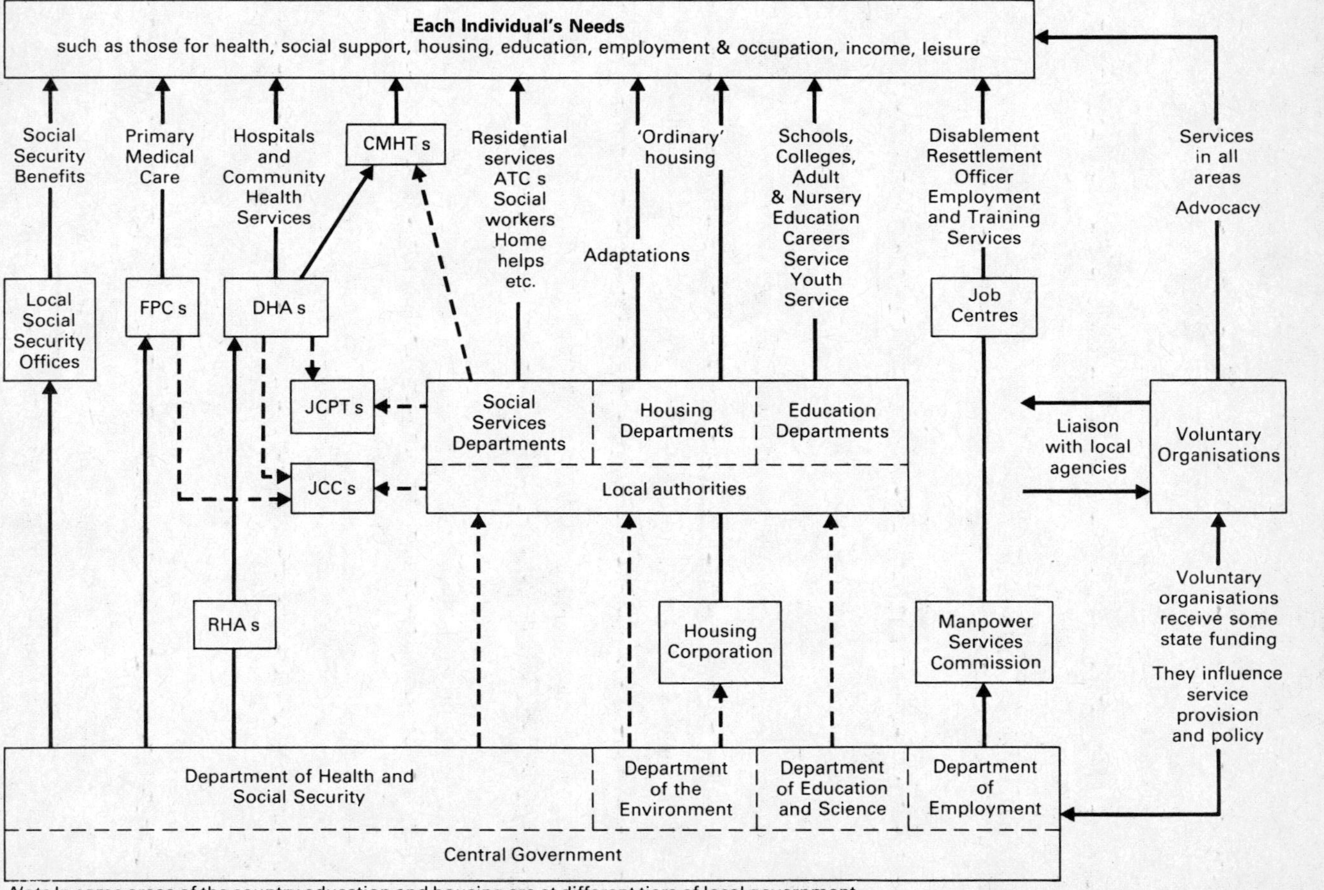

Note In some areas of the country education and housing are at different tiers of local government.

FIGURE 36.2 Services for mentally handicapped people in England. (Office of Health Economics/Mencap, 1986)

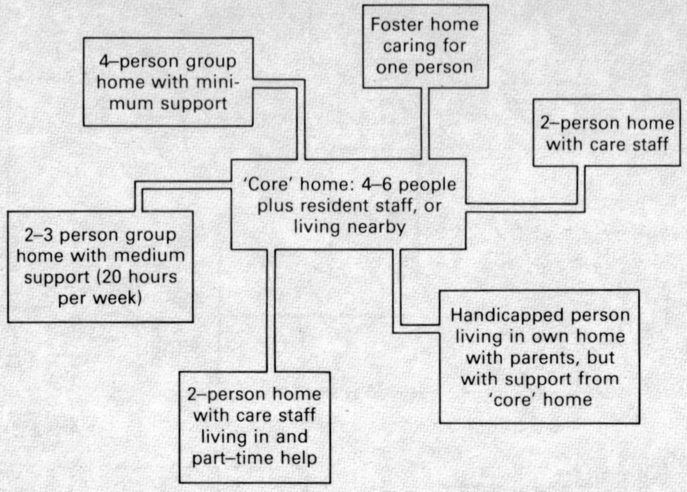

FIGURE 36.3 The 'core and cluster' principle (King's Fund Centre, 1980)

3 **Principles of planning the service** These include:

(a) Planning principles and policies, such as the involvement of local people, and representation on planning groups
(b) The tasks of the team, including agreeing the philosophy, aims and objectives of the service
(c) Operational planning
(d) Forward planning
(e) Costing

4 **Further principles** These include:

(a) The development of individual programme plans for clients
(b) The acquisition of suitable housing
(c) Staffing the service
(d) Monitoring and evaluation of the service provided

7.3 The development of community mental handicap teams

Bicknell (1985), writing from the standpoint of health services, has described such teams,

> The team of health care professionals that is vital to the delivery of health care . . . works under a variety of names but is most frequently referred to as the community mental handicap team (CMHT). Crucial to the functioning of this team is the core membership of the community nurse in mental handicap and of the social worker who, while funded by social services, will have a strong and traditional link

> with the health service. Most teams are supported by clinical psychologists, educationalists, physiotherapists, speech therapists and occupational therapists, while the medical contribution is made by a psychiatrist, a general practitioner and a clinical medical officer . . . the above list is not meant to be complete or unchangeable.

7.4 Further developments

1 **The developments of materials to enhance living** A very encouraging development has been the devising of teaching materials to enhance the opportunities for independent living for handicapped people. These include the Hampshire Assessment for Living with Others (H.A.L.O.) materials, which are gaining increasing attention.

2 **Self advocacy** A further development has been the enabling of handicapped people to speak for themselves and for others in e.g. the provision and design of services. They are thus able to make demands from firsthand knowledge as consumers – rather than as passive recipients of other people's decisions.

References

American Psychiatric Association (1980), *Diagnostic and Statistical Manual of Mental Disorders* (DSM III), Washington: APA.

Bicknell, J. (1985), 'The mental handicap service – modern concepts of care' in D. Sines and J. Bicknell (eds) (1985), *Caring for Mentally Handicapped People in the Community*, London: Harper & Row.

Birch, H. G., Richardson, S. A., Baird, D., Horobin, G. and Illsley, R. (1970), *Mental Subnormality in the Community*, Baltimore: Williams & Wilkins.

Collins, M. and Collins, D. (1976), *Kith and Kids*, London: Souvenir Press.

Cunningham, G. C. and Sloper, P. (1978), *Helping Your Handicapped Baby*, London: Souvenir Press.

DES (1978), *Special Educational Needs* (The Warnock Report), London: HMSO.

Foxen, T. and McBrien, J. (1978), *Training Staff in Behavioural Methods* (Education of the Developmentally Young Project), Manchester: Manchester University Press.

Hampshire Social Services (1980), *Hampshire Assessment for Living with Others*, Winchester.

King's Fund Centre (1980), *An Ordinary Life*, London: KFC.

Masidlover, M. and Knowles, W. (1982), *Derbyshire Language Scheme*, Derbyshire County Council.

Mittler, P. (1979), *People, Not Patients*, London: Methuen.

Mittler, P. (1984), 'Quality of life and services for people with disabilities', *Bulletin of the British Psychological Society* (1984), vol. 37, pp. 218–25.

Mittler, P. and Serpell, R. (1985), 'Services: an international perspective' in A. M. Clarke, A. D. Clarke and J. Berg (eds), *Mental Deficiency. The Changing Outlook*, London: Methuen.

Office of Health Economics (1978), *Mental Handicap: Ways Forward*, London: OHE.

Pugh, G. (1981), *Parents as Partners*, London: National Children's Bureau.

Pugh, G. and Russell, P. (1977), *Shared Care: Support Services for Families with Handicapped Children*, London: National Children's Bureau.

Russell, O. (1985), *Mental Handicap*, Edinburgh: Churchill Livingstone.

Shearer, M. S. and Shearer, D. E. (1972), 'The Portage project: A model for early childhood education', *Exceptional Children*, vol. 39, pp. 210–17.

Weatherall, D. (1983), *The New Genetics and Clinical Practice*, Oxford: Nuffield Provincial Hospitals Trust.

Wilcock, P. (1981), 'The Portage Project in America' in Pugh, G. (1981), *Parents as Partners*.

World Health Organisation (1980), *International Classification of Impairments, Disabilities and Impairments*, Geneva: World Health Organisation.

World Health Organisation (1985), *Mental Retardation: Meeting the Challenge*, WHO offset Publication 86, Geneva: World Health Organization.

PART 10

Research concerning situations in which some people seek help

37 Research concerning bereavement and grief reactions

Consultant:* *Dr Colin Murray Parkes, Senior Lecturer in Psychiatry, The London Hospital Medical College, London.

1 Definition

Averill (1968) has written that bereavement or grief behaviour denotes:

> the total response pattern, psychological and physiological, displayed by an individual following the loss of a significant object, with two components: mourning and grief. Mourning refers to the conventional behaviour as determined by the mores and customs of the society; grief is the stereotyped set of psychological and physiological reactions of biological origin.

2 Some figures concerning bereavement

2.1 Official statistics of conjugal bereavement in the UK

	Males		Females	
	1971	1981	1971	1981
Widowed	762	749	3,139	3,182

TABLE 37.1 Marital condition: census figures. Thousands. (OPCS, General Register Office (Scotland); General Register Office (Northern Ireland), *Annual Abstract of Statistics*, No. 121, 1985 Edition)

2.2 Another way of describing the frequency of bereavement

Nuttall (1980) described the situation thus:

> There are three million widows and eight hundred thousand widowers in the United Kingdom. Two hundred thousand children under the age of sixteen have lost a parent through death. In 1977 over thirteen thousand children under the age of fourteen died. . . . Looking at these statistics in another way, they show that each day in the United Kingdom approximately five hundred and fifty wives become widows, one hundred and fifty husbands become widowers, forty young children lose a parent through death and almost forty children under fourteen die.

3 Research on the nature of grief and bereavement

3.1 Grief as a cross-cultural phenomenon

In a comparative study of grief and its manifestations, Rosenblatt, Walsh and Jackson (1976) examined the impact of and response to bereavement across seventy-eight world cultures. Summarizing some of their many findings, they have written,

> It seems basically human for emotions to be expressed in bereavement. When a person reacts with crying, overt anger, or overt fear, that person is behaving as some people in most societies do. Indeed, in the majority of societies, crying occurs frequently among people who are bereaved. . . .

3.2 The existence of stages or components of the grief response

The best-known charting of the stages of grief is that of Parkes (1972), summarized below by Nuttall (1980).

> (a) The initial shock, numbness and sense of unreality not lasting for any set length of time, in some days whilst weeks in others. There is only a gradual emergence into a state of 'knowing', both emotionally and rationally. (b) A phase in which several things are experienced – pining, searching, crying, restlessness, repeated going over what happened, trying to make sense of things, etc . . . it is often hard to live with regrets, anger, feelings of revenge, loss of confidence and concentration. A good deal of support is needed at this time. (c) Depression. This too can be a very difficult time with a double edge to it. A time of apathy, lack of interest or purpose, often a feeling that you are never going to come through to a point where the load is lifted. As well as being difficult for the bereaved person, it can be hard to live with for the relatives and friends as they see little apparent movement. . . . This highlights again how important it is to offer support to the supporters, whether care-givers or relatives. (d) The beginnings of recovery. . . . Gradually there is the acceptance and adjustment. . . . It is also an elusive recovery as memories and events bring feelings of loss and deprivation.

N.B. Parkes (1985) commented that, first, he would now use the expression 'Disorganization and despair' rather than 'Depression' (see [c], above), and, second, his phases of grief are an adaptation of those formulated by Bowlby (1979).

3.3 The desirability of giving way to grief

Ramsay (1977) has summarized the view of many researchers:

> The grief responses to a significant loss are not always present – the 'normal' reactions of shock, despair and recovery are often distorted, exaggerated, prolonged, inhibited or delayed. . . . However, there is

> reasonable agreement in the literature that grief *has* to be worked through; if it is not, the person will continue to have troubles of some sort.

He went on to quote Hodge (1972):

> The problems must be brought into the open and confronted, no matter how unpleasant it may be for the patient. *The grief work must be done*. There is no healthy escape from this. We might even add that the grief work *will be done*. Sooner or later, correctly or incorrectly, completely or incompletely, in a clear or distorted manner, *it will be done*.

4 Research indicating people at risk following bereavement

Parkes (1985) has summarized these, reporting that the variables indicated have been ranked in their approximate order of importance; thus several factors will together contribute to the overall risk:

> The factors which research has shown to contribute to poor outcome are: I *Type of death* (1) A cause for blame on survivor . . .; (2) sudden or unexpected or untimely . . .; (3) painful, horrifying or mismanaged. II *Characteristics of the relationship* (1) relationship 'dependent' or 'symbiotic' . . .; (2) relationship ambivalent . . .; (3) spouse dies . . .; (4) child under 20 dies . . .; (5) parent dies (especially mother) leaving child(ren) aged between 0 and 5 and 10 and 15 . . .; (6) parent dies leaving older unmarried adult. III *Characteristics of survivor* (1) grief-prone personality (expressed in intense clinging and pining) . . .; (2) insecure, over-anxious (with low self-esteem) . . .; (3) previous mental illness . . .; (4) excessively angry . . .; (5) excessively self-reproachful . . .; (6) physically disabled or ill . . .; (7) previous unresolved losses . . .; (8) inability to express feelings (particularly with strong 'macho' self-image prohibiting expression of grief). IV *Social circumstances* (1) family absent or seen as unsupportive (lack of an intimate other) . . .; (2) detached from traditional cultural or religious support systems (especially if immigrant) . . .; (3) unemployed or unhappy at work . . .; (4) with dependent children at home (though this may be a positive factor in the long run . . .; (5) low socio-economic status . . .; (6) other losses . . .

5 Research concerning the vulnerability of bereaved people

5.1 The link between bereavement and increased mortality rate

Several studies, e.g. Parkes, Benjamin and Fitzgerald (1969), have found an increase in the probability of death following bereavement. They reported: 'the mortality rate during the first six months of bereavement was found to be 40% higher than the expected rate based on national figures for married men of the same age.'

5.2 The link between bereavement and increased ill-health

1. In the 'London Study', involving the detailed investigation of twenty-two widows in the year following the death of their spouses (but which lacked a control group), Parkes (1971) found a correlation between their general health and levels of irritability noted at interviews. 'Passive' responders were characterized by tearfulness, visual memories and a sense of the continued presence of the deceased person: 'active' responders were characterized by greater restlessness, irritability, and tension. It was the latter group who were more vulnerable to ill-health.
2. Parkes and Brown (1972), in the American 'Harvard Study', compared the physical and mental health of sixty-eight young widows and widowers fourteen months after bereavement with that of sixty-eight matched non-bereaved people. The former group reported more hospital admissions, more disturbances of sleep, appetite and weight, more depression, strain, loneliness and restlessness.

   This study also indicated that those who received little or no warning of impending bereavement were more vulnerable than those who had had the opportunity to make some prior adjustment.

6 Research upon supporting the bereaved through counselling

Parkes (1980), in a review of this field (in which he examined only studies with random allocation of subjects to experimental and control groups) investigated:

1. Professional services by trained doctors, nurses, social workers, etc., offering individual support.
2. Professional services offering group support.
3. Trained volunteer workers supported by professionals.
4. Self-help groups.

Each is considered briefly below.

6.1 Professional services by doctors, nurses and others

1. An American study by Gerber (1975) compared the effects of offering telephone counselling mainly to 116 bereaved, mainly elderly, people with the effects of non-intervention with a control group of another fifty-three people. The most helpful effects were noted at five and eight months after bereavement, when the supported people were having less medication and fewer consultations with doctors.
2. An Australian study by Raphael (1977) examined the effect of bereavement counselling with thirty-one 'high-risk' widows, compared with thirty-three other 'high-risk' widows not offered counselling. The former received home counselling of between one and nine sessions following bereavement, when expression of grief, anger, anxiety and despair was facilitated and encouraged. Thirteen months after

bereavement the counselled group had required a further twenty-one consultations with doctors: the non-counselled had required forty-seven.

6.2 Professional services offering group support

1. Jones (1979), in Los Angeles, randomly assigned thirty-six widows and widowers to an experimental or control group. The former participated in three hours weekly of group discussion upon a major aspect of bereavement, led by a therapist, during the six to nine months after bereavement. Parkes (1980) reported that despite no significant general outcome differences between the two groups, high-risk participants did show benefit on several measures.
2. Cameron and Parkes (1983) examined the effects of a 'palliative care' unit in Montreal: twenty bereaved people whose relatives had died there, and who had received support from staff afterwards, were compared with twenty other bereaved people whose relatives had died in different units of the same hospital. Parkes reported that families from the palliative care unit showed fewer health problems than control families, required fewer tranquillizers and were less unhappily preoccupied with the dead person.

6.3 Voluntary services

Parkes's own study (1979), of the service for relatives of patients dying at St. Christopher's Hospice in London, distinguished high risk relatives. These were assigned randomly to an experimental group or a control group. The former, of thirty-two people, was offered the help of a volunteer service: the control group of thirty-five was not. Parkes summarized that no differences were found between the groups during the first year after the service was introduced. Persons visited in the second and third years had better health.

6.4 Self-help groups

Vachon and colleagues (1980) examined the value of self-help in Toronto. Sixty-eight widows were randomly assigned to an experimental group while ninety-six others were controls. The former received one-to-one and group support from other widows who had 'resolved their own bereavement reactions . . .': the latter did not.

No significant differences in psychological health were evident at six, twelve and twenty-four months after bereavement, but a small, high risk group of the supported widows fared better than those receiving no support on five measures at both six and twenty-four months after bereavement. Parkes concluded that these results favour the hypothesis that self-help is a valuable support in bereavement, and particularly to the most distressed.

Since, however, this particular group of volunteers had received great help from the researcher, a nurse counsellor with 'great experience in the care of the bereaved'. Parkes concluded, 'the case for self-help without professional backing must therefore be regarded as unproved.'

6.5 Conclusions from the review by Parkes

1 Parkes considered that the evidence suggests that:

> professional services and professionally supported voluntary and self-help services are capable of reducing the risk of psychiatric and psychosomatic disorders resulting from bereavement. Services are most beneficial among bereaved people who perceive their families are unsupportive or who, for other reasons, are thought to be at special risk.

2 From Parkes's own study it appeared that volunteers take about a year to become competent, and 'thereafter many volunteer counsellors come to rival professionals'.
3 Telephone contacts and office consultations are no substitute for home visits.
4 If help can be provided before, as well as after bereavement, the probability of a positive outcome increases.

6.6 The work of CRUSE

Parkes (1985) reported that he knows of no systematic studies of counselling by workers within CRUSE, the national organization offering bereavement counselling, but he noted elsewhere (Parkes, 1985) of CRUSE counsellors: 'with experience, volunteer counsellors develop a high level of expertise.'

7 Research concerning specific groups among the bereaved

7.1 Counselling parents who have experienced a cot death

Limerick (1976) has offered guidelines in this respect. Crucial areas needing attention include:

1 Explanation and clarification of the cause of death . . . together with information that cot death is a recognized medical problem in many parts of the world.
2 Dispelling unfounded beliefs, based upon discredited theories of causation.
3 Reassurance concerning blame and guilt.
4 The need of the whole family for support, inasmuch as such a death may trigger complex family tensions and reactions.
5 The naturalness of the physiological and psychological responses to the experience of grief.
6 Anxiety concerning other or future children.

7.2 Counselling relatives bereaved by suicide

1 A study by Shepherd and Barraclough (1970) examined the needs of thirty-one bereaved people whose spouses had completed suicide. It was noted that 'need' tended to be understood by respondents as 'unmet need'.
   1 81 per cent of the group felt need of comfort and practical help
   2 44 per cent of the group felt need of advice and information
   3 35 per cent of the group felt need of religious counselling
   4 29 per cent of the group felt need of financial help
   5 16 per cent of the group felt need of other kinds of help.

2 The authors make a number of suggestions on how to help those bereaved by suicide:
   (a) A greater role to be played by the GP in referring such relatives to available resources.
   (b) A greater role to be played by the pathologist in offering advice and counselling to the bereaved where an inquest or a post mortem is required.

References

Averill, J. R. (1968), 'Grief: its nature and significance', *Psychological Bulletin*, vol. 70, pp. 721–48.

Bowlby, J. (1979), *The Making and Breaking of Affectional Bonds*, London: Tavistock.

Cameron, J. and Parkes, C. M. (1983), 'Terminal care: Evaluation of effects on surviving family of care before and after bereavement', *Postgraduate Medical Journal*, vol. 59, pp. 73–8.

Gerber, I., Weiner, A., Battin, D. and Arkin, A. (1975), 'Brief therapy to the aged bereaved' in B. Schoenberg and I. Gerber (eds), *Bereavement: its psychological aspects*, New York: Columbia University Press.

Grindel, P. (1981), 'Help for the bereaved', *Health Visitor*, vol. 54, pp. 330–3.

Hodge, J. R. (1972), 'They that mourn', *Journal of Religion and Health*, vol. 11, pp. 229–40.

Jones, J. (1979), Unpublished dissertation, University of California. Referred to in C. M. Parkes (1980), 'Bereavement counselling: does it work?', *British Medical Journal*, 5 July 1980, pp. 3–6.

Limerick, S. (1976), 'Counselling after a cot death', *Health Visitor*, vol. 49, pp. 256–7.

Nuttall, D. (1980), 'Bereavement', *Health Visitor*, March 1980, pp. 84–6.

Parkes, C. M. (1964), 'The effects of bereavement on physical and mental health. A study of case records of widows', *British Medical Journal*, vol. 2, pp. 274–7.

Parkes, C. M. (1971), 'The first year of bereavement. A longitudinal study of the reactions of London widows to the death of their husbands', *Psychiatry*, vol. 33, pp. 444–7.

Parkes, C. M. (1972), *Bereavement: studies of grief in adult life*, London: Tavistock.
Parkes, C. M. (1979), 'Evaluation of a bereavement service', in A. De Vries and A. Carmi (eds), *The Dying Human*, Ramat Gan: Turtledove.
Parkes, C. M. (1980), 'Bereavement counselling: does it work?', *British Medical Journal*, 5 July, pp. 3–6.
Parkes, C. M. (1985), 'Bereavement', *British Journal of Psychiatry*, vol. 146, pp. 11–17.
Parkes, C. M. (1985), Personal communication.
Parkes, C. M., Benjamin, B. and Fitzgerald, R. G. (1969), 'Broken heart: a statistical study of increased mortality among widowers', *British Medical Journal*, vol. 1, pp. 740–3.
Parkes, C. M. and Brown, R. (1972), 'Health after bereavement; a controlled study of young Boston widows and widowers', *Psychosomatic Medicine*, vol. 34, pp. 00–00.
Parkes, C. M. and Weiss, R. S. (1983) *Recovery from Bereavement*, New York: Basic Books.
Ramsay, R. W. (1977), 'Behavioural approaches to bereavement', *Behaviour Research and Therapy*, vol. 15, pp. 131–5.
Raphael, B. (1977), 'Preventive intervention with the recently bereaved', *Archives of General Psychiatry*, vol. 34, pp. 1450–4.
Rosenblatt, P. C., Walsh, R. and Jackson, D. A. (1976), *Grief and Mourning in Cross-Cultural Perspective*, HRAF Press.
Shepherd, D. M. and Barraclough, B. M. (1979), 'Help for those bereaved by suicide', *British Journal of Social Work*, vol. 9, pp. 67–74.
Vachon, M., Lyall, W., Rogers, J., Freedman, K. and Freeman, S. J. (1980), 'A controlled study of self-help intervention for widows', *American Journal of Psychiatry*, vol. 137, pp. 1380–4.

Research concerning family and marital therapy 38

Consultant: Dr Michael Crowe, Consultant Psychiatrist, The Bethlem Royal Hospital and the Maudsley Hospital, Denmark Hill, London.

Full acknowledgment is made that this chapter draws substantially upon the book by Gurman, A. S. and Kniskern, D. P. (1981), *Handbook of Family Therapy*, Brunner/Mazel.

1 A general definition

Gurman and Kniskern (1978) have written,

> Marital-family therapy is presently a widely diverse and growing field. It includes the therapists from many professions, has no unified theory, and few techniques are specific to it.

They suggested that family therapy is unified only in a belief that relationships are of at least as much importance in the behaviour and experience of people as are individual factors.

2 Statistics

2.1 Some relevant figures: the National Marriage Guidance Council

1 **Those seeking help** While it is impossible to gather data concerning the total number of those seeking help with family or marital difficulties because so much of the help is informal, and those offering help are so varied, Table 38.1 shows the numbers of interviews with people seeking help from the Marriage Guidance Council of the UK.

Interviews with	1981–2	1982–3	1983–4	1984–5	(%)
Women	92,000	93,500	94,000	103,000	(43)
Men	41,000	43,000	42,000	43,000	(18)
Pairs etc.	69,000	74,000	79,000	92,000	(39)
Total interviews	202,000	211,000	215,000	239,000	
New cases	36,000	36,000	38,000	41,000	

TABLE 38.1 Annual interviews during the period 1981–5 (*Annual Report*, 1985, National Marriage Guidance Council)

2 **Those offering help** The Annual Report 1985 noted, 'The average number of counsellors, reception interviews and education workers active during 1984–5 was 1850. This was 5 per cent more than the number in 1983–84.'

2.2 The main approaches in the family and marital therapy field

There exist within this field a number of complementary frameworks of theory and practice: these have been discussed and illustrated by Bentovim, Gorell Barnes and Cooklin (1982). In their review, Gurman and Kniskern (1981) suggest the following groupings, each of which is itself composed of several 'schools':

1 **Psychoanalytic and object relations approaches** These are grounded upon psychoanalytic theory, but draw upon other principles as well. A leading figure in this school is Skynner (1976), and Kniskern and Gurman (1981) suggested that the primary goal of therapy in this approach is to identify how family members are projecting difficulties actually associated with the marriage upon e.g. a child of the family. Thereafter help can be given towards a more constructive resolution.

2 **Intergenerational approaches** These seek to go beyond the immediate family circle and to enlist the co-operation of others in resolving the family's distress. Bowen (1978) and Lieberman (1979) have carried out much work in this area, while Whitaker (1975) has developed experiential methods of practising family therapy.

3 **Systems theory approaches** Such approaches, which are now the dominant ones, are grounded in the notion of the family as a system. A number of 'schools' have developed within this framework: these include the 'structural' school, associated with Minuchin (1974), the 'strategic' school, associated with Haley (1976) and the 'systemic' school, developed by Palazzoli and colleagues (1978).

4 **Behavioural approaches** These are based upon principles of social learning theory (see Chapter 9, page 71) and leading researchers in this field are Alexander and Parsons (1973), Patterson (1976), Jacobson (1978) and Crowe (1984). Kniskern and Gurman (1981) have emphasized the strong emphasis which behavioural therapists place upon empirical evaluation and validating treatment outcome.

3 Research concerning the outcome of family and marital therapy

The next sections draw upon two main sources: the chapter by Kniskern and Gurman in the book, *Advances in Family Intervention: Assessment and Theory*, edited by Vincent (1981), and the *Handbook of Family Therapy* (1981), edited by Gurman and Kniskern.

3.1 Some preliminary considerations

1 **The proliferation of research** Gurman and Kniskern (1981) found over 200 reports concerning about 5,000 families. Reviews, which are themselves critical appraisals of a field of research, have also proliferated in this field. By 1981 thirty-two such reviews were available, and it is these that these authors survey.

2 **Inescapable complicating factors** Gurman and Kniskern concluded,

(a) It is impossible to disentangle treatment effects from therapist effects in the studies done to date.
(b) The treatments that have been studied have almost never followed 'pure' applications of given treatment models.
(c) With infrequent exceptions, it is impossible to be certain just what specific treatment interventions have actually been used, since treatment operations have almost never been described in detail.

Crowe (1986) has also noted,

(d) Difficulties in choosing outcome criteria, and of disentangling improvements in the individual (such as a decrease in symptoms) from family relationship improvements.

3.2 Research concerning the model of intervention employed

1 **Outcome rates of family therapies, excluding behaviourally-oriented approaches**

1 Family therapies produce beneficial outcomes in about two thirds of cases. Gurman and Kniskern (1981) reported that their analysis showed 61 per cent of marital cases and 73 per cent of family cases improved; a different analysis, excluding a small sample of cases, gave an improvement rate of 65 per cent to the marital therapy cases.
2 It is important to note, however, that these studies were uncontrolled; i.e. there were not usually control groups of families who did not receive therapy. Such a research design permits improvement (or deterioration) resulting from circumstances other than the therapy to be recognized.
3 These authors noted, moreover, that the data said little about effective components of the intervention, but suggested that they offer at least a crude empirical basis for the continued practice and teaching of marital and family therapy.

2 **Other indications from this group**

1 Conjoint marital therapy (i.e. involving both partners) is probably more effective than group or collaborative methods. Of forty-four comparisons of conjoint methods and all other marital therapy methods,

conjoint treatment emerged superior in thirty-one comparisons, no different in eleven and inferior in only two.

2 Involving both spouses in therapy probably leads to greater chance of positive outcome than involving only one, although this is not conclusively established.

3 Behaviourally-oriented marital therapy

1 This seems to be about as effective for minimally to moderately distressed couples as do therapies of different kinds.

2 Work is developing in this field: see Hahlweg and Jacobson (1984) for several studies. Two studies, Crowe (1978) and Emmelkamp and colleagues (1984) found behavioural and alternative methods to be equivalent, but in Crowe's study the behavioural approach proved more helpful for sexual difficulties.

4 Marital therapy and severely distressed couples Gurman and Kniskern considered there is little evidence that such couples can be significantly helped by therapy of any kind.

3.3 Research concerning the person of the therapist

1 Variables associated with a positive outcome

1 There is increasing evidence supporting the association between treatment outcome and the therapist's skills of relationship. Gurman and Kniskern (1981) have written,

> The literature suggests that it is generally important for the marital-family therapist to be active and to provide some structure, but not to confront tenuous family defenses very early in treatment. Excesses in directiveness are among the main contributors to premature termination, and to negative therapy outcomes.

2 The importance of relationship skills is as great in behaviourally-oriented interventions as in other approaches.

2 Variables associated with a negative outcome Kniskern and Gurman (1981) reported that there is evidence suggesting that,

> Marital and family therapies, at times, make individual patients and their marital and/or family relationships worse. It appears that about 5–10 percent of couples and families become worse at least during, if not because of, the nonbehavioral family treatment they receive.

They continued,

> There is evidence that a particular therapist style is associated with such negative outcomes. These therapists provide relatively little structuring and guiding of early treatment sessions, use frontal confrontations of

highly affective material and label unconscious motivation early in therapy rather than stimulating interaction, gathering data, or giving support. In particular, these therapists do not actively intervene to moderate interpersonal feedback in families in which one member has very low ego strength.

3 **Other variables** There is no empirical evidence to support the view that therapy practised with a therapist and a co-therapist leads to more beneficial outcomes to the couple or family than that practised by one therapist working alone.

3.4 Components of family and marital therapy which contribute to effectiveness

There is consistent evidence to suggest that approaches which increase a couple's or a family's communication skills contribute to a positive outcome, regardless of the model of therapy employed (Birchler, 1979). Gurman and Kniskern (1981), however, stressed that while increased communication skills are a crucial component of effective therapy, they are not sufficient to achieve beneficial outcome alone.

3.5 Treatment for sexual difficulties as a component of marital therapy

Gurman and Kniskern (1981) noted that the number of well-controlled studies in the area was low, but that there was significant empirical support for conjoint, behaviourally-oriented therapies for sexual dysfunction; they considered these the 'treatment of choice' for such difficulties, especially when there are no severe non-sexual marital problems.

3.6 Other difficulties which respond well to family therapy

Gurman and Kniskern (1981) reported that structural family therapy (Minuchin, 1974) had thus far received encouraging empirical support for the treatment of child and adolescent anorexia (Minuchin, 1978), asthma (Minuchin and colleagues, 1975) and adult drug addiction (Stanton and Todd, 1978).

3.7 Length of treatment by family or marital therapy

There have been good results from both behavioural and non-behavioural family and marital therapies of relatively short duration. The mean number of sessions in studies reviewed by Gurman and Kniskern, as well as by other researchers, was nine.

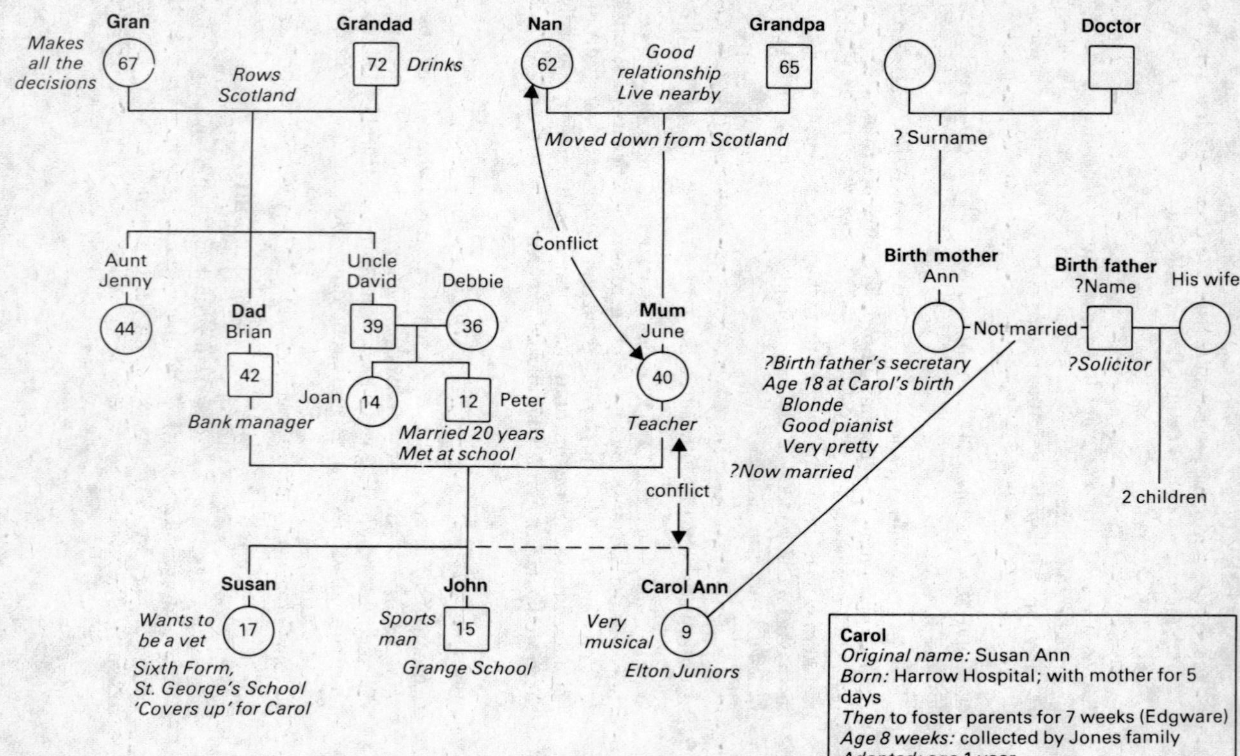

FIGURE 38.1 An example of a geneogram (Finch and Jaques, 1985)

3.8 Other aspects of family therapy requiring investigation

Further studies seem urgently needed in e.g. the following areas:

1 The value of compiling geneograms with families. There is some evidence of their usefulness, particularly in inter-generational work (Lieberman, 1979). Finch and Jaques (1985) have described how therapists can devise them together with families in clarifying relationships and attempting to help with some of the difficulties faced by adopted children and their families. Empirical evidence upon how they may be devised and used most helpfully would be of great value. See Figure 38.1.
2 The value of combining behavioural and non-behavioural approaches within a strategy of helping.
3 The examination of which particular kinds of difficulty within families respond best to which specific models or strategies of intervention.

References

Alexander, J. F. and Parsons, B. (1973), 'Short-term behavioural intervention with delinquent families: impact on family process and recidivism', *Journal of Abnormal Psychology*, vol. 81, pp. 219–25.

Bentovim, A., Gorell Barnes, G. and Cooklin, A. (eds) (1982), *Family Therapy*, New York: Academic Press.

Birchler, G. R. (1979), 'Communication skills in married couples' in S. Bellack and M. Hersen (eds), *Research and Practice in Social Skills Training*, New York: Plenum.

Bowen, M. (1978), *Family Therapy in Clinical Practice*, New York: Jason Aronson.

Crowe, M. J. (1978), 'Conjoint marital therapy: a controlled outcome study', *Psychological Medicine*, vol. 8, pp. 623–36.

Crowe, M. J. (1984), 'The analysis of therapist intervention in three contrasted approaches to conjoint marital therapy' in K. Hahlweg and N. Jacobson (eds), *Marital Interaction*, London: Guilford Press.

Crowe, M. J. (1986), Personal communication.

Emmelkamp, P., Van der Helm, M., Macgillavry, D. and Van Zenten, B. (1984), 'Marital therapy with clinically distressed couples: a comparative evaluation of system-theoretic, contingency contracting and communication skills approaches' in K. Hahlweg and N. Jacobson (eds) (1984), *Marital Interaction*, London: Guilford Press.

Finch, R. and Jaques, P. (1985), 'Use of the geneogram with adoptive families', *Adoption and Fostering*, vol. 9, no. 3, pp. 36–7.

Gurman, A. S. and Kniskern, D. P. (1978), 'Research on marital and family therapy: progress, perspective and prospect' in S. Garfield and A. E. Bergin (eds), *Handbook of Psychotherapy and Behaviour Change*, Chichester: Wiley.

Gurman, A. S. and Kniskern, D. P. (1981), *Handbook of Family Therapy*, New York: Brunner/Mazel.

Hahlweg, K. and Jacobson, N. (1984), *Marital Interaction*, New York: Guilford Press.

Haley, J. (1962), 'Whither family therapy?', *Family Process*, vol. 1, pp. 69–100.
Haley, J. (1976), *Problem Solving Therapy*, San Francisco: Jossey-Bass.
Jacobson, N. S. (1978), 'Problem solving and contingency contracting in the treatment of marital discord', *Journal of Consulting and Clinical Psychology*, vol. 45, pp. 92–100.
Kniskern, D. and Gurman, A. (1981), 'Advances and prospects for family therapy research' in J. P. Vincent (ed.), *Advances in Family Intervention, Assessment and Theory*, vol. 2, Greenwich, Connecticut: Jai Press Inc.
Lieberman, S. (1979), 'Transgenerational analysis: the geneogram as a technique in family therapy', *Journal of Family Therapy*, vol. 1, pp. 51–64.
Minuchin, S. (1974), *Families and Family Therapy*, Cambridge, Mass.: Harvard University Press.
Minuchin, S., Baker, L., Rosman, B., Liebman, R., Milman, L. and Todd, T. (1975), 'A conceptual model of psychosomatic illness in children', *Archives of General Psychiatry*, vol. 32, pp. 1031–8.
Minuchin, S., Rosman, B. and Baker, L. (1978), *Psychosomatic Families*, Cambridge, Mass.: Harvard University Press.
Palazzoli, M. S., Boscolo, L., Cecchin, G. and Prata, G. (1978), *Paradox and Counter-paradox*, New York: Jason Aronson.
Patterson, G. R. (1976), 'Some procedures for assessing changes in marital interaction patterns', *Oregon Research Institute Bulletin*, vol. 16 (7).
Patterson, G. R. and Hops, H. (1972), 'Coercion, a game for two. Intervention techniques for marital conflict' in R. E. Ulrich and P. Mountjoy (eds), *The Experimental Analysis of Social Behaviour*, New York: Appleton.
Skynner, A. R. C. (1976), *Systems of family and marital psychotherapy*, New York: Brunner/Mazel. British edition entitled *One Flesh, Separate Persons*, London: Constable.
Skynner, A. C. R. and Skynner, P. (1978), *Systems, Families and Therapy*. Paper presented at the American Association of Marriage and Family Counsellors meeting, Houston, October 1978.
Stanton, M. D. and Todd, T. C. (1976), 'Structural family therapy with heroin addicts: Some outcome data'. Paper presented at the Society of Psychotherapy Research, San Diego, June 1976.
Stanton, M., Todd, T., Stier, F., Van Deusen, J., Marder, L., Rosoff, R., Seaman, S. and Skibinski, E. (1979), *Family Characteristics and Family Therapy of Heroin Addicts, 1974–1978*. Submitted to the National Institute on Drug Abuse by the Philadelphia Child Guidance Clinic, 1979.
Stuart, R. B. (1980), *Helping Couples Change*, New York: Guilford Press.
Vincent, J. P. (1981), *Advances in Family Intervention, Assessment and Theory*, Greenwich, Connecticut: Jai Press, Inc.
Wells, R. and Dezen, A. E. (1978), 'The results of family therapy revisited: The nonbehavioural methods', *Family Process*, vol. 17, pp. 251–74.
Whitaker, D. A. (1975), 'A family therapist looks at marital therapy' in A. S. Gurman and D. Rice (eds), *Couples in Conflict: New Directions in Marital Therapy*, New York: Jason Aronson.

Research concerning sexual dysfunction and difficulties

***Consultant:* Dr Michael Crowe, Consultant Psychiatrist, The Bethlem Royal Hospital and the Maudsley Hospital, London.**

1 Definition and classification

1.1 One possible definition

Jehu (1979) has suggested, 'Sexual dysfunctions are defined . . . as responses to sexual stimulation that the clients and/or their partners consider to be inadequate.'

1.2 Classification of sexual dysfunctions and difficulties

1 A number of ways of categorizing these have been suggested: one based upon the work of Jehu (1979) is shown in Table 39.1.

Aspect	*Male*	*Female*
Interest or desire	Inadequate sexual interest or desire	Inadequate sexual interest or desire
Arousal or intromission	Erectile dysfunction (impotence)	Vasocongestive dysfunction Vaginismus (involuntary muscular resistance to penetration)
Orgasm or ejaculation	Premature ejaculation Retarded ejaculation Retrograde ejaculation	Orgastic dysfunction
Pleasure	Inadequate sexual pleasure Dyspareunia (pain)	Inadequate sexual pleasure Dyspareunia (pain)

TABLE 39.1 Categories of sexual dysfunction. (After Jehu, 1979)

2 Bancroft (1983), however, noted the dangers of over-simple allocation to categories of dysfunction, and highlighted the need for individualized assessment of difficulties. He noted the importance of

recognizing the 'varied and unique ways in which individuals and couples present with sexual problems'.

2 Prevalence

2.1 Difficulties in obtaining accurate data

Any figures suggested concerning the numbers of those who experience sexual difficulties, or for those who seek help, must be imprecise. There are few studies based on representative samples: some have a bias towards middle-class respondents, such as those attending family planning clinics.

2.2 A Dutch study of a sample of the general population

Bancroft (1983) reported that among the more representative studies in that of Frenken (1976) who sampled 500 married men and women. The analysis of his data revealed two relatively independent factors within the sexual motivation scale: '(a) The ability to enjoy sexual interaction and to become sexually aroused and (b) the ability to experience and be satisfied with orgasm.'

Concerning (a), Bancroft summarized, '26% of men and 43% of women indicated problems with enjoyment and arousal and a further 9% of women expressed actual aversion.'

Concerning (b), he summarized, '12% of men and 33% of women indicated difficulty or dissatisfaction with orgasm with a further 5% of women being anorgasmic.'

3 Origins of sexual dysfunction and difficulties

3.1 Biological factors

1 Physical and medical conditions

1. Kaplan (1974) reported that as many as 10 per cent of those seeking help in her sample had medical disorders or other contributory physical conditions; different workers have suggested a figure of 20 per cent. Such conditions are particularly associated with impotence and dispareunia, and can include early diabetes, neurological disorders and genital irregularities. Variables such as the effects of medication, illness (physical or psychiatric), alcohol and drugs can also be important.
2. Kaplan pointed out that mild medical conditions may interact with psychological ones, such as anxiety, to produce a dysfunction which neither alone would have caused. She also noted the effects of stress and/or depression upon the sexual response, and the importance of recognizing and treating these conditions first.

2 **The effects of ageing**

1 Kaplan reported that both Kinsey et al. (1948) and Masters and Johnson (1970) found evidence that:

> Men experience the peak of sexual responsiveness and capacity around the ages of 17 and 18 and thereafter show a steady decline. Women, on the other hand, attain their sexual peak in the late thirties and early forties and thereafter decline at a slower rate than men.

2 Masters and Johnson (1970) noted that men in later life take longer to establish erection, and need more physical stimulation for this.
3 Most researchers stress, however, that sexual responsiveness at any age is highly individual and variable, and depends on a multiplicity of factors.

3.2 Psychological factors

The need for a multi-variate model.

Kaplan (1974) suggested that while there are many psychological theories of sexual dysfunction, including the psychoanalytic and the behavioural, a single model is inappropriate. She concluded,

> A more satisfying alternative is a synthesis which conceptualises the etiology of sexual dysfunction as being due to both remote and immediate causes. These two sets of causes operate on different levels, but they are not incompatible.

She also described trust and openness as 'indispensable pre-requisites' of full sexual experience.

3.3 Specific sources of difficulty

Kaplan suggested that these include:

1 **Not engaging in effective sexual behaviour** This often stems from genuine ignorance of male and female sexual anatomy and of the activities which may be helpful in promoting sexual responsiveness.

2 **Fear of failure** This is an extremely common condition, especially in men. Anticipatory anxiety, leading to difficulties in performance, can produce a vicious circle which is both very distressing, and a challenging situation in which to intervene.

3 **Defences against erotic feelings** There are many reasons why people do not become sexually aroused: these include lack of trust, self-critical feelings and perfectionism concerning standards expected of the relationship.

4 **Difficulties in communicating sexual needs to the partner** There may be an absence of information and feedback concerning sexual needs and wishes; this absence can, of itself, interrupt and undermine an otherwise satisfying relationship.

3.4 Further issues

1 **The learned nature of many sexual difficulties** Many sexual difficulties can be understood as having been learned according to principles of social learning theory, via patterns of conditioning and socialization. It is thus often possible to employ these same principles of social learning theory to decondition anxiety and to enable people to learn other responses.

2 **The potential for dominance contests between partners** Several writers have noted this problem. It seems that such contests may be fairly frequent, and may lead to some sexual difficulties. As views and social customs about 'appropriate' relationships between men and women change, the prevalence of these contests may increase or decrease.

4 Research on ways of helping people with sexual difficulties

4.1 Helping with sexual difficulties when there are no severe non-sexual problems

1 Gurman and Kniskern (1981) noted that the number of well-controlled studies in this field is low, but that nevertheless there is considerable consensus upon the empirical evidence: namely, the value of conjoint, behaviourally-oriented treatment, associated with counselling support and information-giving.
2 Gurman and Kniskern (1981) and Bancroft (1983) appear to see such approaches as the 'treatment of choice', particularly when there are no severe non-sexual marital difficulties.

4.2 Outcome studies of treating male and female dysfunctions

Researchers such as Jehu (1979) and Bancroft (1983) have summarized the following studies:

1 **The classic study by Masters and Johnson (1970)**

1 This drew upon principles of relaxation, the reduction of anxiety and the gradual building of a repertoire of mutually helpful sexual behaviours, and was conducted from 1959 to 1969. The effectiveness of treatment, with 448 men and 342 women, was evaluated both at the end of treatment and at a five-year follow-up.
2 Findings indicated that 18 per cent of cases showed no response to treatment. The remaining 82 per cent showed varying degrees of success,

and 74.5 per cent showed improvement at the five-year follow-up. No significant differences were found between males and females at either evaluation.

3 Jehu (1979), however, noted the weaknesses of this study:
  (a) The lack of a control group
  (b) The imprecise statement of the criteria by which 'success' was judged.
  (c) Selection bias of the authors.
  (d) Giving treatment in a 'hotel fortnight' rather than in a home setting.

2 Some additional studies

1 Obler (1973) compared three forms of intervention:
  (a) Desensitization therapy, with e.g. confidence training.
  (b) Psychodynamically-based group therapy.
  (c) A no-treatment, control condition.

  The results, on physiological, behavioural and cognitive measures, were consistent in showing the first approach as the most helpful.

2 Matthews and colleagues (1976), working within the National Health Service, examined the contributions of several variables to ways of helping people. Thirty-six couples participated, in three parallel treatment groups, each with a different combination of components:
  (a) Systematic desensitization, plus counselling.
  (b) Directed practice, plus counselling: (this was adapted from the Masters and Johnson approach).
  (c) Directed practice group, with minimal counselling.

  Results indicated trends favouring the second approach.

3 Outcome studies concerning male dysfunction

(a) *Treatment for erection difficulties* Treatment by the Masters and Johnson approach, involving teaching relaxation and anxiety management, was found by three sets of researchers, Masters and Johnson themselves (1970), Kockott (1975) and Ansari (1976), to lead to success rates of 66 per cent, 66 per cent and 67 per cent respectively. The success achieved by Masters and Johnson was generally maintained at five-year follow-up, but had dropped to 33 per cent among participants in the Ansari study.

(b) *Treatment for premature ejaculation* Studies in this area offer encouraging results: Masters and Johnson (1970) and Yulis (1976) report success rates of 97 per cent and 89 per cent respectively.

4 Outcome studies concerning female dysfunctions

(a) *Treatment for vaginismus* Studies here have all reported relatively high success rates after treatment. Masters and Johnson (1970) reported 100 per cent success, and while this level is unusual, other researchers have reported encouragingly high success rates.

(b) *Treatment for difficulties in reaching climax* Studies by, e.g., Wallace and Barbach (1974), are typical of the encouraging work being conducted, while Riley and Riley (1978) have reported the usefulness of the vibrator as an aid in enabling women to reach orgasm.

5 Other aspects of helping to resolve sexual difficulties

5.1 The increasing consensus upon common features of helping

Many researchers, e.g. Jehu (1979) and Bancroft (1983), seem to agree that valuable helping features include:

1 The building of a trusting relationship between the therapist and the persons being helped.
2 Careful assessment of the difficulties being experienced, and of other contributory factors.
3 A carefully planned intervention, involving explaining fully the whole approach to the person being helped.

Each of these will be considered separately below.

1 Building a trusting relationship between therapist and those being helped

1 Mathews and colleagues (1976), (see 4.2, page 373) found this an essential accompaniment to directed practice. Many therapists who now use the Masters and Johnson approach accept the necessity of offering a trustful counselling relationship as well.
2 Researchers agree that features of this relationship include:
   (a) The conveying of respect and empathy for those seeking help.
   (b) The opportunity to speak of subjects seldom discussed in an open and unembarrassed way.
   (c) The opportunity to acknowledge aspects of the couple's relationship which may be contributing to sexual difficulties.
   (d) The giving of accurate information concerning sexual anatomy and behaviour.
   (e) Opportunities to discuss fears e.g. about 'normality'.
   (f) The consideration of moral or religious implications which people may wish to discuss.

2 Careful assessment of the difficulties being experienced

1 Bancroft (1983) suggested that the therapist, who needs specialized training, should consider the following topics, and how they affect each person:
   1 The precise nature of the sexual problem.
   2 The history of the sexual problem.
   3 The nature of the general relationship . . . and other details of the immediate family and children.
   4 Psychiatric history: the recognition of depression is important.

5 Medical history.
6 Contraceptive history.
7 Menstrual history.
8 Atttitudes to the sexual problem and possible treatment.

2 Crowe (1986) has noted the particular importance of medical assessment of any organic factors: e.g. diabetes or neurological disorders in impotence, endocrine disorders in lack of sex drive, pelvic disease in dyspareunia and general psychiatric and relationship factors.

3 Jehu (1979) suggested that essential components of the assessment include the following:

(a) Identifying and specifying difficulties This is likely to include gathering very precise information on the difficulties being experienced, their nature, timing, frequency, duration, onset and history.

(b) Noting the circumstances of the difficulties Clarifying any particular circumstances which affect the relationship. These may include:

(a) understanding of sexual responses
(b) levels of anxiety experienced
(c) other difficulties within the relationship
(d) the impact of patterns of upbringing
(e) the impact of possible traumatic events
(f) levels of communication between the couple
(g) opportunities for privacy at home

(c) Clarifying the implications of offering help This will include consideration of the motivation of the partners to involve themselves in the necessary activities.

3 **A carefully planned treatment intervention** Jehu (1979) and Bancroft (1983) seem to agree that essential features include:

(1) Selecting and specifying goals Jehu suggests that 'these should be chosen largely by the client and his or her partner in accordance with their own wishes and values, although in consultation with the therapist.' The greater the clarity, the simplicity and the attainability of goals, the better; in this way success leads to success.

(2) Planning a suitable programme Jehu and others have suggested that some specific procedures which may be helpful include:

(a) Relaxation training.
(b) Anxiety management training. (See Chapter 32, page 305)
(c) Individualized treatment programmes drawing e.g. on principles from social learning theory.
(d) Assertion training.
(e) Fantasy training.

(f) Planning 'homework': graduated practice.
(g) Enabling people to gain success in simple assignments, in the knowledge that this will motivate them further.

(3) Monitoring the intervention Jehu (1979) has noted,

> Having planned a programme of treatment, its progress and outcome are systematically monitored and evaluated on a continuous basis throughout implementation and follow-up periods. This provides feedback to the client on . . . progress and reveals any necessity for a revision of the treatment plan.

References

Ansari, J. M. A. (1976), 'Impotence: Prognosis, A controlled study', *British Journal of Psychiatry*, vol. 128, pp. 194–8.

Bancroft, J. (1983), *Human Sexuality and its Problems*, Edinburgh: Churchill Livingstone.

Crowe, M. (1986), Personal communication.

Frenken, J. (1976), *Afkeer van seksualiteit*. Van Loghum Slaterus Deventer. (English summary: pp. 219–25)

Gurman, A. and Kniskern, D. (1981), *Handbook of Family Therapy*, Brunner Mazel.

Jehu, D. (1979), *Sexual Dysfunction: A Behavioural Approach*, Chichester: Wiley.

Kaplan, H. S. (1974), *The New Sex Therapy: Active Treatment of Sexual Dysfunctions*, London: Bailliere Tindall.

Kinsey, A. C., Pomeroy, W. R. and Martin, C. E. (1948), *Sexual Behaviour in the Human Male*, London and Philadelphia: Saunders.

Masters, W. H. and Johnson, V. E. (1970), *Human Sexual Inadequacy*, Boston: Little, Brown & Co.

Mathews, A., Bancroft, J., Whitehead, A., Hackmann, A., Julier, D., Bancroft, J., Gath, D. and Shaw, P. (1976), 'The behavioural treatment of sexual inadequacy: a comparative study', *Behaviour Research and Therapy*, vol. 14, pp. 427–36.

Obler, M. (1973), 'Systematic desensitization in sexual disorders', *Journal of Behaviour Therapy and Experimental Psychiatry*, vol. 4, pp. 93–101.

Riley, A. J. and Riley, E. J. (1978), 'A controlled study to evaluate directed masturbation in the management of primary orgasmic failure in women', *British Journal of Psychiatry*, vol. 133, pp. 404–9.

Wallace, D. H. and Barbach, L. G. (1974), 'Preorgasmic group treatment', *Journal of Sex and Marital Therapy*, vol. 1, pp. 146–54.

Yulis, S. (1976), 'Generalization of therapeutic gain in the treatment of premature ejaculation', *Behaviour Therapy*, vol. 7, pp. 355–8.

Research concerning homosexuality

40

***Consultant:* Professor D. J. West, Professor of Clinical Criminology, University of Cambridge, Cambridge.**

1 Definitions

1.1 A general definition

The condition of being sexually and emotionally attracted by a person of one's own sex.

'Homosexuality' refers to both male and female sexes having a relationship with someone of their own sex.

1.2 A psychiatric definition

(according to the Mental Disorders Section of the International Classification of Diseases of the World Health Organisation, 9th edition).

302.0 *Homosexuality*: Exclusive or predominant sexual attraction for persons of the same sex with or without physical relationship.

N.B. The American Psychiatric Association, however, in 1973 deleted homosexuality from the list of mental disorders, and replaced it with a new category of 'sexual orientation disturbance', described as follows:

> This category is for individuals whose sexual interests are directed primarily toward people of the same sex and who are either disturbed by, in conflict with, or wish to change their sexual orientation. This diagnostic category is distinguished from homosexuality, which by itself does not necessarily constitute a psychiatric disorder. Homosexuality per se is one form of sexual behaviour and, like other forms of sexual behaviour which are not by themselves psychiatric disorders, is not listed in this nomenclature of mental disorders.

2 Prevalence

While the secrecy which is still associated with homosexuality and lesbianism makes the gathering of precise data difficult, some indicators are available. West (1977) has drawn attention to the following sources of information.

2.1 The Kinsey reports (1948 and 1953)

1 Concerning males, Kinsey (1948) reported,

> 37% of the total male population has at least some overt homosexual experience to the point of orgasm between adolescence and old age;
>
> 8% of the males are exclusively homosexual for at least three years between 16 and 55;
>
> 4% of white males are exclusively homosexual throughout their lives after the onset of adolescence.

2 Concerning females, Kinsey (1953) reported that by the age of forty-five, 13 per cent of women in his sample had had overt lesbian contacts leading to orgasm, although double that number had had erotic experiences with other women. West (1977) quoted Kinsey (1953),

> contacts which had proceeded to orgasm has occurred in about a third as many females as males. Moreover, compared with the males, there were only a half to a third of the females who were, in any age period, primarily or exclusively homosexual.

2.2 Cross-cultural evidence

West (1977) reported the review by Ford and Beach (1952) who drew upon the Yale Cross-Cultural Survey, and analysed the relevant information from 200 societies. Among the seventy-six societies for which data concerning homosexuality was available, forty-nine allowed some form of homosexual behaviour for some members of the community; the other twenty-seven discouraged it, sometimes gently, sometimes with severe punishment.

3 Research concerning the causation of homosexuality

3.1 Research into gender identity and sexual preference

West (1983) has written,

> In the ordinary course of events gender identity is established in infancy, sexual preferences becoming manifest later. Homosexual preferences arise with particular frequency where there has been difficulty or discontent in childhood with gender identity or gender role, but among the vast majority of individuals with no such problems homosexual preferences still occur quite often. The important determining factors of a homosexual orientation or of homosexual interests almost certainly vary from one person to another.

West (1983) went on to suggest a number of variables as possible contributors to the development of a homosexual or lesbian orientation. These include:

1 **A possible genetic contribution** West (1977) considered that the evidence *may* indicate the involvement of genetic factors, though he views the evidence that there is a direct genetic link to be dubious. In 1983 he concluded, 'Genetic factors may be important, especially where a primary, exclusive orientation is concerned.' Recent research, (Gladue and colleagues, 1984) suggests that foetal hormonal disturbance, resulting in anomalous sex differentiation of the brain, may be an important factor.

2 **The contribution of variables from social learning theory** Of these, West (1983) has written: 'Cross-cultural observations (Carrier, 1980) point to the enormous influence of culture in determining the social implications of homosexual behaviour and in influencing its incidence and manifestations.' There appears to be little evidence of any *simple* acquisition of a homosexual orientation, e.g. by means of conditioning (Bell, 1981). Other researchers, however, have drawn attention to the relevance of other concepts implicit within social learning theory; thus Stoller (1968) has highlighted the non-availability in some instances of clear sex-role models for some children, and the well-documented instances of children deliberately being brought up as members of the opposite sex.

3 **The contribution of variables from psychoanalytic theory** West (1983) commented that psychoanalysts have emphasized their view that the families of some male homosexuals are characterized by the presence of a dominant mother and an unsatisfactory father figure. He commented that evidence for the influence of this particular pattern of relationships in the generality of male homosexuals is uncertain. (West, 1977).

3.2 An American study of variables affecting sexual preference

An extensive survey with about 1,500 homosexual men and women living in the San Francisco Bay area reported by Bell, Weinberg and Hammersmith (1981) examined associations between particular variables and adult sexual preference. Atkinson, Atkinson and Hilgard (1983) have summarized these:

1 By the time both the boys and the girls reached adolescence, their sexual preference was likely to be determined, even though they might not yet have become very active sexually.
2 Among the respondents, homosexuality was indicated or reinforced by sexual feelings that typically occurred three years or so before their first 'advanced' homosexual activity.
3 The homosexual men and women in the study were not particularly lacking in heterosexual experiences during their childhood and adolescent years.
4 Among both men and women in the study, there was a powerful link between gender nonconformity as a child and the development of homosexuality.
5 The respondents' identification with their opposite-sex parents while

growing up appeared to have no significant impact on whether they turned out to be homosexual or heterosexual.

6 For both the men and the women in the study, poor relationships with fathers seemed to play a more important role in predisposing them to homosexuality than the quality of their relationships with their mothers.
7 Insofar as differences can be identified between male and female psychosexual development, gender non-conformity appeared to be somewhat more important for males and family relationships appeared to be more important for females in the development of sexual preference.

3.3 An overview of research and theories of the causation of homosexuality

West (1977) suggested that on the available evidence, homosexuality has multiple roots. He concluded,

> Homosexuality, like any other pattern of human behaviour, is the outcome of a complex interaction between individual needs and dispositions on the one hand, and environmental pressures, constraints and opportunities on the other. No single causal explanation will ever suffice. Moreover, the key influences need not be the same in every case; different people may reach a similar sexual orientation by very different routes. Generalisations for many cases will not apply to all.

It is thus apparent that, as in so many situations referred to in this book, homosexuality has to be understood as a circumstance which is multi-factorial.

4 Research concerning change of sexual orientation

4.1 Research into spontaneous change of orientation

1 The study referred to above, Kinsey (1948), found that a considerable and spontaneous shift in sexual orientation occurred as young males matured: whereas at age twenty, only 80 per cent of males were predominantly heterosexual, by age forty-five this figure had risen to 93 per cent.
2 West (1977) reported that spontaneous reversals of sexual orientation, even among long established homosexuals, both can and do occur (e.g. Aaron, 1972), and West went on to point out the importance therefore of avoiding dismissing the possibility of change to someone who is actively seeking help in changing his or her orientation.

4.2 The effectiveness of therapy

West (1977) commented that systematic studies of people undergoing psychological therapy for a homosexual orientation, with assessment before treatment and evaluation afterwards, are rare. He added that, in general, the more careful the assessment, the more modest the claim of effectiveness.

1 **Psychotherapy** Curran and Parr (1957), when examining the outcome for 100 men who received psychotherapy, compared twenty-five of these with a matched control group of twenty-five homosexuals treated in other ways. Follow-up at four years indicated that the group who had received psychotherapy more often reported having come to terms with their situation, but they showed no greater change towards heterosexuality than did the control group.

2 **Behaviour therapy** A review by Bancroft (1974) of the many studies which draw upon principles of social learning theory, such as desensitization and behavioural rehearsal, in treating homosexuals who sought treatment, found that about a third showed evidence of sustained heterosexual adaptation.

4.2 An overview of the evidence concerning change of sexual orientation

1 West (1977) has concluded that while there is some evidence of the usefulness of some forms of treatment to some people seeking help, no one treatment or combination of treatments seems superior to others, so a therapist can probably best help by choosing approaches that seems most suited to the individual.
2 He has also indicated that the motivation of the individual person seeking help to change his or her orientation is crucial; and while avenues of help are available, it may be the wisest course to try to help troubled people to accept their homosexuality, rather than give ill-founded advice which may lead to severe disappointment. Marriages entered into by persons with strong homosexual urges frequently break down. (Ross, 1983).

References

Aaron, W. (1972), *Straight: A Heterosexual Talks about his Homosexual Past*, New York: Doubleday.

Atkinson, R. L., Atkinson, R. C. and Hilgard, E. R. (1983), *Introduction to Psychology*, 8th edition, New York: Harcourt Brace Jovanovich, Inc.

Bancroft, J. (1974), *Deviant Sexual Behaviour: Modification and Assessment*, Oxford: Clarendon Press.

Bell, A. P., Weinberg, M. S. and Hammersmith, S. K. (1981), *Sexual preference: Its development in Men and Women*, Bloomington, Indiana: Indiana University Press.

Carrier, J. M. (1980), 'Homosexual behaviour in cross-cultural perspective' in J. Marmor (ed.), *Homosexual Behaviour*, New York: Basic Books.

Curran, D. and Parr, D. (1957), 'Homosexuality: an analysis of 100 male cases', *British Medical Journal*, (i) pp. 798–801.

Ford, C. S. and Beach, F. A. (1952), *Patterns of Sexual Behaviour*, London: Eyre & Spottiswoode.
Gladue, B. A., Green, R. and Hellman, R. E. (1984), 'Neuro-endocrine response to estrogen and sexual orientation', *Science*, vol. 225, pp. 1496–9.
Kinsey, A. C., Pomeroy, W. B. and Martin, C. E. (1948), *Sexual Behaviour in the Human Male*, London and Philadelphia: Saunders.
Kinsey, A. C., Pomeroy, W. B., Martin, C. E. and Gebhard, P. H. (1953), *Sexual Behaviour in the Human Female*, London and Philadelphia: Saunders.
Norris, S. and Read, E. (1985) *Out in the Open*, London: Pan Books.
Ross, M. W. (1983), *The Married Homosexual Man*, London: Routledge & Kegan Paul.
Stoller, R. J. (1968), *Sex and Gender*, New York: Science Books.
West, D. J. (1977), *Homosexuality Re-examined*, London: Duckworth.
West, D. J. (1983), 'Homosexuality and lesbianism', *British Journal of Psychiatry*, vol. 143, pp. 221–6.
World Health Organisation (1980), *Glossary of Mental Disorders and Guide to their Classification*, Geneva: WHO.

41 Research concerning people wanting to control their violence or anger

Consultant: Dr Kevin Howells, Senior Lecturer in Clinical Psychology, Department of Psychology, University of Birmingham.

This chapter draws substantially upon the chapter 'Social relationships in violent offenders' by Kevin Howells, in S. Duck and R. Gilmour (eds), *Personal Relationships 3: Personal Relationships in Disorder*, published in 1981 by Academic Press.

1 Some relevant definitions

1.1 Legal definitions

Relevant legal definitions are those concerning 'assault' and 'battery'; Smith and Hogan (1983) give the criminal law definitions:

Assault: An assault is any act by which one person, intentionally or recklessly, causes another person to apprehend immediate and unlawful personal violence.

Battery: A battery is an act by which one person, intentionally or recklessly, inflicts unlawful personal violence upon another person.

N.B. Most violence, however, is probably not labelled as criminal.

1.2 A psychiatric perspective

1 **The notion of people having 'personality problems' or 'life difficulties'** Egdell (1980) has suggested that terms such as 'personality disorder', 'psychopathic personality' and 'sociopathic personality' should be confined to clear-cut, multiple, long-standing features which have been independently confirmed. He himself recommends the notion that people have 'personality problems', or 'life difficulties' – thus avoiding stigmatization. Such people are often characterized by:

1 Problems at school, work, with the police or in marriage
2 Rage or fighting
3 Prostitution
4 Vagrancy
5 Running away from home
6 Persistent lying

2 **Further characteristics of people with personality problems** Egdell (1980) has written: 'Such patients also show irresponsibility (often associated with plausibility), lack of concern for others, inability to profit from past experience and an inability to form and maintain close warm relationships.'

2 Statistics

There is no reliable means of gathering information concerning the extent of violence against others, but one indicator is the number of convictions recorded for relevant offences. See Table 41.1.

2.1 Official statistics: selected data

Offenders of all ages found guilty	1982	1983	1984	1985
Indictable offences				
Violence against the person				
Murder	0.1	0.1	0.2	0.2
Manslaughter	0.2	0.2	0.2	0.3
Wounding	49.6	49.5	45.8	45.3
Other offences of violence	1.7	1.6	1.6	1.7

continued overleaf

Summary offences				
Assaults	11.1	10.7	11.4	10.5

TABLE 41.1 Offenders found guilty: by offence group. Magistrates' courts and the Crown Court. England and Wales. Thousands. (*Annual Abstract of Statistics*, 1987)

3 Research into the origins of violent behaviour

Howells (1981) highlighted the fact that studies of violent behaviour have been conducted primarily with violent offenders – a very unrepresentative group. He also acknowledged the difficulty of defining 'aggression' and 'violence' without making value judgments. He went on to summarize several areas of research:

3.1 Investigations into the nature and circumstances of violent offending

The evidence points to the following tentative conclusions:

1 **Serious violence occurs often in intimate relationships** There are consistent findings in both the UK and the USA that much violence occurs within an established relationship. Home Office studies (1961, 1975) show that nearly 60 per cent of adult female victims of murder are the wife or girlfriend of the aggressor: less than 20 per cent of adult male and female victims are killed by strangers. Howells noted:

> Typically the violence follows from an argument or disagreement between the participants. Family quarrels, petty jealousies and disputes are more frequent precipitants of violent incidents than are financial or sexual acquisitiveness.

2 **Not all violent offenders are habitually violence prone** Howells quoted McClintock (1963) who found that 80 per cent of convicted violent offenders had no history of violent offences – although half had previous convictions for non-violent offences. He also quoted the 1975 Home Office study of homicide, which found that only about 26 per cent of offenders had previous convictions for violent offences. On the basis of these and other studies, Howells concluded: 'The evidence does suggest that explanations are not best sought in terms of internal, individual factors, but perhaps by reference to interpersonal and relational factors.'

3.2 Some investigations concerning violent offenders

1 **Aggressors as over-controlled or under-controlled**

   1 Howells (1981) reported the formulation of Megargee (1966) who, noting that a number of violent offenders were 'meek, mild-mannered, deferential persons', distinguished the following groups:

(a) *Over-controlled aggressors*: highly inhibited individuals, whose control is overcome only by extreme levels of provocation.
(b) *Under-controlled aggressors*: individuals with low levels of inhibition, whose control is readily overcome with low levels of provocation.

2 Howells's own work (1981), using repertory grid techniques with violent offenders in a Special Hospital in the UK, found limited support for the above formulation.

2 Social interaction styles of violent offenders

1 Howells (1981) highlighted the contribution of Toch and his analysis of the sequence of interactions leading to violent social incidents. In his book, *Violent Men*, Toch (1969) analysed in fine detail the escalation of reciprocal provocation between a policeman and someone whom the latter wanted to interview.

2 Toch proposed a series of 'modes of approach to the relationship', which might make violent outcomes more likely. (The groups being studied by Toch were violent offenders, but the formulation could probably be extended to any population.)
(a) The '*self-image promoters*', who value 'toughness and masculine status' and seek confirmation of this image by provoking violence. Demeaning insults and threats to masculinity in group contexts are likely to be the precipitating stimuli.
(b) The '*social skills deficient*' *aggressors*, who use aggression because they do not have the command of language or the confidence to enable them to deal more strategically with a situation.
(c) The '*self-defenders*', who are forever detecting threat, and who use violence in a bid to be the first to eliminate the opposition.

3 Howells (1981) commented that the above categories need testing empirically, and he considered that the contribution of non-verbal variables, as indicators e.g. of threat, may be under-estimated by Toch.

3.3 Studies concerning appropriate assertion training

A number of studies have drawn on the findings from social skills training in order to use relevant findings to help people manage violent behaviour. Howells quoted the work of Ivey (1973), and wrote: 'Sessions involved video-taping typical social interactions and identifying behaviours that created the impression of hostility – in this case, rate of speech and tone.'

3.4 Studies concerning the readiness to perceive threat

1 Howells (1981) highlighted the importance of noting 'cognitive variables' – of how people perceive and 'construct reality' – when seeking to understand violent behaviour. Dyck and Rule (1978) found a readiness on the part of some offenders to attribute aggressive intent

towards themselves more readily than did a control group, and Howells noted: 'A person who is repetitively aggressive may inadvertently organize other people to be hostile towards him, making his hostile attributions realistic.'

2 Howells summarized this research field by suggesting that: 'any therapeutic programme should include efforts to encourage the violent person's cognitive re-structuring of social events and his relationships with other people.'

3 He sees the work of Novaco (1977a and 1977b) as very encouraging, and considers the 'stress inoculation' approach as particularly important. This will be considered later in this chapter.

3.5 A psychological formulation of anger

In the light of the above studies, Howells (1981) considered that the formulation of anger arousal offered by Novaco (1978) is the most helpful. Howells wrote: 'Anger is viewed as a combination of physiological arousal and a cognitive labeling of that arousal as a function of internal and external cues and one's overt and covert behaviour in the situation'. This somewhat unusual formulation may be clarified by Figure 41.1, devised by Novaco (1978). It will be noted that this is a multi-factorial formulation.

4 Research on helping people to control their violence or anger

4.1 Ethical issues

1 Howells reported that there is encouraging evidence that people *can* be taught to manage their inclination to violent behaviour. It is, however, vital to take into account '. . . the relationships that form the context of the violent acts and . . . the violent person's view of relationships and other people.'

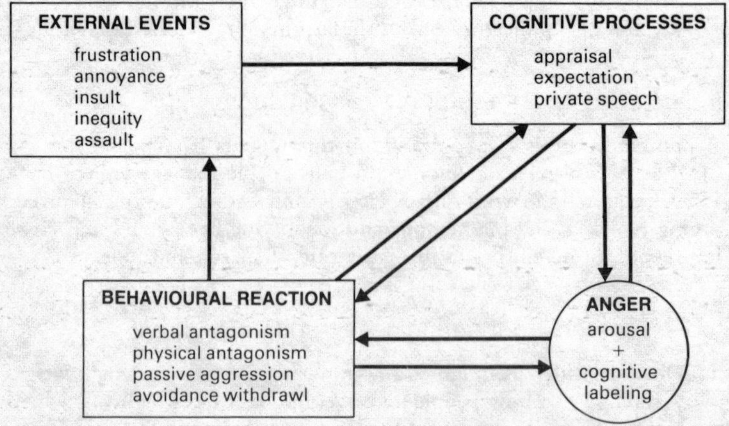

FIGURE 41.1 Determinants of anger arousal (Novaco, 1978)

2 Howells fully accepts that in some instances violent behaviour will be seen by the perpetrators as a 'legitimate and even necessary, form of action' and suggested:

> It is inappropriate, and perhaps unethical, to attempt psychological intervention in such cases. There will also be, on the other hand, very many people who, in a manner which they only dimly understand and feel incapable of controlling, find themselves precipitated into unforeseen and personally unacceptable violence against wives, children, acquaintances and strangers briefly met. The latter group might be a legitimate target for the interventions described.

4.2 Principles of management in the psychiatric context

Egdell (1980) emphasized the importance of:

1 Realistic expectations: violent and impulsive people do not readily form the close and reliable relationships which ideally underpin therapeutic endeavour.
2 Establishing clear goals for work together. Egdell noted 'Priorities set by the patient, such as finance, housing, or police problems, may need to be dealt with as a first step.'
3 Pinpointing triggers to violence; e.g. real or imagined criticism, brooding on the past or current frustrations.
4 Working on impulsiveness as a source of difficulties. Egdell is in sympathy with Howells's idea of supporting the person's view that he *can* control his behaviour, and helping him rehearse doing so.

4.3 'Stress inoculation' and anger management approaches

1 **Some early research** The groundwork of this approach was laid down by Meichenbaum and Cameron (1973); Meichenbaum (1975a) drew attention to 'self-instructions' as a key variable. For example, people seeking to control anger can be taught to say to themselves (as one of a number of strategies), 'Keep calm; don't lose your temper; remember just to ignore him.'

2 **A three stage model** This model, developed by Novaco (1975), has close links with the above: it contains:

(a) *The stage of cognitive preparation* Here those seeking help are taught to recognize their personal anger patterns and violence-provoking situations; e.g. by means of a diary to provide a data base.
(b) *The stage of skill acquisition* Here these personal patterns and habits are re-examined. Trainees are asked to reconsider their tendencies to perceive threat and to develop other ways of reacting to situations: e.g. 'If he wants to get me wound up, he's going to be disappointed.' Trainees are taught to focus upon what they want as an *outcome* of an interaction, and on how to cope in order to achieve this. Trainees

are also taught relaxation skills, to counter-condition tension in difficult situations.

(c) *Application practice* Here participants are taught by role-play, to cope with situations which might be triggers to violence. Competence in dealing with provocative events is developed from the easiest to the most difficult. The range of strategies taught includes relaxation, self-instruction and self appreciation.

3 **A test of this approach** Novaco (1978) conducted a study in which thirty-four people seeking help were allocated to one of four possible forms of training. These were found, by self-report, physiological and other measures to be effective in the following order:

(a) Combined cognitive and relaxation training.
(b) Cognitive training alone.
(c) Relaxation training alone.
(d) Simple trainer attention.

4 **The need for further research** Howells noted the encouraging beginnings, but stresses the need for large-scale, well-controlled studies, with long-term follow up.

References

Duck, S. and Gilmour, R. (eds) (1981), *Personal Relationships. 3: Personal Relationships in Disorder*, London: Academic Press.

Dyck, R. J. and Rule, B. G. (1978), 'Effect on retaliation of causal attributions concerning attack', *Journal of Personality and Social Psychology*, vol. 36, pp. 521–9.

Egdell, H. (1980), 'Problem personalities – recognition and management', *Medicine*, vol. 35, pp. 1789–93.

Foreyt, J. P. and Rathjen, D. P. (eds) (1978), *Cognitive Behaviour Therapy: Research and Application*, New York and London: Plenum Press.

Goldfried, M. (1971), 'Systematic desensitisation as training in self control', *Journal of Consulting and Clinical Psychology*, vol. 37, pp. 228–35.

Home Office (1961), *Murder*, London: HMSO.

Home Office (1975), *Homicide in England and Wales, 1967–1971*, London: HMSO.

Howells, K. (1976), 'Interpersonal aggression', *International Journal of Criminology and Penology*, vol. 4, pp. 319–30.

Howells, K. (1978), 'The meaning of poisoning to a person diagnosed as a psychopath', *Medicine, Science and the Law*, vol. 8, pp. 178–84.

Howells, K. (1981), 'Social construing and violent behaviour in mentally abnormal offenders' in J. Hinton (ed.), *Dangerousness: Problems of Assessment and Prediction*, London: Allen & Unwin.

Howells, K. (1981), 'Social relationships in violent offenders' in S. Duck and R. Gilmour (eds), *Personal Relationships. 3: Personal Relationships in Disorder*.

Ivey, A. E. (1973), 'Media therapy: educational change planning for psychiatric patients', *Journal of Consulting Psychology*, vol. 20, pp. 338–43.

Lazarus, R. (1966), *Psychological Stress and the Coping Process*, New York: McGraw-Hill.

McClintock, F. H. (1963), *Crimes of Violence*, London: Macmillan.

Megargee, E. I. (1966), 'Undercontrolled and overcontrolled personality types in extreme antisocial aggression', *Psychological Monographs*, vol. 80, no. 116.

Meichenbaum, D. (1975a), 'Self instructional methods' in F. H. Kanfer and A. F. Goldstein (eds), *Helping People Change*, New York: Pergamon Press.

Meichenbaum, D. (1975b), 'A self-instructional approach to stress management: A proposal for stress inoculation training' in Spielberger, C. and Sarason, I. (eds), *Stress and Anxiety*, vol. 2, New York: Wiley.

Meichenbaum, D. and Cameron, R. (1973), *Stress inoculation: a skills training approach to anxiety management*, Unpublished manuscript, University of Waterloo, Ontario: Canada.

Novaco, R. W. (1975), *Anger Control: the Development and Evaluation of an Experimental Treatment*, Lexington, Mass.: D. C. Heath.

Novaco, R. W. (1977a), 'Stress inoculation: A cognitive therapy for anger and its application to a case of depression', *Journal of Consulting and Clinical Psychology*, vol. 45, pp. 600–8.

Novaco, R. W. (1977b), 'A stress inoculation approach to anger management in the training of law enforcement officers', *American Journal of Community Psychology*, vol. 5, pp. 327–46.

Novaco, R. W. (1978), 'Anger and coping with stress' in J. P. Foreyt and D. Rathjen (eds), *Cognitive Behaviour Therapy: Research and Application*.

Rimm, D. C., Hill, G., Brown, N. N. and Stuart, J. (1974), 'Group assertive training in treatment of expression of inappropriate anger', *Psychological Reports*, vol. 34, pp. 791–8.

Smith, J. C. and Hogan, B. (1983), *Criminal Law*, London: Butterworth.

Toch, H. (1979), *Violent Men*, Chicago: Aldine Publishing Co.

42 Research concerning the use and misuse of alcohol

Consultant: Dr Douglas Cameron, Consultant Psychiatrist, Leicestershire Community Alcohol and Drugs Services.

1 Definitions

There are major difficulties in establishing definitions and criteria for alcohol-misuse and associated disorders. There is no agreement upon what constitutes such a disorder, nor upon whether the 'alcohol-dependence syndrome' exists. The only responsible course seems to be to report a number of different definitions and formulations.

1.1 A tight formulation

The *International Classification of Diseases* 9 of the World Health Organisation includes:

> 303 *Alcohol dependence syndrome*
>
> A state, psychic and usually also physical, resulting from taking alcohol, characterised by behavioural and other responses that always include a compulsion to take alcohol on a continuous or periodic basis. . . .

1.2 A loose formulation: 'alcohol use giving rise to problems'

Many researchers, e.g. Cameron (1985), recognizing that the use of alcohol occurs in a wide range of social contexts, and encounters differing social sanctions, advocate a 'continuum' formulation which accepts that many people have alcohol-related problems from time to time. This formulation takes account of inconclusive evidence concerning a 'dependence syndrome', allows for individualized responses, and avoids the dangers of labelling.

1.3 An intermediate formulation

Heather and Robertson (1981) gave the position of Edwards and Gross (1976) concerning the alcohol dependence syndrome:

> They . . . stress that by the term syndrome they mean to imply no more than the concurrence of a set of phenomena. . . . The syndrome is described as consisting of seven essential elements: (i) narrowing of the drinking repertoire; (ii) salience of drink-seeking behaviour; (iii) increased

tolerance to alcohol; (iv) repeated withdrawal symptoms; (v) relief or avoidance of withdrawal symptoms by further drinking; (vi) subjective awareness of compulsion to drink; and (vii) reinstatement of the syndrome after abstinence.

2 Some statistics

2.1 A British survey of alcohol consumption

Great Britain							Percentages and numbers
	Type of drinker						
	Abstainer	Occasional	Infrequent light	Frequent light	Moderate	Heavier	Sample size (= 100% (numbers)
Males (%)							
18–24	4	5	9	30	18	34	1,113
25–44	5	6	12	34	17	27	3,062
45–64	7	11	13	42	13	15	2,440
65 or over	14	15	13	47	8	4	1,455
All aged 18 or over	7	9	12	38	14	20	8,070
Females (%)							
18–24	8	12	21	43	10	5	1,177
25–44	7	16	23	45	6	2	3,428
45–64	12	23	18	45	2	–	2,690
65 or over	24	29	14	33	–	0	2,135
All aged 18 or over	13	20	19	42	4	2	9,430

TABLE 42.1 Drinking habits: by sex and age, 1984. (*Social Trends* 1987)

The terms refer to those having drunk, on a typical occasion, in the previous 12 months:

Abstainer:	no alcohol
Occasional:	some alcohol once or twice
Infrequent light:	1–4 units once or twice a month
Frequent light:	1–4 units between 'once' and 'most days' a week
Moderate:	5–6 units between 'once' and 'most days' a week, or 7+ units once or twice a month
Heavier:	7+ units between 'once' and 'most days' a week

A standard unit = half a pint of beer, or
= 1/6 gill spirits (an English single), or
= a glass of wine (4 fluid ozs), or
= a small glass of fortified wine (2 fluid ozs.)
One unit = roughly 9 grammes of absolute alcohol

The authors noted, 'this conversion technique is commonly used for measuring total alcohol consumption, but it must be stressed that in the GHS (General Household Survey) it was used for comparative purposes only'.

2.2 Different figures according to differing criteria

Smith (1981) has highlighted the difficulties of gathering data concerning alcohol related disorders:

> One San Francisco study showed that a strict definition of alcoholism produced a prevalence rate of 3 per 1000, while criteria that included any drinking problem past or present gave a prevalence rate of 272 per 1000 . . . estimates of the number of alcohol-dependent people in England and Wales vary from 70 000 to 240 000 and those for the number of problem drinkers from 500 000 to 1 300 000.

3 Research contributions to understanding the development of alcohol-related problems

3.1 The need for a multi-variate/systems model

Most researchers appear to agree that a simple formulation of the origins of alcohol-related problems is inaccurate and probably misleading. A model accommodating many interacting variables devised by Thorley (1985) is shown in Figure 42.1.

3.2 Variables implicit in a multi-variate/systems model

These include:

1. Constitutional, e.g. genetic and physiological, variables
2. Family and marital variables
3. Cultural and sub-cultural variables and norms
4. Social and situational variables
5. Social learning theory variables

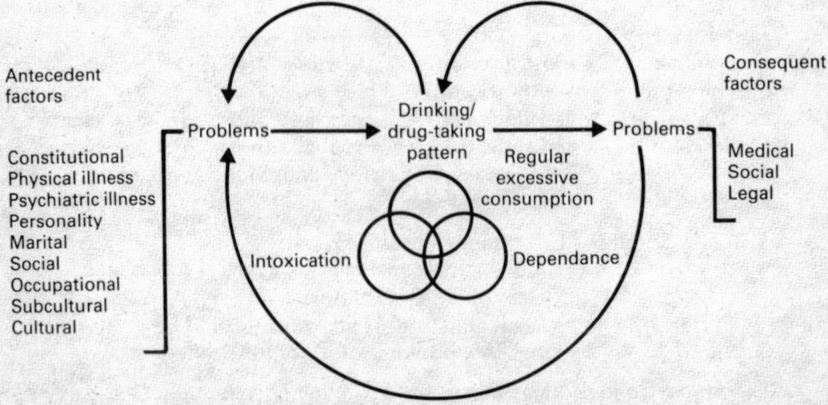

FIGURE 42.1 An explanatory system for problem drinking (Thorley, 1985)

1 **Constitutional variables** Goodwin (1979) has suggested a possible genetic contribution to some alcohol-related difficulties. This arises from Danish longitudinal studies which indicated that sons of people with drink-related problems are four times more likely to have such problems than the sons of people without these problems, whoever brought them up. This was not true, however, of the daughters. A genetic variable could reside in e.g. drink preferences and drink-seeking behaviours.

2 **Family and marital variables** Hawker (1978) found that adolescents *tended* to follow their parents' drinking patterns, while O'Connor (1978) found that the children of teetotal parents, if brought up in societies which permitted drinking, were at increased risk of problem drinking.

3 **Cultural and sub-cultural variables and norms** Nathan (1980) noted the studies by Cahalan (1978) of drinking patterns in America, and found that Italian-Americans and Jewish-Americans, who came from cultures in which drinking occurs in a family or religious context, were unlikely to develop drink-related problems, unlike Irish-Americans, who had lower consumption rates but more drink-related problems.

4 **Social and situational variables** The authors of *Alcohol* (Office of Health Economics, 1981) highlighted the importance of:

> the extent to which an individual's personal life style involves opportunities to drink and/or pressure to do so from peers . . . those who work in bars (and perhaps other branches of the alcohol industry) and those who frequent bars, such as young, single males, all report raised drinking rates.

N.B. Raised drinking rates do not automatically lead to problems. They are, however, variables in a complex multi-variate situation.

5 **Social learning theory variables**

1 Nathan (1980) has emphasized the importance of the *expectancies* that people have of alcohol. If someone believes that alcohol will enhance sexual arousal, or reduce tension and pain, then he or she is more likely to choose to drink, regardless of the evidence that pharmacological effects of alcohol are very unpredictable: to some extent people get from alcohol what they learn to expect.

2 Nathan added that there is evidence that alcohol use is:

> cued and reinforced by factors other than the real or anticipated effects of alcohol itself. To this end, the work of . . . Jessor and Jessor (1975) confirms that introduction to alcohol use is an integral and important part of adolescent peer-group interactions.

3 He also reported that imitation of a role model had been shown by Caudill and Marlatt (1975) to increase drinking in male social drinkers.

4 The prevention of alcohol-related problems

4.1 Research on Health Education campaigns

Smith (1981) described the outcome studies from Health Education campaigns: for example, the national campaign by the Scottish Health Education Unit in 1976 did reach about three quarters of the population, but 'the general level of public knowledge had not significantly increased eight months after the campaign began; and patterns of alcohol consumption had not changed.' (Plant, Pirie and Kreitman, 1979) Smith added, 'Repeated evaluations of the Health Education Council campaign in the north east of England have shown no change in drinking behaviour but some small change in attitudes towards drink and drunkenness.'

4.2 Other strategies

Smith (1981) reported that some researchers, but not all, seem to agree that if the price of alcohol is raised by taxation then consumption will fall, and with it alcohol-related damage. This is because of a view that consumption of alcohol is so distributed in a homogeneous population that the more the whole population drinks, the more very heavy drinkers there will be, and thus the more people there are at risk of bodily damage.

5 Treatment effectiveness for alcohol-related problems

1 'Treatment' is not a unitary concept: different researchers use different goals for treatment. Some assume a goal of controlled drinking: others one of general 'improvement'. It is very important to identify the operational definition of each researcher.
2 Miller and Hester (1980), have conducted an exhaustive review of the research in this field, and have reported their findings under a number of heads. Other studies are also included.

5.1 Average outcomes and spontaneous remission

1 **Average outcome rates** Of these, Miller and Hester reported: 'From the most extensive reviews available, it appears that when problem drinkers are treated, approximately one third become abstinent and an additional one-third show substantial improvement without abstinence.'

They noted, however, that the above figures are based upon short-term follow-up, and longer follow-up studies suggested that on average only 26 per cent of those treated remain abstinent or improved after one year. They also concluded that for untreated problem drinkers about one fifth are abstinent or improved after one year.

2 **Spontaneous remission** Miller and Hester (1980) concluded that among those people with alcohol-related problems, but who did not receive treatment for them, there was a 19 per cent remission rate (abstinent or improved) at one-year follow-up.

3 **Intensive versus minimal treatment** Of particular interest is the study by Edwards and colleagues (1977), who randomly assigned 100 married, healthy men with drinking problems to one of two treatment conditions:

(1) an 'intensive treatment' group including psychotherapy, attending Alcoholics Anonymous, and medication, or
(2) an 'advice' group, who had a single individual session in which the person was told that he should abstain from drinking and was himself responsible for bringing about change.

At both one and two year follow-up, no significant differences were found between the two groups.

5.2 Psychotherapy

Miller and Hester (1980) concluded from their review of the evidence to date that insight-oriented psychotherapy did not represent a treatment of choice for people with drinking problems. They noted: 'Controlled research has pointed to a high drop-out rate and lower or at best equivalent effectiveness in comparison to alternative treatment methods.'

5.3 Alcoholics Anonymous

There are major difficulties in attempting to evaluate research in this field – notably attrition and the shortage of studies with a control group. Miller and Hester (1980) quote the figures of Bebbington (1976) and Jindra and Forslund (1978) as representing minimum and maximum success rates at one-year follow-up respectively: the former arrived at a figure of 26 per cent, the latter at a figure of 50 per cent.

5.4 Group approaches

Miller and Hester (1980) summarized this research as follows:

> In general the outcome for group treatment for alcoholism has been inconsistent, with improvement rates averaging around 40%. Comparative and controlled studies have provided no support for the popular belief that group methods represent a superior approach for treating alcoholics. . . . If any advantage is to be seen for group approaches, it would be a cost-effectiveness advantage.

5.5 Structured family therapy

Miller and Hester (1980) reported from the work of e.g. Steinglass (1979), that despite research design weaknesses, such as small treatment samples, 'Controlled evaluations of family therapies have provided modest support for their efficacy relative to alternative approaches and control conditions.'

5.6 Approaches based on social learning theory principles

1 Such principles include the active use of such well-established principles as contingency management, self-monitoring and cognitive-behavioural analyses. Hodgson and Rankin (1976) and Marlatt (1978) have all made particularly important contributions to this field.
2 The principles themselves are applicable to many approaches and have been employed both in programmes which are abstinence-oriented and in those which aim at controlled drinking. They are particularly relevant in such fields as relapse prevention.

5.7 Controlled drinking as a therapeutic goal

1 Evidence for the effectiveness of controlled drinking

1 Since the initial studies, e.g. Lovibond and Caddy (1970), indicating that the goal of moderate drinking (i.e. non-abstinence-oriented) was attainable, there has been a wealth of research in this field.
2 In particular, Heather and Robertson (1981) have examined the evidence for controlled drinking from two groups of studies: 'clinic alcoholics', already known to clinics and hospitals, and 'problem drinkers', recruited via the media and the courts. Their summaries of the evidence is shown below:

(a) Controlled drinking for 'clinic alcoholics'

1 Many seriously dependent alcoholics respond to certain controlled drinking treatments by successfully controlling their drinking.
2 The most effective treatments used so far appear to be problem-solving skills training, regulated drinking practice and self-management training.

(b) Controlled drinking for 'problem drinkers': tentative conclusions

1 Controlled drinking procedures significantly reduce the level of drinking of many problem-drinkers to non-problem levels.
2 Brief interventions are as effective as intensive ones in achieving this.
3 Self-help manuals together with self-monitoring procedures appear to be the least expensive and simplest effective methods yet devised.
4 Abstinence appears to be an inappropriate goal for most problem drinkers. . . . Such clients also rarely abstain following controlled drinking treatment.

2 The practice of controlled drinking: behavioural self-control

1 Miller and colleagues (1980) are among those who have developed individualized programmes for people seeking to control their drinking. Such programmes tend to include the following components:
   (a) Goal setting: involving the drinkers in setting goals.
   (b) Training in self-monitoring of drinking.

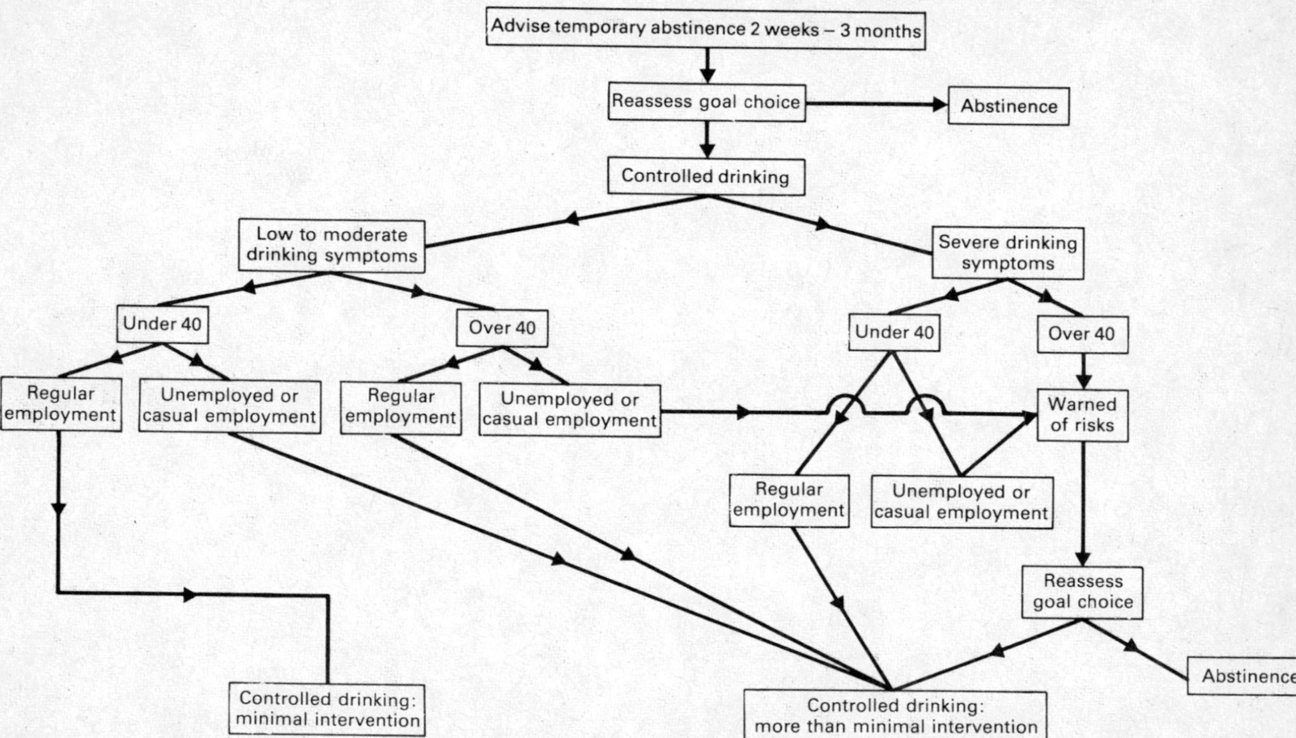

FIGURE 42.2 A tentative decision tree for those male clients wishing to control their drinking (Heather and Robertson, 1981)

(c) Training in monitoring rates of drinking.
(d) Training people to commend themselves for achievement in controlling their drinking.
(e) Detailed analysis of the cues which trigger drinking.
(f) Training in devising alternative strategies to drinking.

2 Miller and Hester (1980) reported that in over five studies (a very low figure), various behavioural self-control approaches have produced total improvement rates averaging around 70 per cent. These findings, however, have tended to be confirmed by other studies: e.g. Sanchez-Craig (1980).

5.8 Apparent areas of increasing consensus among researchers

These areas appear to include:

1 The need for intervention at many levels: educational programmes, publicity about sources of help, price adjustment.
2 The tailoring of treatment strategy to the circumstances of individual people seeking help.
3 The potential for controlled drinking strategies as well as for total abstinence.

References

Bebbington, P. E. (1976), 'The effectiveness of Alcoholics Anonymous: The elusiveness of hard data', *British Journal of Psychiatry*, vol. 128, pp. 572–80.

Cahalan, D. (1978), 'Subcultural differences in drinking behavior in U.S. national surveys and selected European studies' in P. E. Nathan and G. A. Marlatt (eds), *Alcoholism: New Directions in Behavioral Research and Treatment*, New York: Plenum Press.

Cameron, D. (1985), 'Why alcohol dependence – and why now?' in N. Heather, I. Robertson and P. Davies (eds), *The Misuse of Alcohol: Crucial Issues in Dependence, Treatment and Prevention*, Beckenham: Croom Helm.

Caudill, B. D. and Marlatt, G. A. (1975), 'Modelling influences in social drinking: An experimental analogue', *Journal of Consulting and Clinical Psychology*, vol. 43, pp. 405–15.

Costello, R. M. (1980), 'Alcoholism treatment effectiveness: Slicing the outcome variance pie' in G. Edwards and M. Grant (eds), *Alcoholism Treatment in Transition*, London: Croom Helm.

Edwards, G. and Gross, M. H. (1976), 'Alcohol dependence: provisional description of a clinical syndrome', *British Medical Journal*, 1, pp. 1058–61.

Edwards, G., Gross, M. M., Kellar, M., Moser, J. and Room, R. (1977), *Alcohol Related Disabilities*, Offset publication No. 32, Geneva: World Health Organisation.

Edwards, G., Orford, J., Egert, S., Guthrie, S., Hawker, A., Hensman, M., Oppenheimer, E. and Taylor, C. (1977), 'Alcoholism: A controlled trial of "treatment" and "advice"', *Journal of Studies on Alcohol*, vol. 38, pp. 1004–31.

Goodwin, D. W. (1979), 'Genetic determinants of alcoholism' in J. H. Mendelson and N. K. Mello (eds), *The Diagnosis and Treatment of Alcoholism*, New York: McGraw-Hill.

Hawker, A. (1978), *Adolescents and Alcohol*, London: Edsall.

Heather, N. and Robertson, I. (1981), *Controlled Drinking*, London: Methuen.

Heather, N., Robertson, I. and Davies, P. (eds on behalf of the New Directions in the Study of Alcohol Group) (1985), *The Misuse of Alcohol: Crucial Issues in Dependence, Treatment and Prevention*, Beckenham: Croom Helm.

Hodgson, R. J. and Rankin, H. J. (1976), 'Modification of excessive drinking by cue exposure', *Behaviour Research and Therapy*, vol. 14, pp. 305–7.

Jessor, R. and Jessor, S. L. (1975), 'Adolescent development and the onset of drinking: A longitudinal study', *Journal of Studies on Alcohol*, vol. 36, pp. 27–51.

Jindra, N. J. and Forslund, M. A. (1978), 'Alcoholics Anonymous in a Western U.S. city', *Journal of Studies on Alcohol*, vol. 39, pp. 110–20.

Lovibond, S. H. and Caddy, G. (1970), 'Discriminative aversive control in the moderation of alcoholics' drinking behaviour', *Behaviour Therapy*, vol. 1, pp. 437–44.

Marlatt, G. A. (1978), 'Craving for alcohol, loss of control and relapse: a cognitive-behavioural analysis' in P. E. Nathan, G. A. Marlatt and T. Loberg (eds), *Alcoholism: New Directions in Behavioural Research and Treatment*, New York: Plenum Press.

Miller, W. R. (1978), 'Behavioral treatment of problem drinkers: A comparative outcome study of three controlled drinking therapies', *Journal of Consulting and Clinical Psychology*, vol. 46, pp. 74–86.

Miller, W. R. and Hester, R. K. (1980), 'Treating the problem drinker: modern approaches' in W. R. Miller (ed.), *The Addictive Behaviors*, Oxford: Pergamon Press.

Nathan, P. E. (1980), 'Etiology and process in the treatment of narcotic addiction' in W. R. Miller (ed.) (1980), *The Addictive Behaviors*, Oxford: Pergamon Press.

O'Connor, J. (1978), *The Young Drinkers*, London: Tavistock.

Office of Health Economics (1981), *Alcohol: Reducing the Harm*, London: OHE.

Plant, M., Pirie, F. and Kreitman, N. (1979), 'Evaluation of the Scottish Health Education Unit's 1976 campaign on alcoholism', *Social Psychiatry*, vol. 14, pp. 11–24.

Sanchez-Craig, M. (1980), 'Random assignment to abstinence or controlled drinking in a cognitive behavioral program: short-term effects on drinking behavior', *Addictive Behaviors*, vol. 5, pp. 35–9.

Smith, R. (1981), 'Alcohol and alcoholisms: the relation between consumption and damage', *British Medical Journal*, vol. 283, 3 October 1981, pp. 895–8.
Smith, R. (1981), 'Preventing alcohol problems: a job for Canute?', *British Medical Journal*, vol. 283, 10 October 1981, pp. 972–5.
Social Trends (1987) London: HMSO.
(Special Committee of the Royal College of Psychiatrists (1979), *Alcohol and Alcoholism*, London: Tavistock.
Steinglass, P. (1979), 'An experimental treatment program for alcoholic couples', *Journal of Studies on Alcohol*, vol. 40, pp. 169–82.
Thorley, A. (1985), 'The limitations of the alcohol dependence syndrome in multidisciplinary service development', in N. Heather, I. Robertson and P. Davies (eds), *The Misuse of Alcohol: Crucial Issues in Dependence Treatment and Prevention*, London: Croom Helm.

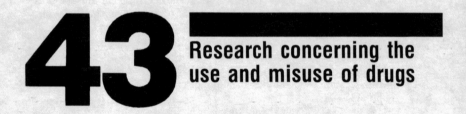

43 Research concerning the use and misuse of drugs

Consultant: Dr Douglas Cameron, Consultant Psychiatrist, Leicestershire Community Alcohol and Drugs Services.

1 The legal position in the UK and some terminology

1.1 The legal position in the UK

Cross and Jones (1984) have written,

> The Misuse of Drugs Act 1971, which replaced earlier legislation, seeks to achieve the two broad objectives of the control of dangerous or otherwise harmful drugs and the prevention of their abuse. . . .
>
> The drugs subject to the Act (the 'controlled drugs') are specified in its second schedule. There are three classes: Class A includes cocaine, LSD, heroin, mescaline and opium; Class B includes amphetamine, cannabis, cannabis resin and codeine; Class C includes benzphetamine and pemoline.

1.2 Some terminology

Drug Misuse: A Basic Briefing (1985) suggested the following descriptions:

> *Tolerance* refers to the way the body adapts to the repeated presence of a drug. . . .
>
> *Withdrawal effects* . . . can be thought of as the body's reaction to the sudden absence of a drug to which it has adapted. . . .
>
> *Dependence* describes a compulsion to continue taking a drug as a result of its repeated administration. In so far as this is to avoid the physical discomfort of withdrawal, we speak of *physical dependence*; in so far as the compulsion has a psychological basis – the need for stimulation or pleasure . . . desire to obliterate reality, etc. then it's referred to as *psychological dependence*. Psychological dependence is recognised as . . . widespread. . . .
>
> *Addiction* implies that a drug dependency has developed which has serious detrimental effects on the individual and on society. As such it is intimately tied up with society's reaction to that dependency, so medical experts now generally avoid the term as carrying too many non-medical connotations.
>
> The term *problem drug use* has been coined to refer to drug use resulting in social, psychological, physical or legal problems associated with dependence, intoxication or regular excessive consumption.
>
> *Drug 'abuse'* and drug '*mis-use*' are terms that are hard to pin down. Essentially they represent the observer's belief that the drug-taking in question is a harmful (abuse) and/or a socially unacceptable way of using that substance (misuse). . . .

2 A classification of the main groups of drugs

The *International Classification of Diseases* (9th edition), (World Health Organisation, 1980) lists several types of drug:

304.0 *Morphine type*

Heroin
Methadone
Opium
Opium alkaloids and their derivatives
Synthetics with morphine-like effects

304.1 *Barbiturate type*

Barbiturates
Nonbarbiturate sedatives and tranquillizers with a similar effect:
  chlordiazepoxide
  diazepam
  glutethimide
  meprobamate

304.2 *Cocaine*

Coca leaves and derivatives

304.3 *Cannabis*

Hemp
Hashish
Marijuana

304.4 *Amphetamine type and other psychostimulants*

Phenmetrazine
Methylphenidate

304.5 *Hallucinogens*

LSD and derivatives
Mescaline
Psilocybin

304.6 *Other*

Absinthe addiction
Glue sniffing

3 Characteristics of the main groups of drugs

3.1 Morphine type

	Heroin	*Chinese heroin*	*Methadone (Physeptone)*
Trade names			
Street names	Junk, stuff, 'H', dope, horse, smack.	'Chinese'	Phy.
Description	Heroin is synthesised from a morphine base, itself a product of raw opium.	A brownish powder, often mixed with talc, sugar or coffee powder.	
Effects	All these drugs are used for the relief of severe pain, . . . but they are particularly dangerous in that they all produce a state of physical and/or psychological dependence upon the drug.		

3.2 Barbiturate type, which depress the central nervous system.

	Barbiturates	*Non-barbiturates* (Tranquillizers)
Trade names	Nembutal, Seconal, Amytal, Luminal	Valium, Librium, Ativan, Mandrax*
Street names	Barbs, reds, blues, downers, sleepers.	*Mandies, knockouts.
Description	These depress the Central Nervous System, and thus reduce anxiety. Because of clear dangers they are less prescribed now than formerly.	These are widely prescribed, despite mounting criticism.

3.3 Cocaine, which stimulates the central nervous system

Street names	Coke, snow
Description	Cocaine is a white powder synthesised from the coca plant.
Effects	Sniffing the powder produces euphoric excitement 15–30 minutes afterwards, but the effects are short-lived.

3.4 Cannabis

	Hashish	*Marijuana*
Street names	Hash, dope, stuff.	Grass, pot.
Description	A brown or black crumbly substance, which may be smoked with . . . tobacco.	Looks like herbal tobacco.
Effects	Both forms, when smoked, produce a feeling of mild intoxication and pleasure. The effects may be similar to alcohol, and can produce disturbances (and enhancements) of perception.	

3.5 Amphetamine type and other psychostimulants

Trade names	Dexedrine, Benzedrine, Preludin.
Street names	Uppers, speed, dexies, bennies, ups.
Description	These are all stimulants to the central nervous system.
Effects	They promote wakefulness, create a sense of well-being, and decrease the effects of fatigue. However, tolerance develops, and they occasionally trigger psychotic episodes. There may be depression on discontinuation.

3.6 Hallucinogens

Trade name	LSD.
Street name	Acid.
Description	LSD stands for lysergic acid/diethylamide, and is a colourless, tasteless, odourless substance derived from ergot.
Effects	The effects vary from ecstacy, sexuality and a state of bliss to horror and terror, with varying effects being experienced by the same individual. The hallucinogenic experiences do not, however, produce withdrawal effects. It is illegal to produce, supply or use this drug.

3.7 Glue sniffing

Street name	Glue
Effects	The sniffing of glue produces a feeling of mild euphoria in the sniffer, which, however, soon passes. A number of side effects, e.g. hallucinations and dizziness, can be more unpleasant than the experience itself, but there are real dangers of asphyxiation if glue is sniffed from, e.g., plastic bags.

TABLE 43.1 A drugs compendium: the trade names, street names and characteristic effects of the main groups of drugs. (After the article in *Observer Magazine*, 21 October, 1973.)

4 The prevalence of drug misuse in the UK

4.1 Some official statistics

It is extremely difficult to establish reliable figures of the prevalence of drug misuse. Table 43.2, however, gives relevant data concerning new narcotic drug addicts over recent years.

United Kingdom Numbers

	Age							
	Under 20	20–24	25–29	30–34	35–49	50 or over	Not known	Total
Males								
1973	149	334	89	23	20	24	5	644
1976	61	315	251	55	35	20	8	745
1981	141	544	511	269	78	15	49	1,607
1982	197	676	593	323	118	16	53	1,976
1983	402	1,011	766	440	192	38	130	2,979
1984	584	1,334	958	570	257	22	115	3,840
Females								
1973	41	79	20	7	8	8	0	163
1976	40	100	55	15	10	12	7	239
1981	91	225	186	84	18	14	23	641
1982	113	271	233	113	41	12	34	817
1983	170	446	315	150	59	18	49	1,207
1984	214	618	405	205	63	19	51	1,575

TABLE 43.2 Narcotic drugs – new addicts notified to the Home Office by age and sex (*Social Trends*, 1986)

4.2 Commentary on Table 43.2

The authors of *Social Trends* (1986) noted,

> One indicator of the increase in drug misuse is the number of new narcotic drug addicts notified by doctors to the Home Office. There were 5,415 notifications of new addicts in the United Kingdom in 1984, nearly 30 per cent more than in 1983 and almost double the number in 1982. . . . Notifications are always highest among 20 to 24 year olds. About 90 per cent of new addicts notified in 1984 claimed addiction to heroin (alone or with other drugs).

4.3 Offenders found guilty of drug offences

	1979	1980	1981	1982	1983	1984
Drug offence	11,864	15,020	15,555	17,585	19,892	20,701

TABLE 43.3 Offenders found guilty (at all courts or cautioned. Numbers of offenders. (*Criminal Statistics*, England and Wales, 1984)

5 Research which contributes to understanding drug abuse

5.1 Differing attitudes to the use of different drugs

As with alcohol, drug-use meets with differing degrees of social acceptance in different cultures. Table 43.1, for example, does not include tobacco but perhaps should do so in view of its harmful effects.

5.2 The variety of those who use drugs

The *Report of the Medical Working Group on Drug Dependence* (1984) lists several groups of users:

a. People, often adolescents, experimenting with drugs or taking them intermittently, who may not be physically dependent at the time of referral, and may have no major problems. They are, however, at risk of increasing the frequency of their use.

b. Psychologically and/or physically dependent misusers whose lives are centred on drugs. They are often involved in a drug subculture, and usually have many related problems.

c. Stable drug users who are psychologically and/or physically dependent on opioids or other drugs which may initially have been prescribed to treat physical disorders.

d. Some long-term drug users may have initially obtained controlled drugs for the treatment of their addiction or may have always obtained their supply from illicit sources. They may nevertheless have maintained stability in their social and working lives.

5.3 Studies of drug users

1 **An early British study** Plant (1975), in his study of drug use in Cheltenham, talked with 200 individuals unknown to 'official agencies': of these, seventy-three were students, forty non-manual workers and eighty-seven manual workers or unemployed. The variety of drugs used is listed in Table 43.4.

Type of drug	No	%
Hallucinogens (including cannabis)	155	77.5
Amphetamines	108	54.0
Hypnotics	93	46.5
Miscellaneous medical (not prescribed)	62	31.0
Raw opiates	33	16.5
Manufactured opiates	30	15.0
Cocaine	30	15.0
Miscellaneous medical (herbs, etc.)	22	11.0

TABLE 43.4 Drugs used by the Cheltenham sample (Plant, 1975)

2 **A study assessing drug misuse in a London borough**

1 Hartnoll, Mitcheson, Lewis and Daviaud (1984) surveyed drug misuse in two areas of London, and the implications for services. Using five independent sources of data, they estimated that the rate per 1,000 of population, aged sixteen to forty-four, had risen from 3.0 in 1977 to 13.4 in 1982 and approximately 14.2 in 1983.
2 One of their conclusions was that for every 'known' regular opioid user who had received treatment at a drug clinic in the previous year, there were six to ten who had not.
3 They concluded that current provision was totally inadequate and called for major investment in new services.

5.4 Overviews of the research on the origins of drug misuse

Plant (1981) considered that two important sociological theories: 'deviancy amplification' and 'anomie', are involved here.

1 **The theory of 'deviancy amplification'** This suggests that the very control which society attempts to exert upon 'deviants' tends to intensify that deviance (e.g. Young, 1971).

2 **The theory of 'anomie'** This body of theory, originating with Durkheim (1954) and developed by Merton (1957), suggested that:

> If people within a society fail to attain their objectives (such as status and influence) by legitimate means, they may use illegal or deviant methods instead. . . . Young people with poor educational opportunities opt out of the work-a-day world and establish a lifestyle (sub-culture) of their own. (Plant, 1981)

Plant criticized the methodology of much of the research upon drug-misuse, and concluded: 'No narrow explanation seems capable of accounting for the range of data and theories. *Drug-taking and drug dependence appear to be influenced by many factors, constitutional, individual and environmental.*' (Teff, 1975)

5.5 A multi-variate/systems, model

1 While there is as yet no evidence of any clear factors which make a vulnerability to drug-abuse more likely, it seems that a multi-factorial model, with many contributory variables, is the most realistic. Figure 43.1 shows the model devised by Cameron (1985), building on the work of Szara and Bunney (1974).
2 Szara and Bunney (1974) made several points, paraphrased below:
(a) the genetic make-up of an individual may play an important part in determining their physical and psychological development.

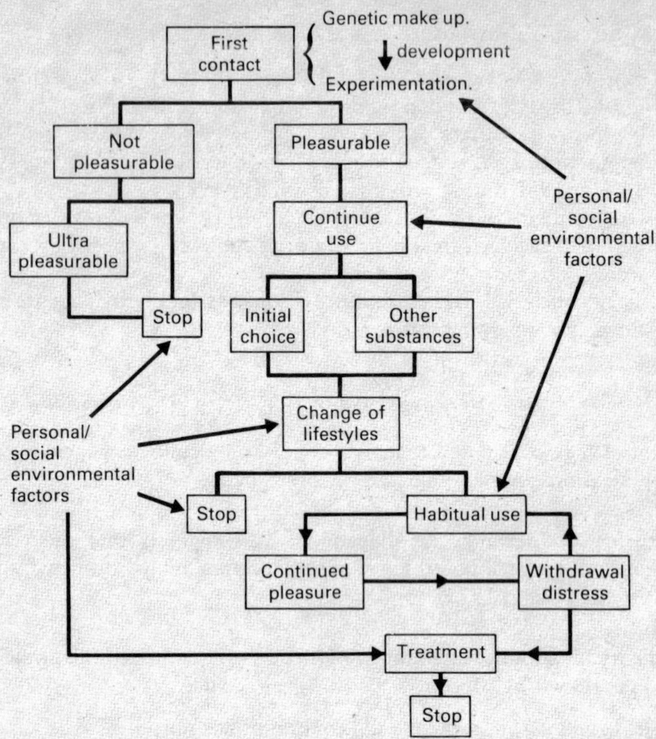

FIGURE 43.1 A multi-variate/systems, model of opiate use and outcomes (Cameron, 1986)

(b) experimentation with drugs may be considered a form of natural exploratory behaviour, affected by availability, peer group pressure, etc.

(c) experimentation with drugs does not necessarily lead to dependence.

6 Research upon prevention of and intervention in drug misuse

6.1 Research upon prevention via education

The authors of *Drugs in Health Education: Trends and Issues* (1982) concluded of the effectiveness of health education programmes:

> The general conclusion that can be drawn from reviewing the available studies (when one concentrates on studies in which the evaluation procedures were rigorous) is that none of the types of drug education so far developed (scare, factual or affective) reduce the rate of experimentation with drugs. However the balance of evidence does not indicate that experimentation is encouraged by drug education.

6.2 A follow-up study of heroin misuse

Gossop (1984) has reported,

> One of the best known follow-up studies of British addicts looked at a group of heroin addicts who approached London drug dependence clinics in 1969. After seven years it was found that 31 per cent were no longer dependent upon opiates (Stimson, Oppenheimer and Thorley, 1978). Most follow-up studies have supported this finding; over a seven-year period, about one-third of any group of addicts will cease to be dependent upon drugs.

6.3 The treatment of heroin misuse

(This section is based substantially upon the chapter by Callahan, 'Alternative strategies in the treatment of narcotic addiction: a review', in the book, *The Addictive Behaviors* edited by W. R. Miller (1980), and published by Pergamon.)

Callahan (1980) reported three main models of the treatment of heroin addiction:

1 The medical model
2 The 'narcotic addiction personality' model
3 The social learning theory model

Callahan's consideration of each model will be considered below:

1 Research within the medical model

1 One form of this assumed that to wean the addict from the drug by reducing the dosage would automatically lead to improvement. Callahan (1980) reported: 'The results of this form of early treatment were disastrous. Most addicts returned to heroin use within hours or days of release.'
2 A second medical model, assuming that patients needed a drug/narcotic in order to function metabolically, prescribed a substitute narcotic, methadone, as a regular maintenance dose. Some evaluations of this approach found positive outcomes: others did not.
3 There seems to be evidence that a drug antagonistic to heroin, naltrexone, is particularly helpful.
4 Simpson (1981) examined variables associated with 1,496 people participating in community drug-treatment agencies, and reported that positive one-year follow-up outcomes were associated with the length of time that patients stayed in methadone maintenance, a therapeutic community, or out-patient drug-free treatment. Outcomes for people who spent less than three months in treatment were least favourable.
5 Attrition (dropping out of treatment) is a difficulty faced by anyone trying to help drug users. Levels of attrition can be somewhat reduced by the use of contracts discussed and agreed and signed at the outset.

2 Research within the 'narcotic addiction personality' model

1 The two main approaches within this model are psychotherapy and the therapeutic community; the study by Platt and Labate (1976) of psychotherapy with drug users suggested that this was not very effective.

2 Therapeutic communities appear to have helped some people, given a lengthy stay. See 1.4, above.

3 Research within the social learning theory model

1 Boudin and his colleagues (1977) reported considerable success using an approach involving,

(a) enabling people to gain self-control, via

stage 1: accurate self-observation, to pinpoint triggers or antecedents to drug taking,

stage 2: self-evaluation, to decide whether drug taking on that occasion is really wanted,

stage 3: planning and carrying out behaviour change on an A.B.C. (Antecedents, Behaviour, Consequences) model.

(b) using 'contingency contracts' (agreements) between the drug user and the helper, in which responsibility, initially in the helper's hands, passes increasingly to the addict.

2 Boudin and colleagues (1977) reported on four levels of adjustment, post-treatment, for the nineteen participants:

(a) work/school performance: 16 had a positive outcome

(b) personal/social adjustment: 13 had a positive outcome

(c) incidence of drug intake, measured by urine analysis: 12 had 'drug-free status'.

(d) frequency of arrests or conviction: 15 had no arrests or convictions.

3 To test both Boudin's model, and the importance of the narcotic antagonist, naltrexone, the Heroin Antagonist and Learning Therapy (HALT) Project was designed. The effectiveness of three approaches was monitored over a two-year period:

a) social learning theory/behavioural approaches alone

b) naltrexone treatment alone

c) combined naltrexone and behavioural approaches.

By the close of the project there were mixed results. At one-year follow up,

a) Four of the fourteen using behavioural approaches were drug-free

b) Ten of the twenty using naltrexone alone were drug-free

c) Eight of the fifteen using a combined approach were drug-free.

Callahan (1980) suggested that despite methodological weaknesses in the study, the value of naltrexone, supported by a behaviourally-based programme, seemed to be apparent.

6.4 The need for a multi-dimensional strategy of intervention

1 This, and other chapters, have advocated a systems approach to understanding situations, so that the impact of many variables is

recognized; a similar approach is needed in intervention. Thus, assessment of the situation of a person with drug-related difficulties will need attention to medical, legal, social psychological and other factors, so that a co-ordinated approach, upon many levels, can be agreed with the person concerned. See also Tether and Robinson (1986).

2 It seems likely that an approach in which the short-term and long-term goals of the intervention are agreed beforehand by the person in need and the helpers, perhaps by means of a written agreement or contract, will offer a useful way of structuring work and evaluating outcome.
3 It is also likely that the personality of the therapist or helper will be an important variable. (See Chapter 10, page 80).

6.5 The treatment of tranquillizer dependence

Petursson and Lader (1984) added to the firm body of evidence concerning dependence upon tranquillizers and the difficulties of withdrawing from long-term use. They concluded that gradual withdrawal is probably the best treatment, under medical supervision, and they suggested that behavioural and other non-pharmacological methods should also be pursued to enable people to deal with their anxieties.

6.6 Responses to glue/solvent misuse

There is little evidence in terms of follow-up studies concerning differing strategies of intervention in this area; however, it seems likely that a multi-dimensional approach, one which involves the families of the young people concerned, is most likely to be helpful.

7 The future of research upon drug misuse

The author of *Treatment and Rehabilitation: The Report of the Advisory Council on the Misuse of Drugs* (1982) suggested that the present shortage of research left them: 'with few ways of judging in what direction current efforts are ineffective and should be curtailed, or of determining the direction in which limited resources can most effectively be deployed or redeployed.' Clearly, further rigorous research is urgently needed.

References

Boudin, H. M., Valentine, V. E., Ingraham, R. D., Brantley, J., Ruiz, M. R., Smith, G. G., Catlin, R. P. and Regan, E. J. (1977), 'Contingency contracting with drug abusers in the natural environment', *The International Journal of the Addictions*, vol. 12, pp. 1–16.

Callahan, E. J. (1980), 'Alternative strategies in the treatment of narcotic addiction: A review' in W. R. Miller (ed.), *The Addictive Behaviors*, Oxford: Pergamon Press.

Cameron, D. (1986); Personal communication.

Cross, R. and Jones, P. (1984), *An Introduction to Criminal Law*, 10th edition, by J. Card, London: Butterworth.

Durkheim, E. (1954), *Suicide: a Study in sociology*, Translated by John Spaulding and George Simpson. (Ed.) G. Simpson. London: Routledge and Kegan Paul.

Edwards, G. and Busch, C. (eds) (1981), *Drug Problems in Britain. A Review of Ten Years*, London: Academic Press.

Gossop, M. (1984), 'Drug and alcohol dependence' in A. Gale and A. Chapman (eds), *Psychology and Social Problems*, Chichester: Wiley.

Hartnoll, R., Mitcheson, M., Lewis, R. and Daviaud, E. (1984), *Assessing Local Drug Problems: A Short Guide*, Drug Indicators Project, 51 Kentish Town Road, London.

Institute for the Study of Drug Dependence (1982), *Drugs in Health Education: Trends and Issues*, London: I.S.D.D.

Institute for the Study of Drug Dependence (1985), *Drug Misuse: A Basic Briefing*, London: ISDD.

Merton, B. K. (1957), *Social Theory and Social Structure*, Toronto: Collier Macmillan.

Miller, W. R. (1980), *The Addictive Behaviours*, Oxford: Pergamon.

Observer Magazine (1978), 'A drugs compendium: What they are, what they look like, what they do, and what the penalties are for misusing them', *Observer*, 21 October 1973.

Petursson, H. and Lader, M. (1984), *Dependence on Tranquillizers*, Maudsley Monograph, Oxford University Press.

Plant, M. (1975), *Drug-takers in an English Town*, London: Tavistock.

Plant, M. (1981), 'What aetiologies?' in G. Edwards and C. Busch (eds), *Drug Problems in Britain. A Review of Ten Years.*

Platt, J. J. and Labate, C. (1976), *Heroin Addiction: Theory, research and treatment*, New York: Wiley.

Report of the Medical Working Group on Drug Dependence (1984), *Guidelines of Good Clinical Practice in the Treatment of Drug Misuse*, London: DHSS.

Simpson, D. (1981), 'Treatment for drug abuse', *Archives of General Psychiatry*, vol. 38, pp. 875–80.

Stimson, G. (1981), 'Epidemiological research on drug use in general populations' in G. Edwards and C. Busch (eds), *Drug Problems in Britain. A Review of Ten Years.*

Stimson, G., Oppenheimer, E. and Thorley, A. (1978), 'Seven-year follow-up of heroin addicts: drug use and outcome', *British Medical Journal*, vol. 1, pp. 1190–2.

Swinson, R. P. and Eaves, D. (1978), *Alcoholism and Addiction. Psychiatric Topics for Community Workers*, London: Woburn Press.

Szara, S. and Bunney, W. E. (1974), 'Recent research on opiate addiction: review of a national program' in S. Fisher and A. Freedman (eds), *Opiate Addiction: Origins and Treatment*, Washington, D.C.: V. H. Winston and Sons, Inc.

Teff, H. (1975), *Drugs, Society and the Law*, Farnborough, Hants: Saxon House.

Tether, P. and Robinson, D. (1986), *Preventing Alcohol Problems: A Guide to Local Action*. London: Tavistock Publications.

Treatment and Rehabilitation. Report of the Advisory Council on the Misuse of Drugs (1982), London: HMSO.

Young, J. (1971), 'The role of the police as amplifiers of deviancy, negotiators of reality and translators of fantasy' in S. Cohen (ed.), *Images of Deviance*, Harmondsworth: Penguin.

INDEX

Action research/service research, 41
Anomie, 407
Adopted children, 247–56;
comparative studies, 249; National Child Development Study, 250; official figures, 239; with special needs, 251,
(mental handicap, 251; older children, 251; physical handicap, 251; sibling groups, 251)
Adopted people, 255; counselling, 255
Adoption, 247–56; adoptive parents, 254; changes in patterns of, 248; continuing contact, 252; definition, 247; planning for permanence, 252, 253; transracial adoption, 253–4
Adoption studies, 249–55; overview of research, 250
Aggression, 20, 197–9
Agoraphobia, 311–12; *see* Anxiety and forms of anxiety, 305–14
Alcohol use and mis-use, 390–400;
definition of mis-use, 390–1;
prevention, 394,
(health education campaigns, 394; other strategies, 394);
statistics, 391; systems model, 392,
(implicit variables, 392–3)
treatment effectiveness, 394–8,
(Alcoholics Anonymous, 395, areas of increasing consensus, 398, average outcomes, 394, behavioural self-control, 396, controlled drinking as goal, 396–7, decision tree, 397, group approaches, 395, intensive versus minimal treatment, 395, psychotherapy, 395, social learning theory approaches, 396, spontaneous remission, 394, structured family therapy, 395)
Anxiety and forms of anxiety, 305–14;
agoraphobia, 306, 311–12,
(prognosis, 312, systems model, 312, treatment, 312);
definitions, 305–7,
(broad, 305, psychiatric, 306);
obsessive-compulsive conditions, 311, 312,
(prognosis, 313, treatment, 312);
phobias, 311–12,
(preliminary considerations, 311, prognosis, 311, treatment, 311)

Baseline, 30, 32, 33
Bed-wetting/enuresis, 205–8;
management, 207–8; origins, 205–7,
(genetic variables, 206, psychological variables, 205, sociological variables, 205, stress, 205);
prevalence, 205;
treatment, 207–8
Bereavement, 353–60; counselling, 356; figures, 353; grief as cross-cultural phenomenon, 354; people at risk after bereavement, 355;
research on support for the bereaved, 356–9
(conclusion from review, 358, professional services, 356–8, professional services giving group support, 357, self-help groups, 357–8, voluntary services, 357, work of Cruse, 358);

specific bereaved groups, 358, 359, (parents experiencing a cot death, 358, relatives bereaved by suicide, 359);
stages of the grief response, 354; vulnerability of bereaved people, 355–6, (increased ill-health, 356, increased mortality, 355)
Borstal, 295, 297; *see* Custodial and other responses to offenders, 294–302
Broken homes, 170; *see* Family life, marriage and divorce, 163–80

Campaigns, 40
Checklists, 93
Child abuse, 225–37; categorization, 225, (multi-variate model, 228–30, sociological-psychological variables, 229, social learning theory variables, 231);
definition, 225;
prevalence, 226–8, (official statistics, 226, Special Unit registers of the NSPCC, 226, studies in the UK, 227, summaries of prevalence in the USA, 227);
prevention, 232–6, (possible symptoms and signs, 232, risk rating scales, 233, social learning theory perspective, 233–4, sociological/community perspective, 232–3)
Child care, 213–24; group care, 215, (across systems, 215)
Child care, residential, 215–19; evaluation, 215, 219, (models, 215, 216);
studies, 219, 220, (consumer surveys, 218, empirical, 217, evaluation of outcome, 219, inter-generational effects, 220, theories, 219);
training for residential work, 222
Child care, statutory, 213–24; description, 213; 'Social Work Decisions in Child Care', 220–1; statistics, 214
Child-rearing variables, (vi)
Child sexual abuse, 225, 227–8, 234–6; characteristics of perpetrators, 234; definition, 225; how revealed, 235; imprisonment for, 235; prevalence, 225–7, (official statistics of incest, 227, other studies, 227–8);
treatment, 235; women's movement response, 236
Claimants' unions, 40
Cognitive variables, 308, 310, 322; anxiety, 308, 310; depression, 322
Cohesiveness, 48–9, 56; intragroup, 48; threat from outside, 56; ways of increasing, 56
Community action, 37; Education model, 38, (example, 39)
Community development, 37; as process, 37;/Education model, 38, (example, 39)
Community organization, 37;/ Education model, 38 (example, 38)
Community work, 35–42; definition, 35; research and evaluation, 40–2; summary of approaches, 40
Community workers, 35; description of work, 35; numbers, 36; organizations employing, 36
Confidentiality, 31, 81
Conciliation, 47, 168
Conduct disorders and young people, 195–204, classification, 195;
intervention, 201–3, (aggressive/destructive behaviour, 201, hyperkinetic/hyperactive behaviour, 203);
origins, 197–200 (aggressive/destructive behaviour, 197–9, hyperkinetic/hyperactive behaviour, 199–200, truancy, 200–1);
persistence studies, 195–6; prevalence studies, 195–6

(Isle of Wight/Inner London Borough, 196, National Child Development Study, 195–6, other, 196–7)
Conflict, 43–50; constructive potential of, 94; effectiveness, 44; intergroup, 44–8,
(characteristics, 45, definition, 43, reduction of, 46–8);
organizational, 43,
(definition, 43);
sources, 94
Conflict analysis, 37
Contracts, 285; family placement of young offenders, 285; foster care, 245; treatment of heroin mis-use, 410
Co-operation, 46–7; promotion between opposing groups, 46
Counselling, 79–85; agreeing goals for, 81–2; contracts, 81, 82; counsellor methods, 82–3; counsellors, 80,
(effective, 80);
definitions, 79; effectiveness, 79; studies with empirical support, 83–4,
(client characteristics, 83, clients receiving help, 84, counsellor persuasiveness, 83, counsellor's own experience, 83, counsellor commitment, 84, lay counsellors, 84, social influence process, 84);
evaluation, 82; gaining an overview, 81; integrated approach, 80; intervention, 82; stages, 81,
(agreeing goals, 81, evaluation, 81, intervention, 81, overview, 81);
traditions, 80,
(behavioural, 80, humanistic, 80, psychoanalytic, 80)
Current life circumstances, (vi)
Custodial and other responses to offenders, 294–302; differing perspectives, 299,
(crime as opportunity, 299, Marxist analysis, 299, prevention is better than cure, 299);
issues arising, 295
(criteria for evaluation, 295, principle of 'parsimony', 296);
official statistics, 294–5; outcomes, 296–9
(borstal, 297, community service orders, 296–7, detention centres, 297, imprisonment, 298–9, probation, 288–9, supervision orders, 296);
reports, 300,
(principles when compiling, 300);
statistics, 294–5

Data, 18–26; pre-measurement, 28; post-measurement, 28; verifiable, 18–26
Delinquency, 272, 273; *see also* Young offenders, 269–79, 280–6
Delinquents, 269–79, 280–6; individual characteristics, 275; impact of socio-economic forces, 278; labelling, 276; major variables, 275, race, 275, sex, 274, social class, 274;
prediction of, 273; cognitive variables, 277; situational variables, 276, 278;
psycho-social variables, 275; sociological contributions, 276, differential association, 276, difficulties in achieving success, 276, level of parental supervision, 276;
statistics, 270–1; systems model, 276
Depression, 315–23; characteristics, 316; classification, 315; cognitive factors, 319; definition, 315; helping depressed people, 320,
(assessment, 321, duration of episodes, 320, subsequent depressive episodes, 320);
models or theories, 317
(biological, 318, developmental predisposition, 318, 319, physiological stressors, 318, psychosocial stressors, 318);

prevalence, 316; stressful events, 318,
(modifying factors, 319);
systems model, 317; treatment, 321,
(cognitive-behavioural approaches, 322, electro-convulsive therapy, 321, medication, 321, social support, 321
Developmental stage, (vi)
Deviancy amplification, 407
Diagnostic and Statistical Manual of
Mental Disorders (DSM III), 5
Disability, 127–37
Disabled Living Foundation, 130
Divorce, 163–71; *see* Family life, marriage and divorce, 163–71
Drugs, use and misuse, 400–13; characteristics of main groups, 402–4; classification, 401; future of research, 411; legal position, 400; offenders found guilty of drug offences, 405; prevention, 408,
(follow-up study, 409, via education, 408);
statistics, official, 404–5; terminology, 401; treatment, 409,
(glue/solvent misuse, 411, models of treatment of heroin misuse, 409, multi-dimensional strategies, 410, tranquillizer dependence, 411);
understanding drug misuse, 406–8,
(differing attitudes to drug use, 406, overview of research on origins of use, 407, sociological contributions, 407, studies of drug use, 406–7, systems model, 408, variety of those using drugs, 406)

Electro-convulsive therapy (ECT), 29, 321
Emotional disorders and young people, 183–94; classification, 183; prevalence, 183–5; resilience, 186–7,
(convergence of evidence, 187);
specific disorders, 187–92,
(anxiety-related, 188, depression, 189, obsessive-compulsive conditions, 189, phobias, 188);
temperamental differences, 187; treatment, 190–2,
(absence of child-adult neurosis link, 192, anxiety, 191, depression, 192, obsessional compulsions, 192, phobias, 191, underlying principles, 190–1)
Empirical approach, 18–34; definition, 18; devising hypotheses, 19; gathering verifiable data, 18–26
(difficulties, 20)
Enuresis, 205–9; *see* Bed-wetting, 205–9
Ethics, 27, 28, 33; ethical acceptability, 28; ethical responsibility, 33
Ethnic minorities, 117–27; education, 122–4,
(Britain as multi-racial, multi-cultural, 123);
employment, 118–20; health, 124; housing, 120–2,
(inner city residence, 122, national survey, 120, standards of amenities, 121, tenure, 121, what sort of housing, 121, where people lived, 121);
racial attacks, 124,
(study by Home Office, 124–5, study by Policy Studies Institute, 125, victims of assault, 126)
Evaluation, 27–34; criteria, 28–9; intervention, 29–33,
(with a single person, 32);
importance, 27; preliminary questions, 27–8; purpose, 27
Experimental method, 23–4, 32–3; example, 24, 32,
(dependent variables, 23, 25);
independent variables, 23, 25

Family life, marriage and divorce, 163–71; breakdown of marriage, 166–7,
(antecedents, 166, processes, 167);

conciliation, 168; divorce/ separation, 167–8, (anti-social behaviour in children, 170, effects of divorce on children, 169, stepfamilies, 168);
marital therapy, 361–8; one-parent families, 172–180; relationships, 165–6,
(expectations, 165, happiness, 165);
statistics, 163–5,
(divorce, 164, households, 163, marriage, 164)

Family/marital therapy, 361–8; definition, 361; geneogram, 366; main approaches, 362; outcome, 362–6,
(aspects of family therapy needing investigation, 367, components contributing to effectiveness, 364, difficulties which respond well, 365, length of treatment, 365; model of intervention employed, 363–4; person of therapist, 364–5; preliminary considerations, 363–4);
statistics, 361–2,
(those offering help, 362, those seeking help, 361)

Feedback, 30, 71, 89–90

Follow-up, 32–3

Foster care, 238–47; children waiting in care, 239–41; classification, 238; definition, 238; foster parents' circumstances, 244; long-term, 241; natural parents of foster children, 241,
('inclusive'/'exclusive' fostering, 243, Length of stay in foster care, 241, 242, maintenance of contact with children, 242–3, planned agreements/contracts, 245, returning home from foster care, 242);
outcomes, 240–1; specialist fostering, 244–5,
(Kent Family Placement project, 245, successful outcomes, 244–5, use of contracts, 245);
statistics of children 'boarded out', 239; success or failure, 244, (breakdown in fostering, 244, pinpointing predictive factors, 244, support for foster parents, 244)

Genetic constitutional factors, (vi), 72; temperament, (vi)

Goal-setting, (vi), 63, 71; anxiety management, 310; anger or violence management, 387; attainability, (vi); 29; definition, 71; sexual difficulties, 375

Groups, problem solving and decision making, 58–64; advantages, 60; conditions for effectiveness, 61; disadvantages, 61; guidelines, 61; leadership, 59–60,
(formal, 59, informal, 59, skills, 59);
participation, 59; risky decisions, 61

Groups, self-help, 62; effects of increased size, 63; features, 62; helper principle, 62; objectives, 63

Groups, small, 51–8; composition, 53, behaviour of dominants, 54, conflicting personalities, 54, size, 53, styles of social behaviour, 53;
dimensions/channels, 51, leaders, 52, sociable behaviours, 51–2, task-related behaviours, 51–2;
formation, 54, hierarchical structure, 55–6, networks of liking and disliking, 56, norms, 55, stages, 54;
verbal and non-verbal communication, 53, categorization, 52

Groups, therapeutic, 64–70; effects, 65,
(global measures of effectiveness, 65, specific measures of effectiveness, 65, specific skills measures, 66, work behaviour, 66);
processes, 66,
(characteristics, 66, composition,

67, leader behaviour, 67, learning mechanisms, 68, phases in development, 67, structure, 67);
group psychotherapy, 69, (children, 69, neurotically ill people, 69, psychotically ill people, 69);
parent counselling, 70; therapeutic communities, 69

Handicapped, physically, 127–37; *see* Physically handicapped, 127–37
Hierarchy/heriarchical structure, 55–60; emergence of leader, 59; fluctuations in, 56; spontaneous emergence, 55
Homosexuality, 377–82; causation, 378–9,
(gender identity and sexual preference, 378–9, overview of research, 380, variables affecting sexual preference, 378–9);
change of sexual orientation, 380, (effectiveness of therapy, 380–1, overview of evidence, 381, spontaneous change of orientation, 380);
definition, 377, prevalence, 377–8
Housing, 40, 120–2; standards of amenities, 121
Hyperactive behaviour, 199–200
Hypothesis, 19, 21, 24, 30

In-group/out-group phenomenon, 44
Inter-disciplinary co-operation, 5, 14
Intergroup conflict, 43–50; characteristics, 45; cohesion, 45; concepts, 44–6,
(in-group/out-group phenomenon, 44, social identity/social comparison theory, 44);
reduction, 46–8
Intergroup contact, 46; effects, 46
Intermediate Treatment, 283; *see* Young offenders, responses to, 280–6
International Classification of Diseases (9th edn) (ICD 9), 5

Justice model, 300; *see* Custodial and other responses to offenders, 294–300

Labelling, 276

Management skills, 86–95; conflict, 94–5,
(constructive potential, 94, resolution, 94, sources, 94);
decision making, 90–1,
(example, 91, stages, 90–1);
definition, 86; enlisting motivation, 93–4,
(consultation, 94, maximizing satisfaction, 93);
objectives approach, 88–90,
(example, 89, features, 88, relevance, 89, research, 89);
organizations/systems, 86–7,
(example, 87);
systems, 87,
(relevance, 87, sub-systems, 87);
use of time, 91,
(additional practices, 93, critical path, 92, examples, 92, forward planning, 92–3)
Marriage, 163–71; *see* Family life, marriage and divorce, 163–71
Maximization theory, 47, 93
Mediation, 48–9
Mental handicaps, 339–50; causation, 341,
(mild, 340, 343, severe, 340);
diagnostic criteria, 339–40; education and development of potential, 343,
(Portage project, 343, studies involving parents, 343–5);
education development in special schools, 345–6,
(developments in Special education, 346, system to replace

categorization, 345, Warnock Report, 345);
prevalence, 340,
(categories based on IQ tests, 340, limitations of IQ based categorization, 341, other estimates, 340, demographic differences, 341);
prevention, 343,
(counselling and screening, 343, maternal age and Down's syndrome, 343);
services, 346–8,
(community mental handicap teams, 348, community based, 346, further developments, 349);
use of terms, 339
Mental impairment, 14
Multi-disciplinary teams, 5

National Association for the Care and Resettlement of Offenders, (NACRO), 270, 271, 291
National Children's Bureau, 3
National Child Development Study, 103, 195, 250
Neuroses, 14
Negotiation, 48–9; principles, 47; systems, 49

Objectives, 29–30; achievement, 29,
(measurement, 30);
advantages of approach, 90;
disadvantages of approach, 90;
see also Management, 86–95
Observational method, 21–2; advantages, 21; disadvantages, 21; example, 22
Obsessive-compulsive conditions, 189, 312–13; *see* Anxiety and forms of anxiety, 305–13
One-parent families, 172–80; circumstances, 174–9,
(employment, 175, housing, 175, income, 174, interaction with social disadvantage, 175, supplementary benefit, 174);
definition, 172; experience within, 178–9; health, 179; impact of financial disadvantage, 179; media images, 177; perceptions, 177; professional attitudes to, 177; statistics, 172–4
Organizations, 86–9; groups in tension, 88,
(example, 88);
objectives, 88–90,
(example, 89, features, 88–9, measuring attainment, 89, relevance, 90, research, 90;)
structure of activities, 87,
(competing for influence, 88, hierarchical tendencies, 87)

Parasuicide (*see also* Suicide), 323–30; characteristics, 325; definition, 323; different groups, 326–7; helping people at risk, 328,
(assessment, 329, further study, 329, risk factors for first episode, 328, risk of repetition, 329, supportive agencies, 330);
identifying those at risk after parasuicide, 327; overlap with suicide, 327–8,
(comparative data, 327–8);
statistics, 324; stressful life events, 326
Participation, 39, 89
People wanting to control their violence, 382–9; definitions, 382–3; helping people to attain control, 386–8,
(cognitive variables, 385–6, ethical issues, 386, goal-setting, 387, pinpointing triggers, 387, principles of management, 387, stress inoculation, 387);
origins of violent behaviour, 384–6,
(aggression as over- or under-control, 384–5, appropriate assertion training, 385, determinants of anger arousal, 386, nature and circumstances of violent offending, 384, readiness

to perceive threat, 385–6, social interaction styles, 385);
statistics, 383–4
Perception, 45; distortion, 45; subjectivity, 3, 20, 45
Personality factors (vi); self-esteem, (vi)
Phobias, 311–12; *see* Anxiety and forms of anxiety, 305–14
Physically handicapped people, 127–37; adjustment to disability, 132,
(adolescents, 132, children, 132);
definitions and terminology, 127–8; housing difficulties, 129,
(families with disabled children, 132, inadequacy of housing, 129);
meaning of disability, 132; needs of families, 132–3,
(information, 133, on-going support, 133, recognising difficulties of adjustment, 133, responses of disabled children, 132, time of diagnosis, 132);
provision of services, 134–5; residential care, 261–2; self-help, 135, professionals, 134; social and emotional problems, 130–1,
(discrimination, 130, emotional strain, 131, financial strain, 131, physical strain, 131, social attitudes, 130, social isolation, 131, stigma, 130);
statistics, 128, 258, terminology, 127–8; transport and mobility difficulties, 129–30
Poverty, social disadvantage, 99–107; definitions and indicators, 99,
(relative concept, 99, society's, 99);
education, 103,
(under-achievement, 103);
extent, 100–1,
(changes in extent, 100–1, numbers, 100–1, rich and control of resources, 101, social class, 101, structure of poverty, 101, survey, 101);
families, 104–5,
(child Poverty Action Group, 105, family Service Units, 105, stresses, 105);
health, 104,
(inequalities, 104, preventive services, 104);
housing, 102; indicators, 99–100; multiple disadvantage, 105,
(index, 105, specific and other problems, 106);
unemployment, low paid employment, 101–2,
(children, 102, class status, 102, impact of low income, 102, inadequate benefits, 101)
Probation, 287–94; areas of consensus, 291,
(limitations of 'treatment' model, 291, provision of help for offenders, 290, trends to reparation and restitution, 291);
definition, 287; diversion from custodial sentences, 290; hostels, 291,
(influence of wardens and matrons, 292);
models of supervision, 289,
(indicators from research, 289–90);
primary aims of service, 288; provision of help for offenders, 288, 290–1,
(studies of after-care, 290–1);
reduction of crime, 288–9,
(differential responses of offenders, 290, holding effect of probation, 289, difficulties of research, 289);
statistics, 287
Psychiatric disorders and young people, 183–94; Family Adversity Index, 185; prevalence studies, 183, 185,
(types of disorder, 184)
Psychiatry, 13–15; range of approaches, 15
Psychology, 12–13, range of approaches, 12–13
Psychopathic personality, 383
Psychoses, 14

Questionnaires, 30–2

Relaxation, 311; anxiety management, 311
'Reliable' data, 20
Research literature, 19, 27
Residential care, 213–24, 257–66; children, 213–24; elderly people, 259–61,
(autonomy for residents, 260, critiques of research, 260–1, dimensions of the social environment, 260, need for privacy, 260, overviews of practice, 259–60, research studies: DHSS, 261–2, statistics, 258–9);
mentally handicapped people, 259, 262–4, 346–9,
(comparative study of group homes, 264, critiques of policy and practice, 263, differences in child management practice, 263, evaluation of provision, 262, principles of researching field, 262, statistics, 259);
mentally ill people, 259, 264–5,
(need for evaluation of provision, 264, range of provision, 264, statistics, 259);
physically handicapped people, 258, 261,
(contrasting models of care, 261, shortage of research, 261, statistics, 258)

Sampling, 20, representativeness, 27
Schizophrenia, 331–9; definitions, 331; origins, 333–6,
(criticism of genetic contribution theory, 334, genetic contribution, 333, neuro-chemical factors, 335, schema for studying origins and development, 336, theories of family causation, 334–5);
prevalence, 332; treatment/management, 337,
(long-term management, 337, medication, 337, milieu therapy, 337, therapeutic communities, 337)
School non-attendance, 189
School phobia/school refusal, 189
Self-help groups (*see also* Groups, self-help), 62–3
Sentencing, 29, 294–302
Sexual dysfunction and difficulties, 369–76; classification, 369; definition, 369; origins, 370–72,
(biological variables, 370–1, further issues, 372, psychological variables, 371, specific sources of difficulty, 371);
prevalence, 370,
(Dutch sample, 370);
ways of helping, 372–3,
(careful assessment, 374, consensus upon common features, 374, outcome studies, 372–3, planned treatment intervention, 375, specifying goals, 375, trusting relationships, 374, when no severe non-sexual problems, 372)
Situation ABC's, (vi), 77
Situational variables, 199; delinquency, 278
Situations political, not personal, 40
Social disadvantage, 99–107 (*see also* Poverty); indicators, 99–100; multiple, 105–6
Social exchange theory, 47
Social isolation, 156
Social learning theory, 71–9; antecedents to learning, 72; applied aspects, 76–8,
(behavioural approaches, 76, child abuse, 233–4, prevention of child abuse, 233–4, contracts, 77, goal-setting, 77);
cognitive processes, 74–5,
(cognitive strategies, 75, competencies, 75, expectancies, 75, personal values, 75);
conduct disorders, 198; convergence of research, 78; definition/description, 71; ethical issues, 78; hyperactive behaviour, 200;

interaction: individual/system, 71, 76; learning by observing/ modelling, 75; partial explanatory framework, 76; principles of reinforcement, 73,
(cognitive processes, 74, continuous positive, 73, differential reward, 74, extinction, 73–4, generalization, 74, intermittent positive, 74, reward, immediate/delayed, 74, reward, large/small, 74, negative, 73, penalty/punishment, 73, positive, 73, social context, 71)
Social Services teams, 29; patch-based, 29
Socialization, 156; conduct disorders, 197–8
Socio-economic variables, (vi), 2, 278; class, 2, 274; race, 275
Sociology, 10, 12; range of approaches, 12
Statistical analysis, 32
Stress, 198; parental, 198
Structural variables, 2; socio-economic variables, 2, 156
Subjectivity, 3, 21
Subjectively expected utility, 47
Suicide (*see also* Parasuicide), 323–30; causation, 324–6,
(behaviour indicating sucidal intent, 326, characteristics of those committing suicide, 325–6, characteristics of those not committing suicide, 325, characteristics among those completing suicide, 325–6, sociological groupings, 324–5);
definition, 323; helping people at risk, 328–30; management of people at risk, 329–30; risk factors, 328; supportive agencies, 330; overlap with parasuicide, 327–8,
(comparative data, 327–8)
Statistics, 324
Supervision orders, 283, 296; *see* Young offenders: responses to, 280–6
Surveys, 21; advantages, 21; disadvantages, 21; examples, 21; stages in, 21
Systems/systems theory, (vi), 2, 9–18; approach, 33,
(disciplines within, 10,/ecological perspective, 9, 41);
approaches, 18; conflict, 43,
(functional, 43–4, dysfunctional, 44);
example of a system, 10; formulations, (vi),
(agoraphobia, 312, alcohol misuse, 392, criminal event, 278, day services, 215, delinquency, 278, depression, 317–18, family, 362, group care, 216, negotiation/ mediation, 48–9, opiate use, 408, suicide, 329, truancy, 200, women and violence, 156);
general systems theory, 9–11; importance, 2; intervening in systems, 15–17,
(process, 17);
models of evaluation, 41–2; sub-systems, 87, thinking in terms of, (vi), 15,
(features, 9, origins, 9–10)

Television violence, 198, 275; conduct disorders, 198; delinquency, 275
Threat, perceived, 48
Trades Unions, 37
Tranquillizers (*see* Drug use and misuse), 411
Truancy, 189, 200; prevalence, 200; systems model, 200

Under-achievement, 103, 122; poor children, 103; West Indian children, 122
Unemployed people, 107–17; definitions, 107–8; effects of becoming, 110–13; factors affecting experience, 112; functions of employment, 110–13,
(work as activity, 110, work as

providing income, 111, work as providing sense of identity, 113, work as providing opportunity for mastery, 111, work as providing opportunity for social contact, 111, work as way of structuring time, 111)

Unemployed people, 107–17; health, 110, 114; individual responses, 114; loss of work as bereavement, 113; mental health, 115; official statistics, 108–9,
(ages of long term unemployed, 109, figures in January 1986, 109, male unemployment, 109, rates of unemployment for selected countries, 108, regional unemployment, 108);
phase model, 113; stages of response, 113; use of Personal Social Services, 115; vulnerable groups, 109;
(older workers, 110, those already unemployed, 110, those on low wages, 110, women, 110, young people, 110)

'Valid' data, 20
Verifiable data, 28
Values, 28; impossibility of value-free research, 28
Violence (*see* Women and rape; Women and violence), 151–9; home, 156
Volunteers, 29, 89

Welfare benefits, 30; take-up, 30
Welfare rights, 40; services, 40
Women's Aid Federation, 157
Women and rape, 157–9; definition, 151–2; responses, 155–7,
(conviction of offenders, 158, imprisonment, 158, re-conviction, 159);
official statistics, 152,
(inadequacy 153)
studies, 157–8,
(American, 157, London, 158);
Women and violence (*see also* Women and rape), 151–7; definitions, 151–2; multi-variate model, 156; Select Committee on Violence in Marriage, 155; statistics, 152; studies, 153–4,
(American, 153, British, 153, family violence, 153, provision for women, 157, Scottish, 154, shortage of research, 155)
World Health Organization, 5, 128, 183, 184

Young offenders (*see also* Delinquency), 269–94; classification, 269; international context, 272; statistics, 269–72,
(changes in rates of offending, 270, females, 274, males, 274, unreliability, 269);
community-based projects, 284–5,
(in the UK, 285, in the USA, 284);
devising strategies of intervention, 281–2,
(variables affecting offending in groups, 281–2);
differing responses, 280–5; diversion from criminal justice system, 280–1,
(outcomes, 282–3);
family placements, 285,
(contracts, 285);
Intermediate Treatment, 283–4,
(goal-setting approaches, 282, shortage of evaluated projects, 283);
statistics, 281; strategies of intervention, 281–3,
(effective strategies, 282, ineffective strategies, 282)
Youth Service, 141–8; description, 141; development, 141; distinguishing features, 142; origins, 141; research, 145–7,
(future, 147, shortage, 146);
statistics, 143–4;

(expenditure, 144, young people involved, 143, youth workers, 143–4);
studies, 145,
(involvement of ethnic minority young people, 146, involvement of young women, 145);
voluntary sector, 146